VETERINARY MEDICINE
Emerging Concepts

VETERINARY MEDICINE
Emerging Concepts

Upasana Saha
Shishir Raj
Mohammed Ali

2025
Agri Horti Press
New Delhi-110 084

ISBN: 978-93-8769-597-9 (Hardbound)

Published By

Agri Horti Press

New Delhi

E-mail: agrihortipress@gmail.com

Preface

“Veterinary Medicine: Emerging Concepts” presents a forward-looking exploration of the evolving landscape of veterinary medicine, incorporating innovative concepts, approaches, and technologies that are reshaping the practice and science of animal health and welfare. This book serves as a vital resource for veterinarians, researchers, educators, policymakers, and students seeking to stay abreast of the latest developments and trends in the field.

The field of veterinary medicine is experiencing rapid transformation driven by advances in science, technology, and societal expectations. From genomics and precision medicine to telemedicine and One Health approaches, new concepts and paradigms are emerging that are revolutionizing how we diagnose, treat, and prevent diseases in animals, as well as how we manage their health and well-being within the context of broader ecosystems and human societies.

The primary objective of this book is to provide readers with a comprehensive overview of emerging concepts in veterinary medicine, covering key topics such as personalized medicine, regenerative therapies, artificial intelligence, telehealth, and sustainable practices. Each chapter explores cutting-edge concepts and their implications for animal health, welfare, and veterinary practice, drawing upon the latest research, case studies, and expert insights.

Contributions from leading experts in the field delve into various aspects of emerging concepts in veterinary medicine, including their scientific foundations, practical applications, and ethical considerations. Special emphasis is placed on interdisciplinary approaches that bridge the gap between traditional veterinary disciplines and emerging fields such as genomics, bioinformatics, bioengineering, and social sciences.

As we navigate the complexities of veterinary medicine in the 21st century, it is essential to embrace innovation, collaboration, and lifelong learning. By staying informed about emerging concepts and leveraging new technologies and approaches, veterinarians can enhance their capacity to address the evolving needs and challenges of animal health, welfare, and society.

We extend our sincere gratitude to the contributors whose expertise and dedication have enriched this book. It is our hope that "Veterinary Medicine: Emerging Concepts" will serve as a thought-provoking resource and catalyst for innovation, dialogue, and excellence in the field of veterinary medicine for years to come.

Upasana Saha

Shishir Raj

Mohammed Ali

Contents

Chapter 1

Dermatology in Dogs and Cats

1. Introduction

The skin is the largest organ of the body with many different functions as thermoregulation, immune protection, sensory perception, vitamin D production and it acts as a barrier between the animal and the environment. Besides all of these important functions and the diseases that affect directly the skin, it may also share or reflect pathologic processes from other tissues. Due to these characteristics, dermatologic problems are among the most commonly seen disorders in veterinary hospitals. It is important for the veterinarian to know and understand about the physiology of the skin and about the most common dermatologic disorders that affects dogs and cats, which will be addressed in this chapter.

2. Skin structure

The skin is divided in three layers: epidermis, dermis and hypodermis (Figure 1). Epidermis, the outermost layer of the skin, is composed by keratinocytes, melanocytes and Langerhans cells. Keratinocytes are also disposed in layers in the epidermis. The deepest one, the stratum basale, is formed by a single row of germinative keratinocytes and also contains melanocytes. These germinative keratinocytes generate the other layers by cell division and differentiation. The next layer, stratum spinosum, differs from stratum basale by the presence of intercellular junctions. Langerhans cells are also present in this layer. Stratum granulosum is characterized by a large amount of keratohyaline granules inside keratinocytes which are important in the skin keratinization process. Stratum corneum, the outer epidermis layer, is composed by keratinocytes in their maximal differentiation degree (corneocytes), interspersed in lipid matrix [1].

Dermis, the layer under the epidermis, is composed by a conjunctive matrix where reticular, elastic and collagen fibers are found. Dermis cellular structure is composed by fibroblasts, mast cells and histiocytes. It also contains epidermal appendages (hair, nails, sebaceous and sweat glands), arrector pili muscles and blood and lymph vessels. Hypodermis or subcutaneous tissue provides support and cushioning against physical trauma. It is composed by a loose connective tissue and elastic fibers interspersed by adipocytes [1]. The hair follicles exhibit activity cycles that result in hair formation. Anagen is a period of active growth when a new hair is being formed. Catagen is when the hair growth stops and degenerative changes occur in the base of the follicle. Telogen represents a period of follicle inactivity, when the hair is shed so that a new one may start to grow [1]. Hair cycle activity, in some dog breeds, is strongly related to temperature variation and photoperiod, leading to decreased hair density in the warmer months, which helps the heat loss in these animals [2].

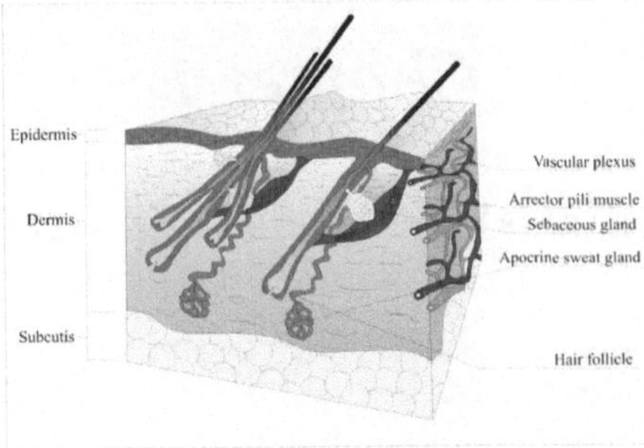

Figure 1. Structure of the skin.

3. Diagnosis techniques

Diagnosis approach for skin diseases depends on obtaining detailed history with thorough physical and dermatological examination. The evaluation offers precious information and guides the investigative process. Specific tests and, occasionally, therapeutic trials should be performed [3].

Skin scrapings, trichogram, fungal and bacterial culture, cytological evaluation and skin biopsy are important diagnosis techniques in dermatology. Skin scrapings are applied in mite detection, and it may be superficial or deep depending on the mite that is suspected. The sample obtained is evaluated under optical microscopy [3]. Fungal culture is recommended for patients that fungal diseases are suspected. Hair samples and skin scales should be collected from the lesion margin. Bacterial culture is not often performed and it is recommended in pyoderma refractory to initial therapy or when rods are observed in cytology [4]. The direct examination of the hairs, the trichogram, is performed by pulling the hairs from the affected area, followed by microscopic evaluation. With this technique it is possible to determinate hair growth phase abnormalities and the presence of follicles parasites and dermatophytes [3]. Cytology is the analysis of tissue cells and it is a highly efficient and valuable exam to evaluate a lesion, after which it is possible to establish the next step in the diagnostic approach. The sample may be obtained by fine-needle aspiration, swab, skin scrapings or lesion imprint [5]. Histopathology associated with clinical findings usually leads to definitive diagnosis. Skin biopsy is recommended in unusual lesions, possibly neoplastic nodules, dermatosis with expensive therapy or when it represents a risk to the patient health, with poor response to previous therapy and to exclude differential diagnoses [4]. To perform the histopathological exam at least three representative samples should be obtained by punch or surgical resection [3].

4. Bacterial skin diseases

Pyoderma is a bacterial skin infection and it is among the most common causes of skin diseases in dogs [6], however, it is less common in cats [7]. Lesions may be superficial and involve only the epidermis or they may affect deeper structures in the dermis or subcutaneous tissue, and it is therefore divided into surface, superficial and deep pyoderma [6]. *Staphylococcus pseudintermedius* is the most commonly isolated bacteria from dog's skin [8] and it is among the main reasons for antimicrobial use in these animals [9].

Surface pyodermas are characterized by superficial erosions of the stratum corneum. The presence of alopecia, erythema and pruritus are common findings [10]. Intertrigo is a surface pyoderma that affects the skin folds found in lips, face, vulva, tail and mammary glands of some breeds, and it may also affect the skin folds of obese animals. Acute moist dermatitis, also known as pyotraumatic dermatitis or hot spots, is of acute onset and rarely occurs as a primary disease in healthy skin, being usually secondary to other diseases [11]. Probably, local irritation due to an underlying cause leads to self-inflicted trauma, which quickly becomes extensive areas of skin damage [10].

Superficial pyodermas are the most common causes of cutaneous bacterial infection in dogs [6]. They affect the superficial portion of the hair follicles (bacterial folliculitis) or the epidermis (impetigo), causing pustules [10, 11]. The most common lesions are crusted papules due to the transient nature of canine pustules. Pruritus, epidermal collarettes, hyperpigmentation and alopecia are also common findings [6]. Impetigo affects sexually immature dogs that may present subcorneal pustules formed in inguinal and axillary areas [10]. Superficial bacterial folliculitis is the most common form of pyoderma in dogs [12]. Papules, pustules associated with hair follicles, epidermal collarettes, alopecia and hyperpigmentation are commonly found [10] (Figure 2).

Deep pyoderma does not occur spontaneously, often starting as superficial pyoderma [6]. Other organisms such as *Proteus* spp., *Pseudomonas* spp. and *E. coli* may be involved [12-14]. The bacterial infection affects the deepest portion of the hair follicle (deep folliculitis), that may lead to follicular wall rupture and to bacterial product release in the dermis (furunculosis), or it can also affect the deeper portion of the dermis and subcutaneous tissue (cellulitis) [10, 15]. The affected skin appears erythematous, hyperpigmented, with the presence of seropurulent debris from the ruptured pustules; variable pruritus, swelling, skin stiffness and evident pain are also noted [6].

Diagnosis is obtained through the evaluation of clinical signs, presence of characteristic skin lesions, elimination of other possible causes of folliculitis and by cytological evaluation of the intact pustules content, exudative lesions and skin debris. In the management of pyoderma, it is important to identify the possible underlying disorder, which may be done through skin scrapings, scabies therapeutic trial, allergy tests, endocrinopathies screenings, hypoallergenic diet trials, strict ectoparasites control and skin biopsies. [16].

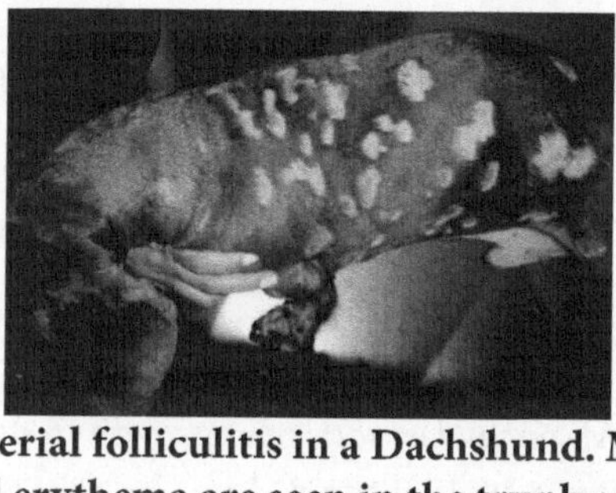

Figure 2. Superficial bacterial folliculitis in a Dachshund. Multiple areas of alopecia and erythema are seen in the trunk area.

The treatment varies depending on presented lesions. Local surface and superficial pyodermas may be treated only with topical antibiotics such as silver sulphadiazine, neomycin or 2% mupirocin ointments applied twice daily over the affected areas. Generalized lesions and deep pyodermas require a combination of oral and topical antibiotics. In patients with severe pruritus it is recommended to use anti-inflammatory doses of prednisone orally for up to two weeks [17]. The antibiotics of choice for oral use include cephalexin (22-33 mg / kg q12h) and amoxicillin associated with clavulanic acid (22 mg/kg q12h) [18]. Recurrent cases require culture and susceptibility testing to access resistance [16].

5. Fungal diseases

5.1. Dermatophytosis

Dermatophytosis is a superficial mycosis caused by *Microsporum*, *Trichophyton* or *Epidermophyton* fungi genera. These fungi are isolated from hair, nails and skin surface since they require keratin for their growth [19]. Dermatophytes are classified into three groups based on their habitat: zoophilic, mostly found in animals, occurring transmission to other animals or to humans; anthropophilic, mostly found in humans, transmitted between humans and rarely to animals and geophilic, dermatophytes, found in the soil, infects humans and animals [20]. *M. canis* is the most frequently isolated fungal species in dogs and cats [21].

Clinically, canine and feline fungal infections differ. Infections in dogs often produce lesions, while it is possible to isolate dermatophytes from clinically healthy cats, which can act as a conidia reservoir of the fungus [22]. The affected animals usually have alopecic, scaly, crusted, erythematous and papular lesions, especially in the face and limbs. Occasionally, dermatophytes may be presented in a nodular form known as kerions. This form of dermatophytosis is characterized by deep, inflammatory and suppurative lesions [23]. Pruritus may vary from absent to severe [24].

The direct microscopic examination of hairs and scales can reveal the presence of fungal hyphae or spores. The fungal culture is the diagnostic test of choice and the sample may be obtained by brushing the animal with a toothbrush or by skin scrapings [25].

The best strategy for the treatment of dermatophytes is the association of systemic and topical antifungal therapy. The aims of the treatment with topical products are the elimination of the fungi present at the epidermis and hair surface, while systemic treatment aims to eliminate infection within the hair shafts [26]. Lime sulfur rinse at 6.5 % twice a week showed good results in cats infected with *M. canis* [27, 28]. Systemic treatment options include itraconazole orally at 10 mg/kg once a day, griseofulvin 50 mg/kg once a day or terbinafine 5 mg/kg once a day [27-29]. The treatment must be extended over 2 to 4 weeks after clinical cure and after obtaining two or more negative fungal cultures [23].

5.2. *Malassezia* dermatitis

Malassezia pachydermatis is a commensal skin yeast, commonly isolated from lips, interdigital skin, anal mucosa and external auditory canal [30]. It is an opportunistic yeast, which usually manifests itself after the installation of other diseases. It is very common in dogs and least frequent in cats [31]. Previous antibiotic therapy is associated with the development of cutaneous *M. pachydermatis* over growth in dogs [32], as well as disorders of keratinization and hypersensitivity diseases [33]. Basset Hounds, Cocker Spaniels and West Highland White Terriers are more predisposed to this type of infection [32].

The most common clinical manifestation of *Malassezia* dermatitis is the presence of moderate to intense pruritus [34]. Erythema, lichenification, oily skin, malodor, alopecia and erosions are also common clinical findings [35] that can be generalized or localized [34].

Cytology is the diagnostic method of choice and allows microscopic identification of the increased number of yeasts. Samples can be obtained by skin scrapings, swabs, direct imprint or by tape preps. Fungal culture is not recommended as a diagnostic procedure because it is not a quantitative assessment [36].

Identification and correction of the predisposing diseases are essential for the successful treatment of *Malassezia* dermatitis [23]. Mild cases can be treated with miconazole, chlorhexidine, ketoconazole or acetic acid shampoos. Baths should be given, two times per week, for a minimum of six weeks [36]. Patients requiring systemic treatment should receive oral antifungals such as ketoconazole, itraconazole or fluconazole 5 mg/kg once a day for a minimum of 30 days [36]. Terbinafine 30 mg /kg every 24 hours on two consecutive days in a week, for six weeks, may also be an effective treatment [37]. In order to prevent recurrences of the disease, regular maintenance therapy may be needed in many dogs [23].

5.3. Sporotrichosis

Sporotrichosis is a subcutaneous mycosis caused by a dimorphic fungus, *Sporothrix schenckii*, which can infect animals and humans [39]. It is a zoonotic disease and transmission to humans occurs through bites or scratches, and contact with cats ulcers [40]. *S. schenckii* is present in the decaying vegetation and soil and animal contamination occurs by skin open lesions such as perforations, bites and scratches. Once in the host organism, the fungus may cause local lesions and possibly systemic signs [41].

Clinically, sporotrichosis has three forms: cutaneous, lymphocutaneous and generalized, and more than one form can occur simultaneously in the same animal. The cutaneous form is usually confined to the area of fungus inoculation and manifests after an incubation period of one month. If this lesion is not treated, the progression to lymphocutaneous form can occur. The lymphocutaneous form is characterized by the development of nodules that evolve into ulcers, affecting skin, subcutaneous tissue, lymph vessels and regional lymph nodes [41]. History of lethargy, anorexia, depression and fever on physical examination suggest the presence of the disseminated form [42].

The diagnosis is based on clinical history, physical examination, cytological evaluation, fungal culture and histopathological findings [43]. Cytological evaluation usually reveals oval to elongate yeast cells consistent with *S. schenckii* form and inflammatory cells may also be present [45]. On histopathology, the presence of deep pyogranulomatous dermatitis, cellular infiltration of polymorphonuclear and mononuclear cells, and the presence of PAS positive structures compatible with *S. schenckii* may be observed [44]. Oral administration of itraconazole 10 mg/kg every 24 hours is the treatment of choice [46].

5.4. Cryptococcosis

Cryptococcus spp. is a saprophytic fungus present in the environment and in the feces of pigeons, capable of causing systemic infection in dogs and cats, with a higher incidence in felines. The species of interest in veterinary medicine are *C. neoformans*, which has a global distribution and *C. gattii* that has a limited distribution [47]. *C. neoformans* typically infects animals by inhalation and may cause ophthalmic, upper respiratory tract and central nervous system lesions. Ulcerative lesions in the nasal, oral or pharyngeal mucosae, or a nasal masse may be present (Figure 3) [31]. Mycotic rhinitis and cutaneous nasal bridge and nasal plan involvement are the most frequent findings. In cats with positive serology for feline immunodeficiency virus (FIV) cryptococcosis tends to manifest itself in a disseminated or advanced form [48].

Cryptococcosis diagnosis is based on fungal culture, cytological, histological and serological exams [49]. Cytological examination may reveal the presence of leukocytes, macrophages and numerous encapsulated structures (yeast) of different sizes (Figure 3) [50, 51].

Drug therapy leads to patient healing in most cases [49] and it consists of oral antifungal use until complete remission of clinical signs, usually in 3 to 12 months. It is strongly recommended not to interrupt the treatment until the titers of antibodies against cryptococcosis are reduced to zero [52]. Drugs commonly used include fluconazole 50 mg/cat every 12 hours [48] and itraconazole 50-100 mg/cat every 24 hours [52], or 10mg/kg for dogs and cats every 24 hours [49]. Patients with nasopharyngeal masses benefit from surgical resection, for upper airway patency and reduction of infected tissue to be treated medically [52].

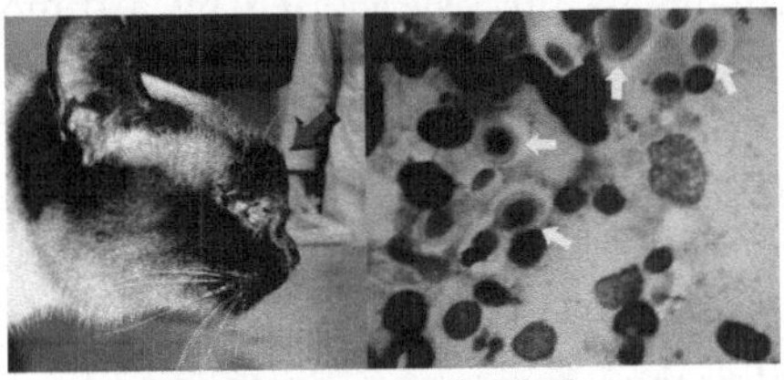

Figure 3. Feline cryptococcosis. Figure on the left: a cat presenting a nasal masse (red arrow). Figure on the right: Cytology by fine needle aspirate of the nasal masse showing several encapsulated structures (yellow arrows) compatible with C. neoformans (microscopic image viewed with a 100x oil objective).

6. Parasitic skin diseases

6.1. Demodicosis

Demodicosis is a very common skin disease in dogs but rare in cats [53]. It is an inflammatory disease, in which large amounts of *Demodex* mites are found in the skin [54]. Mites proliferate in the hair follicles and sebaceous glands causing the disease [55]. It is a common condition and it is often serious in dogs. Besides *Demodex canis*, two less common species were reported [54, 55], *Demodex* sp. *cornei* and *Demodex injai* [55]. Feline demodicosis may be caused by two different kinds of mites, *Demodex cati* and *Demodex gatoi* [53].

The mites are transferred from the mother to the offspring in the early life [56]. *D. canis* is considered a commensal in canine skin. It is believed that this disease is a consequence of a specific immunosuppression, which allows the proliferation of the mites [57]. Genetic factors are probably very important in the development of generalized disease and therefore, breeding of affected animals is contraindicated [54].

Erythema, comedones, scaling, partial or complete alopecia, papules, follicular casts, pustules, and in severe cases, furunculosis, crusting, exudation and ulceration with focal draining tracts can be clinical sings. Generally the lesions begin on the face and limbs, but they may become generalized. Demodicosis can be classified into generalized or localized. The involvement of one complete body region, five or more focal areas, or the involvement of the legs is considered generalized demodicosis. The diagnosis is made by deep skin scrapings or trichogram. In some rare cases, in the legs or certain breeds such as Shar-peis, these tests may be negative, requiring biopsies for mite detection [58].

In most dogs, localized demodicosis resolves spontaneously, thus mite-specific therapy is not necessary until the disease generalizes [53]. The treatment of generalized demodicosis involves several approaches. In addition to the acaricidal treatment, the concurrent secondary infections and underlying diseases should be also accessed [58]. As an acaricidal treatment, ivermectin is recommended at 0.3 to 0.6 mg/kg orally once a day, however, it is recommended to begin the treatment with a lower dose and gradually increase the amount of drug administered. The animal should be monitored for the appearance of adverse effects. Therapy with moxidectin 0.2-0.5 mg/kg orally once a day and doramectin 0.6 mg/kg orally or subcutaneously once a week were proven effective in the treatment of generalized demodicosis. The same careful institution of a gradual dose taken with ivermectin should be applied for these two other drugs. Milbemycin oxime can also be used at 1 to 2 mg/kg orally, once a day, with good results [58]. In cats weekly baths with 2% lime sulfur are indicated for the treatment of demodicosis. There is remote evidence to indicate weekly application of 0.025% amitraz and for the use of doramectin 0.6 mg/kg once a week subcutaneously [53]. Treatment should continue for one month after getting the third consecutive negative scraping [58].

6.2. Canine scabies

Canine scabies is a common condition in dogs and humans, but rare in cats, in which the skin is colonized by *Sarcoptes scabiei* mite after contact with a donor host. The infestation with this mites results in intense pruritus [59, 60]. Female mites dig galleries in the stratum corneum in order to lay their eggs that hatch, releasing larvae forms that migrate to the skin surface, where they reach the adult stage [61].

Extremely irritating and pruritic papular eruption, skin thickening, erythema, alopecia, exudation with crust formation and secondary bacterial infection with pustules are common clinical findings (Figure 4). Chronic lesions are usually confined to the margins of the pinna, elbows and hocks that may present skin thickening, minimal crust formation and persistent pruritus [61].

Skin scraping with microscopic identification of *S. scabiei* is a valuable diagnostic method, although mites are hardly seen in many cases. Diagnosis is usually based on the animal's history, clinical signs and a positive pinnal-pedal reflex (pinna margings are gently scratched and the dog will reflexively use an ipsilateral hind limb to scratch the source of the irritation) [62, 63].

The treatment is recommended to the patient and other animals in their household. Bathing with 0.025% amitraz solution once weekly or twice weekly is recommended as an effective treatment. The therapy should be continued for two weeks after clinical signs remission. Adverse side effects should be monitored during the treatment [64]. Fipronil spray 0.25% can be applied three times with three weeks intervals on puppies [65]. Ivermectin can be administered at 0.2 to 0.4 mg/kg, orally every seven days, or subcutaneously every 14 days. The treatment usually takes four to six weeks [66].This drug is contraindicated in

Collies and their crosses [67]. An effective alternative treatment of scabies is a spot-on application of selamectin at 6-12 mg/kg every 15 to 30 days, for at least three applications and it is apparently, well tolerated in different breeds [67, 68]. Milbemycin oxime at 2mg/kg in a weekly dose, administrated for up to five times has also a good efficacy [69].

NOTE: The permission for the use of macrocyclic lactones in the treatment of cats and dogs is different for each country. The rules concerning its use should be checked before treatment institution and the owners must be warned in order to authorize any extra-label use of these medications.

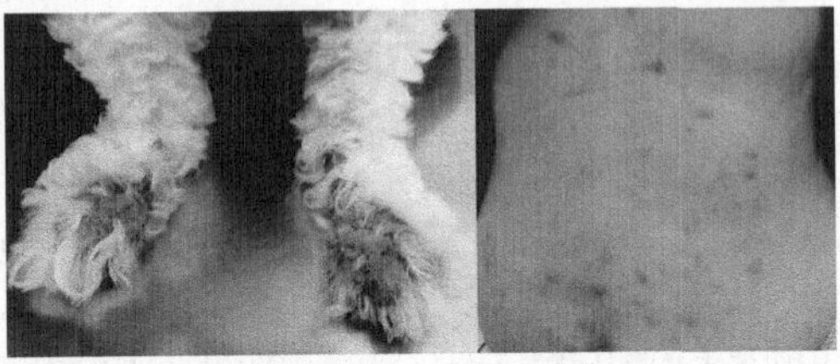

Figure 4. Scabies. Figure on the left: a dog with erythematous, alopecic and lichenified pruritic lesions in the distal aspect of the hind limbs. Figure on the right: the animal's owner presenting abdominal pruritic papular lesions, highlighting the zoonotic aspect of scabies.

7. Allergic diseases

7.1. Flea allergy dermatitis

Ctenocephalides felis felis is the most important ectoparasite in dogs and cats in several countries [70]. Its infestation may cause intense pruritus, self-inflicted trauma and even severe symptoms as anemia. Some animals will develop a severe condition known as flea allergy dermatitis (FAD). After the sensitization, the lesions may be initiated by only a few flea bites [71]. Flea allergy is one of the most frequent conditions in dogs, especially in humid and warm weather countries, where fleas are commonly found [72]. The most common clinical signs are erythema, excoriation, crusting, and pustules that usually affect the medial caudal aspect of forelegs and ventral abdomen; pyotraumatic dermatitis may also be observed [73].

Diagnosis is based on circumstantial evidence, such as clinical response to flea control. A successful treatment for FAD depends on eliminating the allergy source, the flea. Therapy goals are the total elimination of flea population in the patient's body and environment, as well as in contact animals. It is also important to prevent new infestation, what is not always simple, once fleas have a high reproductive capacity and a complex life cycle [71]. Flea control advances with modern insecticides and insect growth regulators markedly decreased the number of affected animals. Products as fipronil, imidacloprid, metaflumizone, nintempiram, selamectin e spinosad proved to be efficient to control fleas in animals with FAD [74]. These products are available in several presentations as shampoo, collars, spray, powder, spot on and oral medication [71].

7.2. Adverse food reaction

Adverse food reactions are described in veterinary medicine since 1920, reporting the occurrence of gastrointestinal signs and skin reactions in response to food allergens [75].

Adverse food reaction refers to any abnormal clinical response assigned to consumption of food or its additives [76]. This reaction is classified as food allergy (immune-mediated) or food intolerance (non-immune-mediated). The majority of reactions in animals are food intolerances and they can be of pharmacological or metabolic origin, poisoning, idiosyncrasy [76, 77], toxicity or anaphylactic reaction to the food [77]. There are some dogs with pruritic skin diseases or otitis which resolves with restrictive diet, but it remains unproved the immunologic cause or hypersensitivity (allergy) associated with cutaneous adverse food reactions (CAFR). Once the etiopathogenesis was not elucidated yet, the term food allergy should be avoided, and CAFR is more appropriate [76, 78]

There are no breed, sex or age predisposition to the occurrence of clinical signs. Pruritus is the most important sign reported and it affects mainly the face, perineum and ears (otitis externa). Gastrointestinal signs as vomiting and diarrhea can also be observed. The best diagnostic approach for CAFR in dogs and cats is feeding them with a diet, with only one source of protein that the animal has never been in contact before (novel protein). The diagnosis is obtained with the resolution of clinical signs after the diet trial and with the return of these signs when the previous diet is offered again. The diet trial should be implemented for at least six weeks. Homemade diets are more appropriate for the CAFR trial described above, but there are also commercially available prescription and hydrolyzed diets [75].

Prescription diets, commercially available in some countries, are made of an unusual protein source and a non-allergenic carbohydrate source such as potato or oat meal. Lamb, duck, rabbit and Kangaroo meat are protein sources usually found in these diets [77]. Another option considered really hypoallergenic is the hydrolyzed diet. For humans it is known that most food allergens are glycoproteins with molecular weight higher than 12,000 d. The hydrolyzed food has smaller peptides what makes them potentially less allergenic [75]. However, a small percentage of allergic dogs show poor response to hydrolyzed food. The possibility of adverse food reaction to hydrolyzed food in sensitive dogs is rare but should be considered [79].

CAFR differential diagnoses are other hypersensitivities as FAD, atopic dermatitis, diseases caused by ectoparasites, and yeast or bacterial infections. These infections can also appear as complications of a pruritic process. Therapy should include secondary infections and otitis externa. Some cases also demand severe pruritus control while the diet trial is applied. Any drug therapy should be interrupted at least three weeks before the end of the diet trial, so that the clinician can access the animal response to the diet [75]. It is still unknown if animals develop tolerance to food allergens after a long period without contact, as reported in humans, however, natural hyposensitization is apparently rare [77].

7.3. Atopic dermatitis in dogs

Canine atopic dermatitis (CAD) is an allergic, hereditary, inflammatory and pruritic skin disease, with characteristic clinical signs associated with immunoglobulin E (IgE) production against environmental allergens [80]. Atopic dermatitis also affects cats, but its incidence is lower than in dogs [81].

Most dogs with atopic dermatitis begin to manifest signs between six months and three years of age [82, 83]. There is no sex predisposition and clinical signs may or not be seasonal, depending on the allergen involved. Usually, patients have a history of pruritus with or without secondary skin or ear infections. Primary lesions include macules and papules, but frequently, patients are presented with secondary lesions from self-inflicted trauma as excoriations, alopecia, lichenification and hyperpigmentation. Lesions affect the face, concave part of the pinna, ventral aspect of the neck, axilla, groin, abdomen, perineum, ventral aspect of the tail, limbs joints, medial aspects of limb extremities, feet and ears [85].

In dog as in human beings there is no pathognomonic sign of atopic dermatitis that could provide a diagnosis based only in history and physical examination. Diagnosis depends on patient fitting in several criteria associated with the condition and on elimination of differential diagnoses. Following clinical diagnosis, laboratory or clinical tests as allergy tests and histopathology, reinforces the diagnosis. However, these tests should not be used to establish the diagnosis but to confirm it [82]. It is important to highlight the fact that some dogs with inflammatory and pruritic skin diseases, displaying clinical signs identical to those found in CAD, may have no IgE production in response to environmental allergens. This condition is known as "canine atopic like dermatitis" [80]. Other dermatosis might share similar signs with canine atopic dermatitis or could be concurrent diseases and it is why they should be eliminated or controlled before the conclusive diagnose of CAD. Differential diagnoses for CAD are FAD, CAFR, pruritic parasitic diseases, bacterial pyoderma, *Malassezia* dermatitis and other allergic diseases [82, 83]. Allergy tests goals are to determinate allergens, to contact avoidance and to be included in the allergy specific immunotherapy [83]. No allergy test is completely sensitive or specific, therefore, clinically normal animals can have positive responses and animals with negative results can have clinical characteristics of the disease [82]. Allergens generally related to CAD pathogenesis are domestic dust mites, mold spores, trees and grasses pollens, antigens from insects and epidermis [84].

Atopic dermatitis is one of the most common skin diseases in dogs, however, its pathogenesis is not completely understood, so there is no curative therapy available yet [85]. Diverse topical and systemic therapies are currently available for CAD treatment such as specific allergy immunotherapy, corticosteroids, calcineurin inhibitors, anti-histamines and essential fatty acids. Unfortunately, these therapies are not effective in all cases or show adverse effects with long term use [86]. For most dogs with atopic dermatitis, the elimination or prevention of the contact with allergens is extremely difficult and drug therapy is not always satisfactory, in these cases the possibility to modulate the immune response to allergens is a good option. Specific allergy immunotherapy, also known as hyposensitization, desensitization or allergy vaccines [85], is defined as the act of administrating increasing amounts of allergen extracts to an allergic patient, in order to minimize the symptoms related to allergen exposure. Immunotherapy is not an option for patients that do not produce IgE against allergens with clinical relevance [87]. As a result, 50 to 100% of dogs submitted to immunotherapy may show improvement in clinical signs after four months of treatment, and some of these animals remain with no clinical sign for long periods [88]. Despite broadly applied in the treatment of human atopic dermatitis, there are just a few studies of the topical corticosteroids use in veterinary medicine. Triamcinolone 0.015% spray was used with good results during a month with minimal side effects [89]. Recently, hydrocortisone aceponate 0.0584% spray applied once daily in affected areas, in the dose of two sprays for each 100 cm2, during 84 days was markedly effective, showing results similar to those obtained with cyclosporine therapy, although with no adverse effects [90]. Frequently used oral glucocorticoids are prednisone, prednisolone and methylprednisolone, considered efficient and with rapid anti-allergic effect, at 0.5 to 1.0 mg/kg once or twice daily. Once desired effect is achieved, the dose may be decreased maintaining efficiency. Often observed adverse effects are related to dose and duration of the treatment [89]. Calcineurin inhibitors as tacrolimus 0.1% ointment applied twice daily on localized lesions is efficient in CAD treatment [91]. Good efficacy can also be observed with oral cyclosporine 5 mg/kg once daily during four to six weeks. When using cyclosporine the dose is usually reduced to half after obtaining improvement in clinical signs, maintaining the efficiency. Side effects as vomiting and transient diarrhea can occur. Oral anti-histamines has been used for decades in CAD treatment, however, there is no study showing conclusive evidences of its efficacy. Adverse effects of anti-histamines may be sedation and lethargy but this signs are uncommon. Omega 3 and 6 essential fatty acids from vegetal or from fishes source has been used for longer than 20 years in the treatment of atopic dermatitis. They are commercially available in capsules, liquid or enriched diet. The benefits of fatty acids therapy for CAD, is not clear despite the many studies in the area, however, they might reduce the corticosteroids dose, after 8 weeks of concurrent therapy [89].

8. Immunologic skin diseases

8.1. Pemphigus complex

Pemphigus complex diseases result from the production of autoantibodies directed against epidermal intercellular content, resulting in cell separation with intraepidermal bullae formation. The deposition of antibodies promotes the physical separation of the cells; moreover, it is believed that the release of cell proteases occur, which digests the intercellular substance, further aggravating the condition. Among the forms observed in dogs and cats are pemphigus erythematosus, pemphigus vulgaris, pemphigus vegetans and pemphigus foliaceus, the latter being the most common autoimmune skin disorder in these species [92], which will be discussed in this chapter.

Pemphigus foliaceus is observed more frequently in middle-aged animals, especially in domestic short haired cats and in dogs of some predisposed breeds such as Bearded Collies, Japanese Akitas, Chow Chows, Doberman Pinschers and Newfoundlands [93, 94]. It is a vesiculobullous, erosive disorder, which produces evident footpad hyperkeratosis. The face, trunk and abdomen are also frequently affected [95, 96]. Pustules, crusted lesions, erythema, alopecia and secondary pyoderma may also be present [94, 96]. Cachexia and sepsis secondary to infection may be observed in severe cases [97].

When present, pustular lesions can be evaluated cytologically and can reveal non degenerated granulocytes and acanthocytes [94]. Histologically intraepidermal and intrafollicular pustules are observed, with the presence of superficial perivascular dermatitis and acanthocytes [92, 93, 98]. The histologic presence of acantholysis is the Hallmark of the pemphigus complex [98].

Therapy requires the use of immunosuppressant or immunomodulators. Prednisone, prednisolone and methylprednisolone are commonly used in the treatment of pemphigus. Initially it is recommended a dose of 2.2 to 4.4 mg/kg, every 24 hours, for all three drugs. If therapeutic response is seen in 14 days, the dosage should be reduced gradually over 30 to 40 days. After this, an alternate day dose should be implemented, reaching a final protocol of 1 mg/kg every 48 hours or less [98]. In resistant cases of canine pemphigus, the use of prednisolone can be combined with azathioprine (2.2 mg/kg q12h or q24h) or cyclophosphamide (50 mg/m2 q48h). Feline pemphigus normally responds well to prednisolone, although resistant cases may benefit from a combination of prednisolone and chlorambucil (0.1-0.2 mg/kg every 24 hours or every other day) [94]. Topical glucocorticoids can be used as a single therapy, in localized forms of pemphigus or used for persistent lesions, as adjunctive therapy to the systemic treatment [98]. The occurrence of deaths in cases of pemphigus foliaceus are mainly from side effects of the drugs, secondary infections or in many cases, the pet owner requests euthanasia [97].

8.2. Discoid lupus erythematosus

Discoid lupus erythematosus (DLE) is an immune-mediated disease in which the lesions are similar to those of systemic lupus erythematosus (SLE), although, without the presence of the fluorescent antinuclear antibody and without the involvement of other body systems, as occurs in SLE [99]. The etiology is unknown, however, sunlight can precipitate or exacerbate the lesions. The most commonly affected regions of the body are the face and ears. Initially, there are depigmentation, erythema and desquamation. The lesions progress to scaly and swollen plaques. Definitive diagnosis is made by characteristic histopathology or immunofluorescence. Affected animals usually have a good response to systemic therapy with glucocorticoids, but topical presentations are also an option to the treatment [100]. Topical tacrolimus 0.1% can be an alternative therapy to the treatment with glucocorticoids, and was effective and safe for the treatment of DLE in dogs [101].

9. Metabolic and endocrine diseases

9.1. Hypothyroidism

Hypothyroidism is an endocrine disorder associated with a reduced production of T4 and T3 hormones by the thyroid gland [102]. Rarely affects cats [103], however, is the most common endocrinopathy in dogs [104]. The primary destruction of the thyroid gland occurs in more than 95% of adult dogs with hypothyroidism [104,105]. Thyroid hormones are extremely important in the maintenance of normal skin function, and dermatologic conditions are reported in 60 to 80% of hypothyroidism cases [106,107]. Usual findings are changes in coat quality and color, alopecia (in most cases, bilaterally symmetric and sparing head and limbs), superficial pyoderma, dry and desquamated skin, dry or oily seborrhea, brittle and easily pulled hairs, hyperkeratosis, hyperpigmentation, comedones, otitis, deficient healing of wounds, pruritus, myxedema and obesity [108].

Diagnosis is based on clinical signs, and on serum total TSH and free T4 [109]. Histopathology may show highly suggestive signs of hypothyroidism as follicle atrophy, hyperkeratosis, epidermal melanosis, many follicles in telogen phase [110], hypertrophy and vacuolization of arrector pili muscles, increased dermal mucine and thickened dermis [111].

Oral sodium levothyroxine (T4), 20 µg/kg twice daily, is the drug of choice for hypothyroidism [108]. The patient should receive appropriate treatment for dermatologic conditions presented, although they tend to disappear with the sodium levothyroxine administration.

9.2. Hyperadrenocorticism

Hyperadrenocorticism, also known as Cushing syndrome, results from chronic excessive cortisol secretion by the adrenal glands. It occurs iatrogenically, after synthetic glucocorticoids administration, or spontaneously, as a consequence of pituitary or adrenal gland primary hyper function. In dogs and cats, 80 to 85% of spontaneous hyperadrenocorticism are hypophysis-dependent [112]. Poodles, Dachshunds, Boston Terriers and Boxers are the more often affected dog breeds, and it rarely occurs in cats [113].

Symptoms as polyuria, polydipsia, polyphagia, hepatomegaly and abdominal swelling (pot-bellied appearance) are commonly observed. Dermatological signs include hypotrichosis, alopecia along the back tending to be symmetrical and bilateral, comedones, pyoderma and seborrhea [112]. Hyperpigmentation, thinner skin and calcinosis cutis occurs less frequently [114]. Clinical signs associated to laboratorial evaluation and diagnostic imaging findings, leads to the diagnosis. Plasma ACTH, low dexamethasone dose suppression test, ACTH stimulation test [113, 115] and urinary cortisol/creatinin ratio [116] confirms hyperadrenocorticism. It is also important to obtain the history of glucocorticoids use to eliminate iatrogenic cause [117].

Hyperadrenocorticism therapy depends on etiology, severity degree, tumor malignancy and availability of treatment options [118]. In hypophysis-dependent cases of adrenal dysfunction, surgical resection of the pituitary gland can be performed with low mortality rate. Adrenalectomy is recommended in cases of adrenal neoplasms. Drug therapy to control hypercortisolism involves the oral use of mitotane (o, p'-DDD), 50 mg/kg once a day [113] or oral trilostane, 2 to 3 mg/kg once a day. Some dogs may show a transient worsening of dermatological signs, especially with mitotane use. Complete resolution of dermatological signs usually takes months to be achieved [118].

10. Acquired alopecia

10.1. Canine pattern baldness

Canine pattern baldness is a common condition that affects short coated dog breeds with the development of acquired alopecia in specific body regions as, post-auricular, ventral cervical, chest, abdomen and caudomedial aspect of the thighs [119] (Figure 5). Canine pattern baldness is an aesthetic problem, with no consequences to patients health however, treatment may be required by the owners. Treatment may be tried with oral melatonin 5 mg (one capsule), once daily during 30 days to promote hair growth in alopecic regions [119,120].

10.2. Canine follicular dysplasia

Follicular dysplasia is an inherited condition characterized by an abnormal development of the hair follicle, leading to hair structural abnormalities and alopecia [121]. Neck, back and hind limbs can be affected and secondary pyoderma and comedones are common clinical findings [122]. The diagnosis confirmation through histopathology revel a great number of dysplastic follicles, dysplastic hair shafts and melanin aggregates within the hairs [123]. Patients can experiment spontaneous remission of follicle dysplasia, however, oral administration of 3 mg melatonin twice daily may help hair regrowth [124].

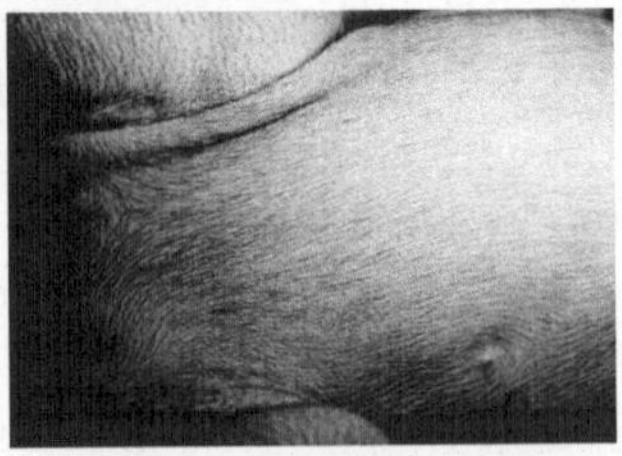

Figure 5. Canine pattern baldness. A Doberman pinscher with alopecia of the chest, which is characteristic of pattern alopecia (Veterinary Hospital of the Federal University of Viçosa).

10.3. Post clipping alopecia

Post clipping alopecia or post clipping hair follicles arrest [125] is a common but poorly understood syndrome in dogs, characterized by the absence of hair in consequence to a deficient growth in a previously clipped area [126]. In some cases the hair may take years to grow back. On clinical exam, the skin is normal with well delimited alopecic areas. Diagnosis is closed by the history of alopecia after clipping with no other dermatologic sign. If any systemic sign or other skin disorders are present, it is recommended to perform appropriate laboratory procedures to search for the endocrinopathies [125]. Usually no treatment is required [122]

10.4. Alopecia X

Alopecia X is a disease previously known as adrenal congenital hyperplasia, Cushing-like disease, dermatosis responsive to castration and adult-onset hyposomatotropism [127]. It is a condition associated with abnormalities on the hair cycle, affecting mainly the German Spitz breed. Affected animals display hairs in telogen phase what prevents new hair growth [128]. These animals are clinically healthy and show progressive hair loss, symmetric and non-pruritic, with variable degree of hyperpigmentation [129]. Histopathology findings are similar to those found in endocrinopathies, such as comedones, superficial and infundibulum hyperkeratinization, however, the presence of catagenization with flame follicle formation, confirms alopecia X diagnosis [127].

Therapies with sex hormones, growth hormone, mitotane and castration usually do not produce consistent results. Trilostane 10.5 mg/kg once a day, or twice a day, may produce complete hair growth in affected animals after four to eight weeks of treatment [129].

11. Keratinization disorders

11.1. Seborrhea

Seborrheic dermatitis is a skin keratinization disorder which can be primary or secondary. Primary keratinization disorders are inherited and exhibits breed predisposition. Usually, clinical signs appear before two years of age [130]. About 90% of the cases are secondary to an underlying disease [131,132] such as metabolic, hereditary or nutritional disorders [133] that causes excessive skin desquamation [131,132].

Seborrhea is classified in seborrhea sicca or oleosa according to hair and skin appearance [131,132]. In seborrhea sicca the coat is opaque and dry, containing aggregates of white to greyish scales, and in seborrhea oleosa there are adhesions of yellowish to brown lipid material, with greasy appearance [130]. Animals often exhibit pruritus, folliculitis, pyoderma, inflammation and hyperkeratosis plaques formation [131,132].

Diagnosis is based in history, clinical signs, physical examination findings and complementary exams to eliminate differential diagnosis or to determinate the primary disease. Frequently, it is necessary to perform skin scrapings, fungal and bacterial cultures, allergy tests, endocrine function evaluation, skin biopsy and evaluation of therapy response to close the diagnosis. Histopathology reveals abnormal keratinization of the epidermis and hair follicles, orthokeratotic and parakeratotic hyperkeratosis, follicular hyperkeratosis, dyskeratosis and perivascular superficial dermatitis [130].

Seborrhea treatment goals are scales and crusts removal and oil, pruritus and inflammation reduction [131,132]. Cases of primary idiopathic seborrhea could be treated with oral Vitamin A (600 to 800 UI/kg, twice daily) or with retinoids as isotretinoin and etretin (1 a 2 mg/kg a q12h) [134]. Salicylic acid and sulfur shampoos are recommended and might have positive results in moderate cases. Tar shampoos are recommended to severe cases of seborrhea oleosa in dogs, however, they are contraindicated in cats [135]. Secondary cases have an excellent prognosis when the underlying disease is eliminated, while primary keratinization disorders demand lifelong control and treatment [130].

11.2. Acne

Acne is a common disorder in cats and it may result from an idiopathic keratinization defect or a secondary reaction pattern to another disorder [136]. The most common skin changes are found in the chin and lip margin, and they include comedones, crusts, papules, erythema, alopecia and variable pruritus. Usually this disorder courses with secondary bacterial pyoderma and in some cases, with *M. pachydermatis* infections [137]. Papules, pustules, furunculosis and cellulitis might be signs of a secondary infection. Changes in hair follicle cycle, immunosuppression, stress, deficient grooming and concurrent viral infections are possible causes for this disorder [136]. Histology shows periductal linfoplasmocitary inflammation, sebaceous gland duct dilatation and follicular keratosis with obstruction and dilatation of the follicles [137]. Mild cases can be treated with anti-seborrheic shampoo; however, severe cases require association with systemic antimicrobial therapy or systemic corticoids [136]. Mupirocin 2% ointment is efficient when applied on lesions twice daily [138]. Topical tretinoin 0.01 to 0.025% (lotion or ointment) improves the clinical signs in chronic cases [139,140]. Proper recognition and treatment of secondary infections contribute to a successful therapy [137]. Feline acne has a good prognosis, however, symptomatic lifelong treatment is often necessary to control the condition [140].

12. Psychogenic diseases

12.1. Acral lick dermatitis

Acral lick dermatitis is characterized by ulcerated, proliferative, firm and alopecic plaques, derived from compulsive licking of the distal portion of the limbs [141] (Figure

6). Secondary bacterial infection is frequent and contributes to the sorely pruritic nature of the lesions [142]. This condition may originate from psychogenic (fear, and/or anxiety-based conditions), dermatologic (secondary to hypersensitivity, demodicosis, neoplasms and fungal or bacterial infections), traumatic, neuropathies or articular diseases [141,142].

Diagnosis requires complete clinical evaluation (anamnesis, physical, neurological and dermatological exams), complete blood cell count, serum biochemical profile and urinalysis. Only after the elimination of possible organic causes for acral lick dermatitis, it can be considered a behavioral disorder. In this case, the animal behavior should be evaluated, with the observation of its environmental and social stimuli and their motivational status. Treating acral lick dermatitis is notoriously challenging. The animal's environment should be modified to eliminate or minimize their exposure to stress factors [142], and the use of anti-depressives as fluoxetine 20 mg/day may help significantly in compulsion control which improves the lesions [143].

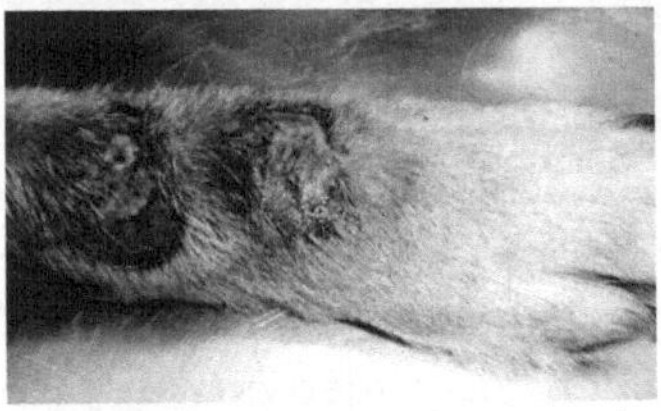

Figure 6. Acral lick dermatitis. Ulcerated plaques with tissue necrosis in the distal potion of a dog's forelimb.

13. Nutritional skin diseases

13.1. Vitamin A responsive dermatosis

Vitamin A is essential to the maintenance of epithelial tissue integrity and is especially important in the keratinization process [144]. Vitamin A responsive dermatosis is an uncommon condition, observed mainly in properly fed Cocker Spaniels [145] that may exhibiting skin desquamation, pruritus, oily skin, characteristic hyperkeratotic plaques and secondary pyoderma [144]. Histopathology reveals follicular oriented exuberant hyperkeratosis [145].

Lesions do not improve with anti-seborrheic therapy, but oral supplementation of vitamin A (retinol), at 10.000 UI once a day, provides clinical improvement in 5 to 8 weeks of treatment. Lifelong treatment is usually necessary [144].

13.2. Zinc responsive dermatosis

Zinc is essential in the cellular metabolism and also in hair and skin health maintenance [144]. Zinc responsive dermatosis is an unusual disorder in dogs and it is characterized by scaling, focal erythema, crusts and alopecia, mainly over the head [146].

Two syndromes are recognized in dogs. Syndrome I affect young adult dogs fed with balanced diets, especially Siberian Huskies and Alaskan Malamutes, however, it was reported in other breeds [146,147]. Affected animals have a diminished ability to absorb zinc from the intestinal tract, due to some subclinical disease or to genetic factors [144]. Syndrome II is observed in rapidly growing puppies, especially of giant breeds, fed with zinc deficient diets or with excessive calcium phytate [144,146].

The diagnosis is based on history, clinical signs, characteristics lesions, breed, skin biopsy and response to zinc supplementation. The histopathological abnormalities found are papillary epidermal hyperplasia, confluent spongiotic parakeratosis and suppurative crusts [146].

Syndrome I control requires lifelong oral zinc supplementation with zinc methionine 1.7 mg/kg once a day, zinc gluconate 5 mg/kg once a day or zinc sulfate 10 mg/kg once a day [14]. Refractory cases to oral supplementation could receive intravenous administration of zinc sulfate at 10 to 15 mg/kg once a week, initially during four weeks and later each one, to six months [144]. Prognosis is good in most cases, although, lifelong supplementation may be required. Affected animals should be removed from breeding [147].

Syndrome II has an excellent prognosis and only requires food balancing to supply the zinc deficiency, however, signs remission occur faster with oral zinc supplementation [144].

13.3. External ear diseases

The external ear is divided in three parts: inner, middle and outer ear. External or outer ear comprises the pinna, vertical canal and horizontal canal, formed by auricular and annular cartilages. The diameter of the external ear canal varies according to the age, breed and size of the animal and it is separated from the middle ear by the tympanum, a thin semitransparent membrane with an elliptic shape [148]. External ear diseases are particularly important in veterinary dermatology, since the outer ear is formed in the embryo life through a skin invagination, being susceptive to a number of dermatologic conditions [149]. Otitis externa is the most frequent disorder of the outer ear canal in dogs and cats, consisting in the inflammation of its epithelium [150,151].

In order to achieve the correct diagnosis and a successful therapy, it is essential to recognize and understand the primary predisposing and perpetuating causes. Primary causes are factors or processes that trigger the inflammation in the outer canal [152]. The most frequent trigger factors are parasitic infestation (*Octodetes cynotis, Demodex canis, Sarcoptes scabiei, Notroedes cati*), foreign body, allergic diseases and hypersensitivities (atopic dermatitis, food allergy, contact allergic dermatitis), keratinization disorders (seborrhea, sebaceous adenitis), hormonal disorders and autoimmune diseases (pemphigus, lupus erythematous). Predisposing causes are factors and process that increases the risk of otitis development, such as the ear conformation (narrow ear canal, excessive hair in the ear canal, long and pendulous ears), excessive humidity (baths, swimming habit), iatrogenic factors (use of cotton swab to clean the ear, use of irritant cleaning solutions) and the occurrence of obstructive ear diseases (polyps and neoplasms) [151].

Factors that help to perpetuate otitis are bacterial infection (*Staphylococcus pseudintermedius, Pseudomonas aeruginosa*), yeast infection (*M. pachydermatis*) and complications of otitis media, as ear canal narrowness due to hyperplasia and calcification of the cartilage structures [151,153,154].

The initial sign of otitis externa is erythema of the pinna and outer ear canal. Worsening of symptoms can lead to head shake, ear pruritus, malodorous purulent or ceruminous discharge, edema, pain and evidences of self-inflicted trauma as aural hematoma and acute moist dermatitis in the base of ears. Chronic or recurrent otitis can lead to soft tissue hyperplasia, ear canal stenosis and occlusion [151].

Diagnosis requires physical and dermatological examination, knowledge of the dermatological history and clinical signs development. Otoscopic examination is the first choice technique to evaluate the outer ear canal [155] and it should be performed in every patient with signs of otitis [156]. It is important to notice that a healthy ear canal might have small amounts of yellowish or brown cerumen [150]. Through otoscopy the clinician can access the presence of inflammation, exudate, hyperplasia, stenosis, foreign body, neoplasms and evaluate the tympanic membrane. Depending on the degree of pain, inflammation and stenosis, it might be necessary to use topical or systemic corticoids for two to three weeks before performing an otoscopic examination [156].

Cytological analysis is required for the diagnosis, and samples should be obtained from both pinna and the outer vertical and horizontal canal. Cytology can provide early information about the inflammatory response and microbial organisms or parasites involved in the process [150].

A successful therapy is based on: removing or controlling the primary cause and predisposing factors; eliminating bacterial and yeast infection, parasite infestation and foreign bodies on ear canal; cleaning the pinna, vertical and horizontal canal; eliminating debris, exudates and cerumen. It is also extremely important to instruct the owner about cleaning techniques and administration methods for topical medications [150].

Gram positive bacterial infections can be treated with topical steroidal antibiotics (fusidic acid) and topical fluoroquinolones (marbofloxacin and orbifloxacin). Gram negative infections could also be treated with fluoroquinolones or with topical cationic polipeptides (polymyxin B) and aminoglycosides (neomycin, framycetin, gentamicin) [154]. Aminoglycosides are contraindicated in cases of tympanic membrane rupture due to their ototoxicity [150]. *Malassezia* species are usually susceptible to azoles (clotrimazol and myconazol) and polyene macrolides (nistatin) [154].

The use of topical drugs such as moxidectin 1% and imidacloprid 10% (0.1 mg/kg, two applications with two weeks interval) is effective for *Otodectis cynotis* infestation in cats [157].

Animals with acute otitis should be treated twice daily during 7 to 14 days. Chronic or recurrent cases should be treated for, at least 4 weeks, and systemic anti-inflammatory drugs are recommended in association to the topical therapy (prednisone or prednisolone 0.5 mg/kg q12h) [158]. Glucocorticoids efficiently control the inflammation and may prevent or reverse tissue hyperplasia and canal stenosis [154].Therapy should be discontinued only when cytology is negative for microorganisms, if there is no ear canal edema and if the epithelium has a normal appearance [158].

References

1. Thomsett LR. Structure of Canine Skin. The British Veterinary Journal 1986; 142 (2) 116-23.
2. Favarato ES, Conceição LG. Hair Cycle in Dogs with Different Hair Types in a Tropical Region of Brazil. Veterinary Dermatology 2008; 19(1) 15-20.

3. Beale K. Dermatologic Diagnostic Techniques. In: Florida Veterinary Medical Association: proceedings of FVMA's 82nd Annual Conference, April 29-May 1, 2011, Orlando, EUA.

4. Mueller RS (Ed.). Specific Tests in Small Animal Dermatology. In: Dermatology for the Small Animal Practitioner. Ithaca: IVIS; 2006. http://www.ivis.org/advances/Mueller/part1chap3/chapter.asp?LA=1 (accessed 01 August 2012).

5. Shelly SM. Cutaneous Lesions. Veterinary Clinics of North America: Small Animal Practice 2003; 33(1) 1-46.

6. Ihrke PJ. An Overview of Bacterial Skin Disease in the Dog. British Veterinary Journal 1987; 143(2) 112-8.

7. Moriello KA. Pyoderma. In: Kahn CM. (ed.) The Merck Veterinary Manual. Whitehouse Station: Merck Sharp & Dohme Corp.; 2011. Avaliable from: http://www.merckvetmanual.com/mvm/index.jsp?cfile=htm/bc/70900.htm (accessed 12 August 2012).

8. Devriese LA, Vancanneyt M, Baele M et al. Staphylococcus pseudintermedius sp. nov., a coagulase-positive species from animals. International Journal of Systematic and Evolutionary Microbiology 2005; 55(4) 1569–73.

9. Guardabassi L, Loeber ME, Jacobson A. Transmission of Multiple Antimicrobial-resistant Staphylococcus intermedius Between Dogs Affected by Deep Pyoderma and their Owners. Veterinary Microbiology 2004; 98(1) 23-7.

10. Mason, I.S. Canine Pyoderma. Journal of Small Animal Practice 1991; 32(8) 381–6.

11. Cobb MA, Edwards HJ, Jagger TD, Marshall J, Bowker KE. Topical Fusidic Acid/Betamethasone-Containing Gel Compared to Systemic Therapy in the Treatment of Canine Acute Moist Dermatitis. Veterinary Journal 2005; 169(2) 276-80.

12. Ihrke, P.J. Bacterial Skin Disease in the Dog: A Guide to Canine Pyoderma. Newark: Bayer/Veterinary Learning Systems, 1996.

13. Hill PB, Moriello KA. Canine Pyoderma. Journal of American Veterinary Medical Association 1994; 204(3) 334–40.

14. Scott, D.W., Miller, W.H., Griffin, C.E. Muller & Kirk's Small Animal Dermatology. 6th edition. Philadelphia: W.B. Saunders; 2001.

15. Lloyd, D. Dealing with Cutaneous Staphylococcal Infection in Dogs. In Practice 1996;18(2) 223-31.

16. Coyner, KS. Challenges & New Developments in Canine Pyoderma - Disease Overview & Diagnosis. Today's Veterinary Practice 2012; 2(1) 31-38.

17. Coyner, KS. Challenges & New Developments in Canine Pyoderma - Topical & Systemic Treatment. Today's Veterinary Practice 2012; 2(2) 36-44.

18. May, E.R. Bacterial Skin Diseases: Current Thoughts on Pathogenesis and Management. Veterinary Clinics of North America: Small Animal Practice 2006; 36(1) 185-202.

19. Hainer BL. Dermatophyte Infections. American Family Physician 2003; 67(1) 101-8.

20. Georg LK. Dermatophytes: New methods in classification. Atlanta: Public Health Service; 1957.
21. Lewis DT, Foil CS, Hosgood, G. Epidemiology and Clinical Features of Dermatophytosis in Dogs and Cats at Louisiana State University: 1981–1990. Veterinary Dermatology 1991; 2(2) 53–8.
22. Sparkes AH, Werret G, Stokes CR, Gruffydd-Jones TJ. Microsporum canis: Innaparent Carriage by Cats and the Viability of Arthrospores. Journal of Small Animal Practice 1994; 35(8): 397-401.
23. Bond R. Superficial Veterinary Mycoses. Clinics in Dermatology 2010; 28(2) 226-36.
24. Moriello KA. Treatment of Dermatophytosis in Dogs and Cats: Review of Published Studies. Veterinary Dermatology 2004; 15(2) 99-107.
25. Moriello KA, Newbury S. Recommendations for the Management and Treatment of Dermatophytosis in Animal Shelters. Veterinary Clinics of North America: Small Animal Practice 2006; 36(1): 89-114.
26. Borgers M, Xhonneux B, Van Cutsem J. Oral Itraconazole Versus Topical Bifonazole Treatment in Experimental Dermatophytosis. Mycoses 1993; 36(3-4) 105-15.
27. Newbury S, Moriello KA, Verbrugge M, Thomas C. Use of Lime Sulphur and Itraconazole to Treat Shelter Cats Naturally Infected with Microsporum canis in an Annex Facility: an Open Feld Trial. Veterinary Dermatology 2007; 18(5) 324-31.
28. Newbury S, Moriello KA, Kwochka KW, Verbrugge M, Thomas C. Use Of Itraconazole and Either Lime Sulphur or Malaseb Concentrate Rinse to Treat Shelter Cats Naturally Infected with Microsporum canis: an Open field Trial. Veterinary Dermatology 2010; 22(1) 75-9.
29. Balda AC, Otsuka M, Gambale W, Larsson CE. Comparative Study of Griseofulvin and Terbinafine Therapy in the Treatment of Canine and Feline Dermatophytosis. Veterinary Dermatology 2004; 15(Issue Supplement s1) 44.
30. Bond R, Saijonmaa-Koulumies LEM, Lloyd DH. Population Sizes and Frequency of Malassezia pachydermatis at Skin and Mucosal Sites on Healthy Dogs. Journal of Small Animal Practice 1995; 36 (4) 147–50.
31. Hirsh DC, Biberstein, EL. Yeasts - Cryptococcus, Malassezia and Candida. In: Hirsh DC, MacLachlan NJ, Walker RL (eds). Veterinary Microbiology 2nd ed. Ames: Blackwell Publishing; 2004. p265-72.
32. Plant JD, Rosenkrantz WS, Griffin CE. Factors Associated with and Prevalence of High Malassezia pachydermatis Numbers on Dog Skin. Journal of the American Veterinary Medical Association 1992; 201(6) 879-82.
33. Bond R, Ferguson EA, Curtis CF, Craig JM, Lloyd DH. Factors Associated with Elevated Cutaneous Malassezia pachydermatis Populations in Dogs with Pruritic Skin Disease. Journal of Small Animal Practice 1996; 37(3) 103-7.
34. Mason, K.V.: Malassezia: Biology, associated diseases and treatment. In: Annual Members' Meeting AAVD & ACVD, vol.12: proceedings of American Academy of Veterinary Dermatology/ American College of Veterinary Dermatology 1996, Las Vegas, EUA. Harrisburg: American Academy of Veterinary Dermatology; 1996.

35. Machado ML, Ferreiro L, Ferreira RR, Corbellini LG, Deville M, Berthelemy M, Guillot J. Malassezia dermatitis in Dogs in Brazil: Diagnosis, Evaluation of Clinical Signs and Molecular Identification.Veterinary Dermatology 2011; 22(1) 46-52.

36. Ihrke, PJ. Malassezia dermatitis: diagnosis & management. In: proceedings of 33rd World Small Animal Veterinary Association Congress, 20-24 August 2008, Dublin, Ireland.

37. Berger DJ, Lewis TP, Schick AE, Stone RT. Comparison of Once-Daily Versus Twice-Weekly Terbinafine Administration for the Treatment of Canine Malassezia Dermatitis - a Pilot Study. Veterinary Dermatology 2012; Early View (Online Version of Record published before inclusion in an issue).

38. Bond R, Guillot J, Cabañes FJ. Malassezia Yeasts in Animal Disease. In: Boekhout T, Guého-Kellermann E, Mayser P, Velegraki A (eds). Malassezia and the Skin: Science and Clinical Practice. Heidelberg: Springer; 2010. p.271-92.

39. Lacaz, C. S.; Porto, E.; Martins, J. E. C.; Heins-Vaccari, E. M.; Melo, N. T. Esporotricose e Outras Micoses Gomosas. In: Lacaz, C. S.; Porto, E.; Martins, J. E. C.; Heins-Vaccari, E. M.; Melo, N. T. (eds.). Tratado de Micologia Médica Lacaz 9ª. ed. São Paulo: Sarvier; 2002. p.479-97.

40. Kauffman CA. Sporotrichosis. Clinical Infectious Diseases 1999; 29(2) 231-6; quiz 237.

41. Welsh, RD. Sporotrichosis. Journal of the American Veterinary Medical Association 2003; 223(8) 1123-6.

42. Rosser EJ, Dunstan RW. Sporotrichosis. In: Greene C (ed.). Infectious Diseases of the Dog and Cat 3nd ed. Canada: Elsevier; 2006. p.609-27.

43. Larsson CE. Esporotricose. Brazilian Journal of Veterinary Research and Animal Science 2011; 48(3) 250-9.

44. Madrid, I. M.; Xavier, M. O.; Mattei, A. S.; Carapeto, L. P.; Antunes, T. A.; Júnior, R. S.; Nobre, M. O.; Meireles, M. C. A. Esporotricose Óssea e Cutânea em Canino. Brazilian Journal of Veterinary Research and Animal Science, 2007; 44(6) 441-3.

45. Cagnini DQ, Rodrigues MMP, Palumbo MIP, Heckler MCT, Peixoto AS, Amorim RL, Machado LHA. Cytologic Diagnosis and Treatment of Feline Sporotrichosis: Case Report. Veterinária e Zootecnia 2012; 19(2) 186-91.

46. Boothe DM, Herring I, Calvin J, Way N, Dvorak J. Itraconazole Disposition After Single Oral and Intravenous and Multiple Oral Dosing in Healthy Cats. American Journal of Veterinary Research 1997; 58(8) 872-7.

47. Grace SF. Cryptococcosis. Norsworthy GD, Grace SF, Crystal MA, Tilley LP (eds). The feline patient 4th. ed. Iowa: Blackwell Publishing; 2011. p.97-9.

48. Malik R, Wigney DI, Muir DB, Gregory DJ, Love DN. Cryptococcosis in Cats: Clinical and Mycological Assessment of 29 Cases And Evaluation of Treatment Using Orally Administered Fluconazole. Journal of Medical and Veterinary Mycology 1992; 30(2) 133-44.

49. Chiesa S. C., Castro R. C., Otsuka M., Michalany N. S., Larsson Jr C. E., Larsson C. E. Cryptococcosis in São Paulo (Brazil): Clinical and Epidemiological Features (1992–2003). Veterinary Dermatology 2004; 15(Supplement s1) 46.

50. Martins DB, Barbosa ALT, Cavalheiro A, Lopes STA, Santurio JM, Schossler JE, Mazzanti A. Diagnóstico De Criptococose Canina pela Citologia Aspirativa por Agulha Fina. Ciência Rural 2008; 38(3) 826-9.

51. Trivedi SR, Malik R, Sykes JE. Feline Cryptococcosis: Impact of Current Research on Clinical Management. Journal of Feline Medical Surgery 2011; 13 (3) 163-172.

52. Hunt GB, Foster SF. Nasopharyngeal Disorders. In: Bonagura JD, Twedt DC (eds). Kirk's Current Veterinary Therapy XIV. St. Louis: Saunders Elsevier, 2009; 624-25.

53. Mueller RS. Treatment Protocols for Demodicosis: an Evidence-Based Review. Veterinary Dermatology 2004; 15(2) 75-89.

54. Gortel, K. Update on Canine Demodicosis. Veterinary Clinics of North America: Small Animal Practice 2006; 36(1) 229-41.

55. Rojas M, Riazzo C, Callejón R, Guevara D, Cutillas C. Molecular Study on Three Morphotypes of Demodex Mites (Acarina: Demodicidae) from Dogs. Parasitology Research 2012, Online First™, 16 August 2012. http://www.springerlink.com/content/h0357h6867775g66/fulltext.pdf (acessed 20 August 2012).

56. Baker KP. The Histopathology and Pathogenesis of Demodecosis of the Dog. Journal of Comparative Pathology 1969; 79 321-7.

57. Mason I, Mason K, Lloyd D. A Review of the Biology of Canine Skin with Respect to the Commensals Staphylococcus intermedius, Demodex canis and Malassezia pachydermatis. Veterinary Dermatology 1996; 7(3)119-32.

58. Mueller, RS, Bensignor E, Ferrer L, Holm B, Lemarie S, Paradis M, Shipstone MA Treatment of Demodicosis in Dogs: 2011 Clinical Practice Guidelines. Veterinary Dermatology 2012; 23(2): 86-96, e20-1.

59. Arther RG. Mites and Lice: Biology and Control. Veterinary Clinics of North America: Small Animal Practice 2009; 39(6) 1159-71.

60. Currier RW, Walton SF, Currier BJ. Scabies in Animals and Humans: History, Evolutionary Perspectives, and Modern Clinical Management. In: The Evolution of Infectious Agents in Relation to Sex: proceedings of Annals of the New York Academy of Science 2011; New York, USA.

61. Thomsett LR. Structure of Canine Skin. The British Veterinary Journal 1986;142(2) 116-23.

62. Mueller RS, Bettenay SV, Shipstone M. Value of the Pinnal-Pedal Reflex in the Diagnosis of Canine Scabies. Veterinary Record 2001; 148(20) 621-3.

63. Greiner E. Diagnosis of Arthropod Parasites. In: Zajac AM, Conboy GA. Veterinary Clinical Parasitology. 8th ed. Hoboken: Wiley-Blackwell, 2012: 217-303.

64. Folz SD, Kratzer DD, Kakuk TJ, Rector DL. Evaluation of a Sponge-On Therapy for Canine Scabies. Journal of Veterinary Pharmacology and Therapeutics 1984; 7(1) 29–34.

65. Curtis, C.F. Use of 0.25 Per Cent fipronil Spray to Treat Sarcoptic Mange in a Litter of five-Week-Old Puppies. Veterinary Record 1996; 139(2) 43–44.

66. Paradis M. Ivermectin in Small Animal Dermatology. Part II. Extralabel Applications. Compendium of Continuing Education for the Practicing Veterinarian 1998; 20: 459–69.

67. Curtis CF. Current Trends in the Treatment of Sarcoptes, Cheyletiella and Otodectes Mite Infestations in Dogs and Cats. Veterinary Dermatology 2004; 15(2) 108-114.

68. Six RH, Clemence RG, Thomas CA, Behan S, Boy MG, Watson P, Benchaoui HA, Clements PJ, Rowan TG, Jernigan AD. Efficacy and Safetyof Selamectin Against Sarcoptes scabiei on Dogs and Otodectes cynotis on dogs and Cats Presented as Veterinary Patients. Veterinary Parasitology 2000; 91(3-4) 291–309.

69. Miller Jr WH, Jaham C, Scott DW, Cayatte SM, Bagladi MS, Buerger RG. Treatment of Canine Scabies with Milbemycin Oxime. Canadian Veterinary Journal 1996; 37(4) 219–21.

70. Rust MK, Dryden MW. The Biology, Ecology, and Management of the Cat Flea. Annual Review of Entomology 1997; 42 451-473.

71. Carlotti DN, Jacobs DE. Therapy, Control and Prevention of Flea Allergy Dermatitis in Dogs and Cats. Veterinary Dermatology 2000; 11(2) 83-98.

72. Gross TL, Halliwell REW. Lesions of Experimental Flea Bite Hypersensitivity in the Dog. Veterinary Pathology 1985; 22(1) 78-81.

73. Wilkerson MJ, et al. The Immunopathogenesis of the Flea Allergy Dermatitis in Dogs, an Experimental Study. Veterinary Immunology and Immunopathology 2004; 99 (3-4) 179-92.

74. Dryden MW. Flea and Tick Control in the 21st Century: Challenges and Opportunities. Veterinary Dermatology 2009; 20 (5-6) 435-440.

75. Jackson HA. Diagnostic Techniques in Dermatology: The Investigation and Diagnosis of Adverse Food Reactions in Dogs and Cats. Clinical Techniques in Small Animal Practice 2001; 16(4) 233-235.

76. Hillier A, Griffin CE. The ACVD Task Force on Canine Atopic Dermatitis (X): Is There a Relationship Between Canine Atopic Dermatitis and Cutaneous Adverse Food Reactions? Veterinary Immunology and Immunopathology 2001; 81(3-4) 227-231.

77. Hensel P. Nutrition and Skin Diseases in Veterinary Medicine. Clinics in Dermatology 2010; 28(6) 686-693.

78. Bloom P. Cutaneous Adverse Food Reactions in Dogs: Something New to Chew On. The Veterinary Journal 2011; 187(3) 289.

79. Ricci R, et al. A Comparison of the Clinical Manifestations of Feeding Whole and Hydrolysed Chicken to Dogs with Hypersensitivity to the Native Protein. Veterinary Dermatology 2010; 21(4) 358-366.

80. Halliwell R. Revised Nomenclature for Veterinary Allergy. Veterinary Immunology and Immunopathology 2006; 114(3-4) 207-208.

81. Scott DW, Paradis M. A Survey of Canine and Feline Skin Disorders Seen in a University Practice: Small Animal Clinic, University of Montréal, Saint-Hyacinthe, Québec (1987-1988). Canadian Veterinary Journal 1990; 31(12) 830-835.

82. DeBoer DJ, Hillier A. The ACVD Task Force in Canine Atopic Dermatitis (XV): Fundamental Concepts in Clinical Diagnosis. Veterinary Immunology and Immunopathology 2001; 81(3-4) 271-276.

83. Olivry T, DeBoer DJ, Favrot C, Jackson HA, Mueller RS, Nuttall T, Prélaud P. Treatment of Canine Atopic Dermatitis: 2010 Clinical Practice Guidelines from the International Task Force on Canine Atopic Dermatitis. Veterinary Dermatology 2010; 21(3) 233-248.

84. Hill PB, DeBoer DJ. The ACVD Task Force in Canine Atopic Dermatitis (IV): Environmental Allergens. Veterinary Immunology and Immunopathology 2001; 81(3-4) 169-86.

85. Olivry T, Sousa CA. The ACVD Task Force in Canine Atopic Dermatitis (XIX): General Principles of Therapy. Veterinary Immunology and Immunopathology 2001; 81(3-4) 311-16.

86. Bloom P. Atopic Dermatitis in Dogs – Hitting the Moving Target. The Veterinary Journal 2006; 171(1) 16-7.

87. Bousquet J, et al. Allergen Immunotherapy: Therapeutic Vaccines for Allergic Diseases A WHO Position Paper. Journal of Allergy and Clinical Immunology 1998; 102(4) 558-62.

88. Griffin CE, Hillier A. The ACVD Task Force in Canine Atopic Dermatitis (XXIV): Allergen-specific Immunotherapy. Veterinary Immunology and Immunopathology 2001; 81(3-4) 363-83.

89. Olivry T, Foster AP, Mueller RS, McEwan NA, Chesney C, Williams HC. Interventions for Atopic Dermatitis in Dogs: a Systematic Review of Randomized Controlled Trials. Veterinary Dermatology 2010; 21(1) 4-22.

90. Nuttall TJ, McEwan NA, Bensignor E, Cornegliani L, Löwenstein C, Rème CA.. Comparable Efficacy of a Topical 0.0584% Hydrocortisone Aceponate Spray and Oral Ciclosporin in Treating Canine Atopic Dermatitis. Veterinary Dermatology 2011; 23(1) 4-e2.

91. Bensignor E, Olivry T. Treatment of Localized Lesions of Canine Atopic Dermatitis With Tacrolimus Ointment: a Blinded Randomized Controlled Trial. Veterinary Dermatology 2005; 16(1) 52-60.

92. Gorman NT, Werner LL. Immune-Mediated Diseases of the Dog And Cat. III. Immune-Mediated Diseases of the Integumentary, Urogenital, Endocrine and Vascular Systems. British Veterinary Journal 1986; 142(6) 491-7.

93. Day MJ, Hanlon L, Powell LM. Immune-Mediated Skin Disease in the Dog and Cat. Journal of Comparative Pathology 1993; 109(4) 395-407.

94. Day MJ, Shaw SE. Immune-Mediated Skin Disease. In: Day MJ. Clinical Immunology of the Dog and Cat. 2nd ed. London: Manson Publishing; 2008. p.148-55.

95. Scott DW, Manning TO, Smith CA, Lewis RM. Pemphigus and Pemphigoid in Dogs, Cats, and Horses. Annals of the New York Academy of Sciences 1983; 420 (Defined Immunofluorescence and Related Cytochemical Methods) 353-60.

96. Mueller RS, Krebs I, Power HT, Fieseler KV. Pemphigus Foliaceus in 91 Dogs. Journal of the American Animal Hospital Association 2006; 42(3) 189-196.

97. Tater KC, Olivry T. Canine and Feline Pemphigus Foliaceus: Improving Your Chances of a Successful Outcome. Veterinary Medicine 2010; 105(1) 18-30.

98. Rosenkrantz WS. Pemphigus: Current Therapy. Veterinary Dermatology 2004; 15(2) 90-98.

99. Gershwin LJ. Autoimmune Diseases in Small Animals. Veterinary Clinics of North America: Small Animal Practice 2010; 40(3) 439-457.

100. Griffin CE, Stannard AA, Ihrke PJ, Ardans AA, Cello RM, Bjorling DR. Canine Discoid Lupus Erythematosus. Veterinary Immunology and Immunopathology 1979; 1(1) 79-87.

101. Griffies JD, Mendelsohn CL, Rosenkrantz WS, Muse R, Boord MJ, Griffin CE. Topical 0.1% Tacrolimus for the Treatment of Discoid Lupus Erythematosus and Pemphigus Erythematosus in Dogs. Journal of the American Animal Hospital Association 2004; 40(1) 29-41.

102. Scott-Moncrieff JC, Guptill-Yoran L. Hipotireoidismo. In: Ettinger SJ, Feldman EC. Tratado de Medicina Interna Veterinária. 5.ed. Rio de Janeiro: Guanabara Koogan; 2004. p.1496-506.

103. Ferguson D.C. Update on Diagnosis of Canine Hypothyroidism. Veterinary Clinics of North America: Small Animal Practice 1994; 24(3) 515-39.

104. Meeking SA. Thyroid Disorders in the Geriatric Patient. Veterinary Clinics of North America: Small Animal Practice 2005; 35(3) 635-53.

105. Graham PA, Refsal KR, Nachreiner RF. Etiopatologic Findings of Canine Hypothyroidism.. Veterinary Clinics of North America: Small Animal Practice 2007; 37(4) 617-31.

106. Panciera DL. Hypothyroidism in Dogs: 66 Cases (1987–1992). Journal of the American Veterinary Medical Association 1994; 5 (204) 761-7.

107. Dixon RM, Reid SWJ, Mooney CT. Epidemiological, Clinical, Haematological and Biochemical Characteristics of Canine Hypothyroidism. Veterinary Record 1999; 145(17) 481–7.

108. Scott-Moncrieff JC. Clinical Signs and Concurrent Diseases of Hypothyroidism in Dogs and Cats. Veterinary Clinics of North America: Small Animal Practice 2007; 37(4) 709-22.

109. Lust E. Thyroid Disease in Canines and Felines. US Pharmacist 2005; 30(06) 41-9.

110. Arias PT. Hipotiroidismo canino. Virbac al Día Animales Compañía. 16: 1-6 http://www.webveterinaria.com/virbac/news19/hipotiroidismo.pdf (accessed 08 August 2012).

111. Panciera DL. Canine Hypothyroidism. Part II. Thyroid Function Tests and Treatment. Continuing Education Article – The Compendium Small Animal 1990; 12(6) 843-58.

112. Peterson M.E. Hyperadrenocorticism. Veterinary Clinics of North America 1984; 14: 731-49.

113. Kaufman J. Diseases of the Adrenal Cortex of Dogs and Cats. Modern Veterinary Practice 1984; 65(6) 429-34.

114. Peterson ME. Diagnosis of Hyperadrenocorticism in Dogs. Clinical Techniques in Small Animal Practice 2007; 22(1) 2-11.

115. Peterson, M.E. Diagnosis of hyperadrenocorticism in dogs. In: Cavender A, Davidson M, Gibbs S, Green C, Holley C, Johnston D, Kovacs S. Proceedings of the 16th Annual North Carolina Veterinary Conference, 4-6 November 2011, Raleigh, USA.

116. Goossens MMC, Meyer HP, Voorhout G, Sprang EP. Urinary Excretion of Glucocorticoids in the Diagnosis of Hyperadrenocorticism in Cats. Domestic Animal Endocrinology 1995; 12(4) 355–62.

117. Ghubash R, Marsella R, Kunkle G. Evaluation of Adrenal Function in Small-Breed Dogs Receiving Otic Glucocorticoids. Veterinary Dermatology 2004; 15(6) 363-68.

118. Peterson ME. Treatment of canine hyperadrenocorticism. In: Cavender A, Davidson M, Gibbs S, Green C, Holley C, Johnston D, Kovacs S. Proceedings of the 16th Annual North Carolina Veterinary Conference, 4-6 November 2011, Raleigh, USA

119. Paradis M. Melatonin Therapy for Canine Alopecia. In: Kirk's Current Veterinary Terapy XIII Small Animal Practice. Philadelphia: W.B. Saunders; 2000. p.546-9.

120. Paradis M. Melatonin Therapy in Canine Pattern Baldness. In: Kwochka KW, Willemse T, Von Tscharner C. Advances in Veterinary Dermatology: proceedings of the Third World Congress of Veterinary Dermatology, 11-14 September 1996, Edinburgh, Scotland. London: Elsevier Health Sciences; 1996.

121. Ferrer, L. Follicular dysplasias. In: 4th European Federation of European Companion Animal Veterinary Associations, Società Culturale Italiana Veterinari per Animali da Compagnia Congress: conference proceedings of the 4th European FECAVA SCIVAC Congress, 18-21 June 1998, Bologna, Italy.

122. Cerundolo R. Symmetrical Alopecia in the Dog. In Practice 1999; 21(7) 350-9.

123. Rothstein E, Scott DW, Miller WH Jr, et al. A Retrospective Study of Dysplastic Hair Follicles and Abnormal Melanization in Dogs with Follicular Dysplasia Syndromes or Endocrine Skin Disease. Veterinary Dermatology 1998; 9(4) 235-41.

124. Rachid MA, Demaula CD, Scott DW, Miller WH, Senter DA, Myers S. Concurrent Follicular Dysplasia and Interface Dermatitis in Boxer Dogs. Veterinary Dermatology 2003; 14(3) 159-166.

125. Scott DW, Miller WH Jr. Retrospective Record Review of Canine Postclipping Hair Follicle Arrest. Veterinary Dermatology 2012; 23(3) 248–9.

126. Diaz SF, Torres SMF, Dunstan RW, Lekcharoensuk C. An Analysis of Canine Hair Re-Growth After Clipping for a Surgical Procedure. Veterinary Dermatology 2004; 15(1) 25-30.

127. Rest JR, Lloyd DH, Cerundolo R. Histopathology of Alopecia X. Veterinary Dermatology 2004; 15(Supplement s1) 23.

128. Frank LA. Growth Hormone-Responsive Alopecia in Dogs. Journal of the American Veterinary Medical Association 2005; 226(9) 1494–7.

129. Cerundolo R, Lloyd DH, Persechino A, Evans H, Cauvin A. Treatment of Canine Alopecia X with Trilostane. Veterinary Dermatology 2004; 15(5) 285-93.

130. Campbell KL. Seborrheic Skin Disorders and Their Treatment in Dogs. Clinics in Dermatology 1994; 12(4) 551-8.

131. Halliwell RE. Seborrhea in the Dog. Compendium on Continuing Education for the Practicing Veterinarian 1979; 1 227-36.

132. Ihrke PJ. Canine Seborrheic Disease Complex. Veterinary Clinics of North America 1979; 9 93-106.

133. Gross TL, Ihrke PJ, Walder EJ, Affolter, VK. Diseases with Abnormal Cornification. In: Gross TL, Ihrke PJ, Walder EJ, Affolter, VK. Skin Diseases of the Dog and Cat: Clinical and Histopathologic Diagnosis, Second Edition. Oxford: Blackwell Science; 2005. p.161-98.

134. Noli, C. Seborrhea: why and how does it happen? World Small Animal Veterinary Association: proceedings of the 28th World Congress of the WSAVA 24-27 October 2003, Bangkok, Thailand. Ontario: World Small Animal Veterinary Association, 2003.

135. Rosenkrantz, W. Practical Applications of Topical Therapy for Allergic, Infectious, and Seborrheic Disorders. Clinical Techniques in Small Animal Practice 2006; 21(3)106-16.

136. Rosenkrantz WS. The Pathogenesis, Diagnosis, and Management of Feline Acne. Veterinary Medicine 1991; 86(5) 504-12.

137. Jazic E, Coyner KS, Loeffler DG, Lewis TP. An Evaluation of the Clinical, Cytological, Infectious and Histopathological Features of Feline Acne. European Society of Veterinary Dermatology 2006; 17(2) 134-40.

138. White, S, Bordeau P, Blumstein P, Ibisch C, Re EG, Denerolle P, Carlotti DN, Scott KV. Feline Acne and Results of Treatment with Mupirocin in an Open Clinical Trial: 25 Cases (1994–96). Veterinary Dermatology 1997, 8(3): 157-64.

139. Werner AH, Power HT. Retinoids in Veterinary Dermatology. Clinics in Dermatology 1994; 12(4) 579-86.

140. Hnilica KA. Keratinization and Seborrheic Disorders. In: Hnilica KA. Small Animal Dermatology: A Color Atlas and Therapeutic Guide, 3rd edition. Canadá: Elsevier; 2011. p360-1.

141. MacDonald JM, Bradley DM. Acral Lick Dermatitis. In: Bonagura JD (ed). Kirk's Current Veterinary Therapy XIV: Small Animal Practice. St Louis: WB Saunders; 2009. P468–73.

142. Virga V. Behavioral Dermatology. Veterinary Clinics of North America: Small Animal Practice 2003; 33(2) 231-51.

143. Wynchank D, Berk M. Fluoxetine Treatment of Acral Lick Dermatitis in Dogs: a Placebo-Controlled Randomized Double Blind Trial. Depression and Anxiety 1998; 8(1) 21-3.

144. Watson TDG. Diet and Skin Diseases in Dogs and Cats. Journal of Nutrition 1998; 128(12) 2783S-2789S.

145. Dethioux F. Nutrition, Skin Health and Coat Quality. Veterinary Focus 2008; 18(1) 40-6.

146. Colombini S., Dunstan RW. Zinc-Responsive Dermatosis in Northern-Breed Dogs: 17 Cases (1990-1996). Journal of the American Veterinary Medical Association 1997; 211(4) 451-3.

147. Hall, J. Diagnostic Dermatology. Zinc Responsive Dermatosis. Canadian Veterinary Journal 2005; 46(6) 555-7.

148. Getty R, Foust HL, Prestley ET, Miller ME. Macroscopic Anatomy of the Ear of the Dog. American Journal of Veterinary Research 1956; 17(64) 364-75.

149. Goth GM. Doenças do Ouvido Externo no Cão e no Gato. Veterinary Focus 2011; 21(3) 2-9.

150. McKeever PJ. Otitis Externa. Compendium on Continuing Education for the Practicing Veterinarian 1996; 18(7) 759-73.

151. Rosser EJ Jr. Causes of Otitis Externa. Veterinary Clinics of North America: Small Animal Practice 2004; 34(2) 459-468.

152. August JR. Otitis Externa: a Disease of Multifactorial Etiology. Veterinary Clinics of North America: Small Animal Practice 1988; 18(4) 731–42.

153. Merchant SR. Medically Managing Chronic Otitis Externa and Media. Veterinary Medicine 1997; 92(6) 515-34.

154. Bond R. Selecting Ear Drops for Dogs with Otitis Externa. In Practice 2012; 34(7) 392–9.

155. Paterson S. Diagnostic Approach to Otitis in Dogs. Today's Veterinary Practice 2011; 1(2): 27-32.

156. Cole LK. Otoscopic Evaluation of the Ear Canal. Veterinary Clinics of North America: Small Animal Practice 2004; 34(2) 397-410.

157. Fourie LJ, Kok DJ, Heine J. Evaluation of the Efficacy of an Imidacloprid 10% / Moxidectin 1% Spot-on Against Otodectes cynotis in Cats. Parasitology Research 2003; 90(3) S112-S113.

158. Morris DO. Medical Therapy of Otitis Externa and Otitis Media. Veterinary Clinics of North America: Small Animal Practice 2004; 34(2) 541-55.

Chapter 2

Immunohistochemical Analysis of Progesterone Receptor and Proliferating Cell Nuclear Antigen in Canine Inflammatory Mammary Carcinoma

1. Introduction

Cancer constitutes a major problem in animal pathology and is a subject of intensive research. Canine mammary tumors are common neoplasms and have been reported to account for up to half of all tumors in female dog [1]. All malignant canine mammary tumors have the potential to metastasize and in general, metastasis tends to occur via the lymphatic system to the inguinal lymph nodes or hematogenously to the lungs or to more distant body sites including the liver, spleen, heart, bone [2]. Canine mammary tumors share many similarities with breast cancer in human beings, including the high prevalence of adenocarcinomas, frequency of metastasis and progressive disease [1].

Inflammatory mammary carcinoma is a special type of locally advanced mammary cancer that is associated with particularly aggressive behaviour and poor prognosis in women - in which case it is termed *inflammatory breast carcinoma* (IBC), and in the dog - in which case it is termed inflammatory mammary carcinoma (IMC) [3-8]. In both species, this uncommon type of tumors corresponds to a locally invasive mammary cancer that can be clinically misdiagnosed as a dermatitis or mastitis owing to its special inflammatory phenotype [9,10]. Although the pathogenesis of the disease remains obscure, some special clinical, genetic, biologic and hormonal characteristics have been found to be specific for inflammatory breast carcinoma and inflammatory mammary carcinoma [9,11-13].

Inflammatory mammary carcinoma is a very specific type of rare, very aggressive and highly metastatic mammary cancer in dogs [7,8]. Clinical features include the presence of pain, erythema, edema and ulceration in the skin of the mammary gland region. These features are similar to symptoms of inflammatory diseases such as mastitis and dermatitis [2,7,8]. Histologically there is evidence of a poorly differentiated carcinoma with extensive evidence of both mononuclear and polymorphonuclear cellular infiltrates and often edema. Dermal lymphatic invasion also can be seen histologically. Clinically, these neoplasms grow and metastasize extremely rapidly and invade lymphatics in the skin, resulting in marked edema and inflammation [14].

Two clinical forms of inflammatory mammary carcinoma have been described in women and dogs [8,9,15-17]: primary and secondary. Primary inflammatory mammary carcinoma occurs suddenly in dogs without previous detection of lesions of mammary tumors while the secondary inflammatory mammary carcinoma accompanies mammary tumors [8]. Secondary inflammatory mammary carcinoma is further classified into two types: postsurgical whenever it develops after surgical excision of a previous mammary tumors, and non-postsurgical when developing from a previous mammary tumor not surgically treated that leaded to inflammatory mammary carcinoma [9,18,19].

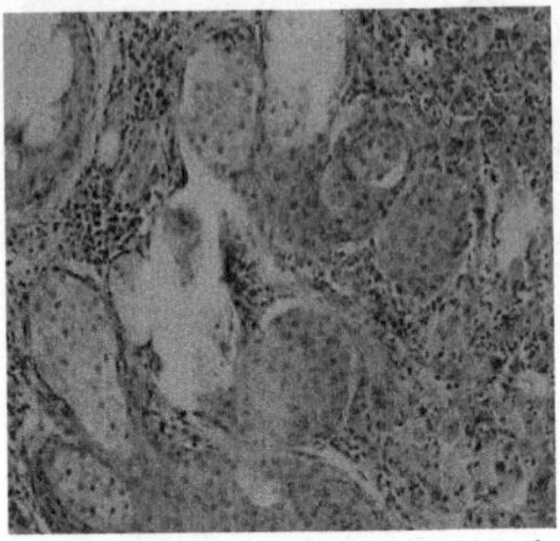

Figure 1. Inflammatory mammary carcinoma (IMC), Hematoxylin-eosin (H&E); Bar = 100μm.

Inflammatory mammary carcinoma occurs most often in female dogs, but it can strike male dogs too. Most dogs that develop this form of reproductive cancer are females who have never been spayed, or who were spayed after they were two years old. Hormone therapy can also increase your female dog's risk of developing mammary cancer. Spaying your dog before she undergoes her first reproductive cycle at six months of age is the best way to prevent inflammatory carcinoma. Rarely, this type of cancer occurs in male dogs, which also have mammary glands. Dogs who develop a mammary carcinoma will have one or more tumors in their mammary glands. More than half of dogs with this type of cancer develop tumors in more than one mammary gland. Malignant tumors grow quickly, are often irregular in shape, may attach themselves to the surrounding skin or tissue, and may cause painful inflammation and even ulceration of the affected area [8,12,13,20,21].

Inflammatory mammary carcinoma in dogs often causes pain and swelling in the affected area. The tumors may be hard or soft. You will be able to feel them under the skin, and often they may be visible to the naked eye as well. The area will be warm and tender to the touch. It is advised to take tissue biopsies of the tumors to determine if they are cancerous and if they are inflammatory carcinoma. Blood tests and urinalysis can help the practitioner to determine if the cancer has spread, and how it may be affecting other body organs [22].

Surgery is sometimes used to remove inflammatory carcinoma tumors, though this is not always advisable in dogs. If the cancer has not yet spread, or if ulceration and infection has occurred, it may be indicated to remove the tumor and affected mammary gland surgically. If the dog has not yet been spayed, your vet may want to perform this procedure as well. Inflammatory mammary cancer in dogs is an aggressive disease that spreads rapidly, and surgery alone often does little to slow or stop its progression [21,22].

The clinician may recommend chemotherapy and radiation therapy to treat your dog's cancer, even if the cancer has not yet spread. The prognosis for inflammatory carcinoma in dogs will depend upon the size of your dog's tumors at the time of diagnosis, and whether or not the cancer has already spread to other parts of the body. Survival time after treatment can range from nine months to two years. Prevent inflammatory carcinoma by having your dog spayed before she is six months old. Dogs who are obese, or who eat diets high in beef and pork, are at an increased risk of developing inflammatory carcinoma [22].

In the clinical evaluation of inflammatory mammary carcinoma observed a strong resemblance to the inflammatory process, so it is often confused with dermatitis [23-25]. Construction of histological inflammatory mammary carcinoma is not uniform - they can be all forms of cancer (Figure 2). Often these are tumors of low maturity. The lymphatic vessels of the skin congestion states of cancer cells. The prognosis is bad.

The purpose of this study was to evaluate of proliferating cell nuclear antigen (PCNA), cytokeratin 19 (CK19), and progesterone receptor (PgR) in two cases of canine inflammatory mammary carcinoma and whether or not these markers might be useful in tumor identification or prognosis.

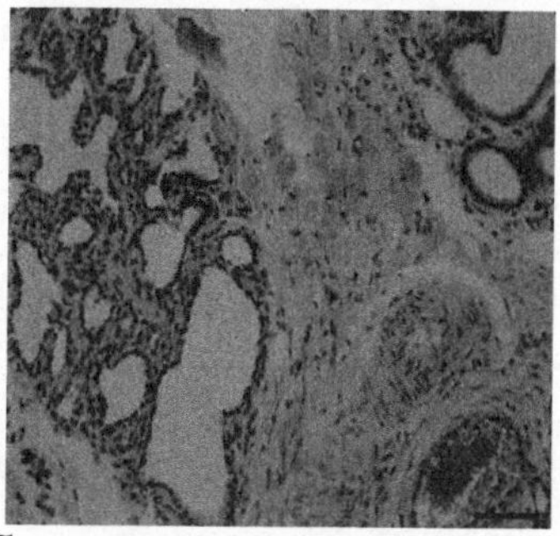

Figure 2. Inflammatory mammary carcinoma (IMC), Hematoxylin-eosin (H&E); Bar = 100µm.

2. Materials and methods

2.1. Materials

A total of 135 samples from canine mammary tumours were used in this study, from which 80 were parafine-embeded archive samples from a period running from 2006 to 2008, and 55 were fresh samples obtained from mastectomy surgery, performed at Warsaw Veterinary Clinics and Small Animal Clinic of the Department of Clinical Sciences, Faculty of Veterinary Medicine, Warsaw University of Life Sciences – SGGW. Through three years period, only two cases of inflammatory mammary carcinoma (IMC) were diagnosed, which were further confirmed by clinical signs and histopathology were selected for further immunohistochemical studies.Investigated material contained 14 adenomas, 66 complex carcinomas (adenocarcinomas), 47 simple carcinomas (adenocarcinomas), 6 solid carcinomas and 2 inflammatory mammary carcinoma (IMC). The number of cancers with a defined grade amounted to, respectively, 1st grade – 48, 2nd grade – 39 and 3rd grade – 34. Mammary gland neoplasms were excised from female dogs belonging to 9 breeds in the ages between 3 and 16 years. There were 106 mixed-breed dogs, 10 German Shepherd Dogs, 5 Boxers, 3, Rottweilers, 2 Beagles, 6 Yorkshire Terrier and 1 each of the following breed: English Springer Spaniel, Labrador Retriever, Doberman Pinscher.

2.2. Methods

Specimens were fixed in 8% buffered formalin, dehydrated and embedded in paraffin. 4μm thick sections were cut from each mammary neoplasm. The sections were mounted onto slides coated with 3-amino-propyltrietoxysilane (Sigma), deparaffinized in xylene and rehydrated in graded ethanol concentrations. Antigen retrieval was performed in 10mM citrate buffer in a microwave oven at 600W for 5 minutes and 300W for 10 minutes. The slides were left to cool at room temperature immersed in the buffer. Thereafter they were washed for 10 minutes in running tap water and rinsing in distilled water. Endogenous peroxidase was quenched by immersion in a solution of 30% hydrogen peroxide and methanol (50 ml of H_20_2 and 50 ml of methanol) for 10 minutes. The slides were washed in distilled water then with TRIS (pH 7.4) for 10 minutes, and then incubated with the primary monoclonal antibodies in humid chamber for 1 hour at room temperature. Primary antibody clones and dilutions used for progesterone receptor (PgR), proliferating cell nuclear antigen (PCNA), and for cytokeratin 19 (CK19) presented (table 1).

Table 1. The antibodies used for immunohistochemistry

Antibody	Type	Dilution	Antigen Retrieval	Incubation	Source
Cytokeratin 19 (CK19)	Mab *	1:50	HTAR **	1 hr, room temp	DakoCytomation
Progesterone Receptor (PgR)	Mab *	1:50	HTAR **	1 hr, room temp	Novocastra
Proliferating cell nuclear antigen (PCNA)	Mab	1:50	HTAR **	1 hr, room temp	DakoCytomation

(*) Mab - mouse monoclonal antibody; (**) HTAR – high-temperature antigen retrieval (with 10 mM citrate buffer, pH 6.0).

The slides were washed in TRIS for 10 minutes. The EnVision +™ System (DakoCytomation) was used for visualization. Visualization was achieved with 3,3'diaminobenzidine tetrahydrocloride (DAB – DakoCytomation) in Tris-HCl buffer, and after rinsed slides were counterstained with hematoxylin Ehrlicha, dehydrated in graded alcohol concentrations and xylene and closed in DPX mounting medium (Gurr®).For progesterone receptor (PgR), proliferating cell nuclear antigen (PCNA), and cytokeratin 19 (CK19), a canine mammary adenocarcinoma was used as positive control. Computer image analysis and Lucia v. 4.21 software were used for interpretation of the results of PCNA, CK19, PgR, expression; using those facilities we could count the number of neoplastic cells featuring stained cytoplasm and nucleus per 1,000 neoplastic cells. Results were analyzed using the SPSS 12.0 program. To determine whether differences for a few independent traits were significant, Kruskal-Wallis test was used. This test is an equivalent to the test of variance for traits without normal distribution. Two-sided correlations were performed using Spearman correlation test. The differences were deemed statistically significant at $p \leq 0.05$.

3. Results and discussion

3.1. Relationship between age of bitches and the grade of malignancy and histological type of tumor of epithelial origin

Dogs were divided into three age groups: <8 years, 8 -12 years and >12 years. In the group of bitches below the age of 8, majority (61.1%) consisted of tumors with the lowest histological grade of malignancy (1st). In the oldest group, 1st and 2nd grade tumors in the 1st and 2nd accounted for 77.8%. In the entire pool of studied tumors in all age groups, the largest share consisted of tumors with the lowest degree of histological malignancy (40.4%) (Table 2). Assessment of the contribution of individual types of tumors at different ages showed that in bitches younger than 8 years the most common findings were adenomas (21.7%) and complex carcinomas (56.5%) and in those over 12 years simple carcinomas occurred most often (55.0%) (Table 3).

Table 2. Incidence of malignancies of various grades in bitches in different age groups

Year of bitches	Tumor grade			Total
	I°	II°	III°	
<8 lat (n=18)	11 (61.1%)	3 (16.7%)	4 (22.2%)	18
8-12 lat (n=85)	30 (36.0%)	29 (35.0%)	26 (30.5%)	85
“/>12 (n=18)	7 (38.9%)	7 (38.9%)	4 (22.2%)	18
total (n=121)	48 (40.4%)	39 (32.8%)	34 (28.1%)	121

Table 3. Occurrence of individual types of epithelial neoplasms in different age groups in bitches

Year of bitches	Types of tumors					Total
	Adenoma	Carcinoma solidum	Adenocarcinoma simplex	Adenocarcinoma complex	Canine inflammatory mammary carcinoma (IMC)	
<8 lat	5 (21,7%)	1 (4,3%)	4 (17,4%)	13 (56,5%)	0	23
8-12 lat	7 (7,8%)	4 (4,4%)	32 (35,6%)	47 (52,2%)	2 (2.2%)	92
“/>12 lat	2 (10,0%)	1 (5,0%)	11 (55,0%)	6 (30,0%)	0	20
Total	14 (10,5%)	6 (4,5%)	47 (35,3%)	66 (49,6%)	2 (1.5%)	135

In our study, two inflammatory mammary carcinoma came from the dogs between the ages of 8 and 9 years (case 1 - 8 year, case 2 - 9 year) (Table 2). These dogs had a clinically diagnosis of IMC at the time of initial examination. The most important findings during physical examination included: erythema and warmth, generalized induration of the involved mammary glands, cutaneous nodules affecting the overlying skin, edema of the proximal portion of the hind limbs.

3.2. Results of proliferative activity in inflammatory mammary carcinoma

The value of mitotic index differed significantly between types of tumors. The lowest proliferative activity was observed in adenomas, the highest in simple carcinoma, solid carcinoma and inflammatory mammary carcinoma. The highest proliferative activity was found in tumors in the 3rd grade of malignancy, the lowest in the tumors in the 1st grade. Expression of PCNA was observed in the nuclei of neoplastic cells that have undergone division (Figure 3). Statistical analysis shows significant differences between particular types of tumors. The lowest number of cells exhibiting PCNA expression was observed in adenomas, the highest in the solid carcinoma, simple carcinoma, inflammatory mammary carcinoma and in tumors with the highest histological grade of malignancy (3rd).

In the two cases canine inflammatory mammary carcinoma on the basis of H&E histopathology found a high mitotic index (3.4 in the first case in the second case 4.1).PCNA index was similarly and markedly elevated in the two animals: in case 1 inflammatory mammary carcinoma was 82%, in case 2 the inflammatory mammary carcinoma was 85% (Figure 3).

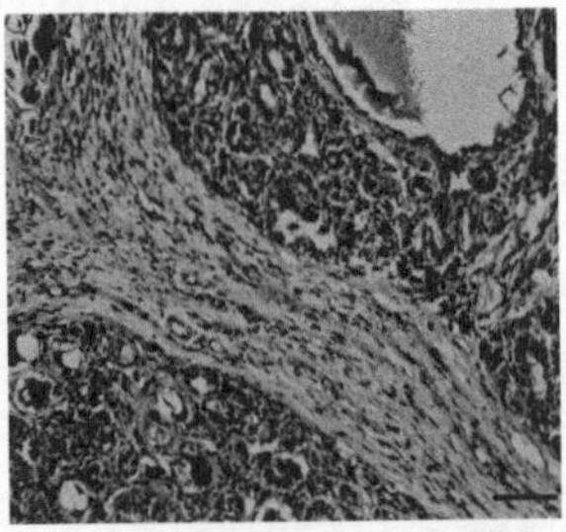

Figure 3. Inflammatory mammary carcinoma – ICM, immunostaining for PCNA in a case of IMC; Bar=100μm

3.3. Results of cytokeratin 19 expression in inflammatory mammary carcinoma

Expression of cytokeratin 19 was observed in the neoplastic cell cytoplasm. Positive CK19 reaction was found in all tumors of epithelial origin. The high expression of CK19 was found also in inflammatory mammary carcinoma (case 1 – intensity level of expression CK19 – 92%; case 2 – intensity level of expression CK19 – 98%) (Figure 4 and 5).

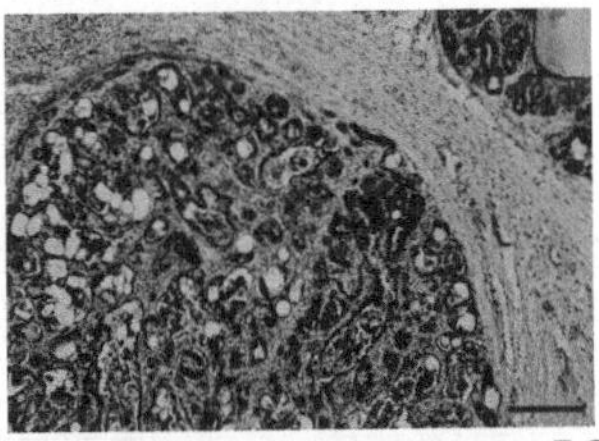

Figure 4.Inflammatory mammary carcinoma – ICM, immunostaining for cytokeratin 19 (CK19) in a case of IMC; Bar=100 μm

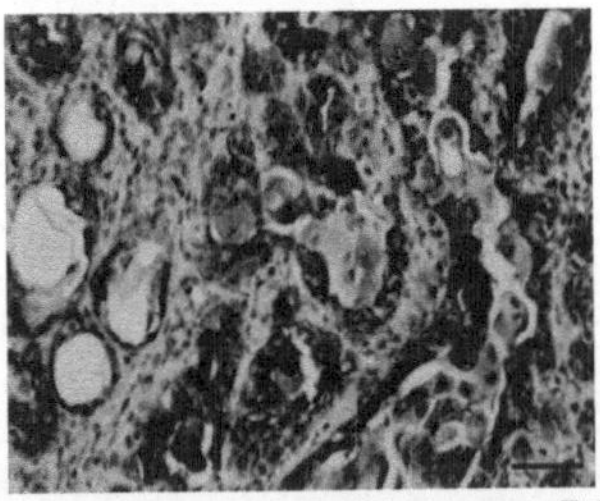

Figure 5. Inflammatory mammary carcinoma – ICM, immunostaining for cytokeratin (CK19) in a case of IMC; Bar=50 μm

3.4. Results of progesterone receptor expression in inflammatory mammary carcinoma

Progesterone receptor expression was detected in the nuclei of tumor cells, but it was also seen in the cytoplasm. Cytoplasmic reaction was considered to be nonspecific. Among all tumors of epithelial origin, expression of progesterone receptors was found in 56 (41.4%), and no reaction was noted in 79 (58.5%). Expression of progesterone receptors was most commonly found in complex cancers (43.9%), simple cancers (42.6%), adenomas (28.6%), while solid cancers rarely expressed them (16.7%). The high expression of progesterone receptors was found also in inflammatory mammary carcinoma 2 (100%) (Figure 6 and 7). Analysis of the average number of cells showing positive expression of progesterone receptors reveals that the level of expression increases with the histological grade of malignancy. It was also found that most tumors expressing progesterone receptors came from dogs younger than 8 years. A positive correlation was found between mitotic index and expression of progesterone receptors in specific types of cancer and statistically significant differences between tumor characteristics were demonstrated (p=0.042).

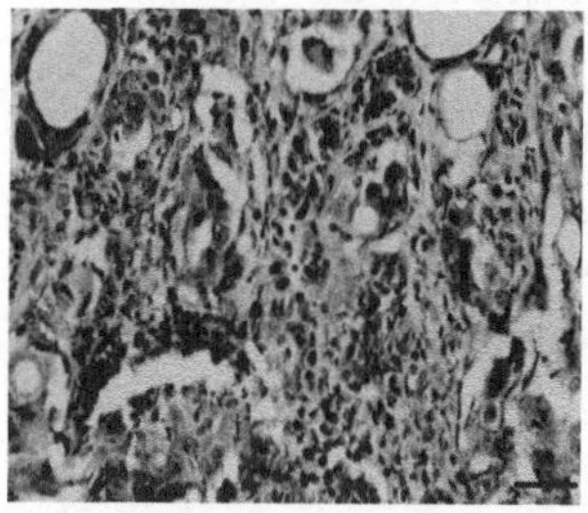

Figure 6.Inflammatory mammary carcinoma – ICM, nuclear expression of progesterone receptor (PgR); Bar=50 μm

Clinical signs and histopathological findings are necessary for the accurate diagnosis of inflammatory mammary carcinoma. Our studies have suggested that inflammatory mammary carcinoma is an aggressive malignancy because in our studies, the percentage of PCNA positive cells within the tumor was high in the two cases. An important marker of malignancy is the proliferative activity. Proper evaluation of proliferative activity of tumor cells is crucial for the evaluation of its biological activity and is used in determining the treatment of cancer. In our study, proliferative activity depended on both, the type of tumor and the degree of histological malignancy. The highest values of mitotic index were recorded in simple carcinomas, solid carcinomas and in two cases of inflammatory mammary carcinoma and in tumors with the highest histological grade of malignancy. Similar results were reported for the expression of PCNA. The highest expression of PCNA was seen in solid carcinomas, simple carcinomas and in inflammatory mammary carcinoma and in 3rd grade tumors.

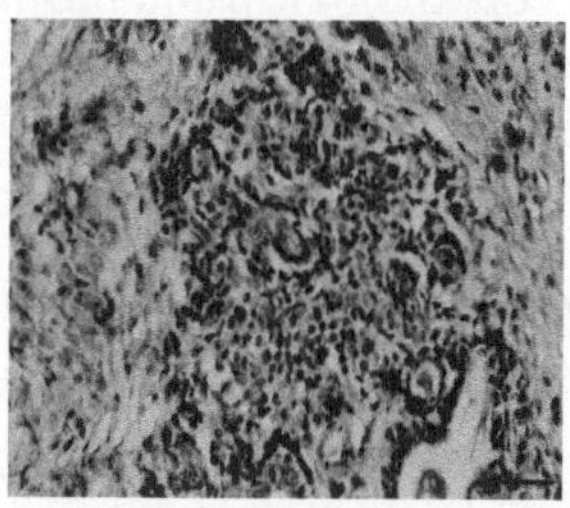

Figure 7.Inflammatory mammary carcinoma – ICM, nuclear expression of progesterone receptor (PgR); Bar=100 μm

In our studies among all tumors of epithelial origin, expression of progesterone receptors was found in 41.4%. Amorim *et al.* (2008) in their study found no expression of PgR in 9 cases inflammatory mammary carcinoma [26]. However, Pen *et al.* (2003) found in their study high positive immune reaction to PgR in inflammatory mammary carcinoma [12].

The high positive immune reaction to PgR in canine inflammatory mammary carcinoma suggests,the possible involvement of special endocrine mechanisms in inflammatory mammary carcinoma development.

During the three years in the research material collected was diagnosed only two cases of canine inflammatory mammary carcinoma, therefore it can be said that canine inflammatory mammary carcinoma is a rare cancer in dogs [8]. Perez *et al.* showed that inflammatory mammary carcinoma is rare in dogs (17,7% of all cases within 4 years) [8]. Yet Susaneck *et al.* [13] claimed that the incidence of canine inflammatory mammary carcinoma has doubled in the past 15 years [7]. Pena *et al.* [12,13] in their research work diagnosed 33 of canine inflammatory mammary carcinoma cases in a 5 years period.

All these authors described this type of cancer as a rare, unusual and different. Authors investigated the relationship between clinical and histopathological characteristics of canine inflammatory mammary carcinoma specifying nuclear antigen expression of PCNA, and expression of progesterone receptor [7,8,12,13].

4. Conclusion

Based on the literature and our own experience it can be concluded that canine inflammatory mammary carcinoma is a rare tumors with poor prognosis. Our research suggests that inflammatory mammary carcinoma is an aggressive malignancy, with a tendency to metastasize at an early stage.

References

1. Rutteman GR, Withrow SJ, MacEwen EG. Tumors of the mammary gland. W: Small Animal Clinicae Oncology Withrow SJ, MacEwen EG. (edit), 3rd ed., Philadelphia 2001; 455-477.
2. Jong-Hyuk K, Keum-Soon I, Na-Hyun K, Seung-Ki C, Alan RD, Jung-Hyang S.. Inflammatory mammary carcinoma with metastasis to the brain and distant organs in a spayed Shih Tzu dog. Journal of Veterinary Diagnostic Investigation 2011; 23(5): 1079-1082.
3. Perez-Alenza MD, Jimenez A, Nieto AI, Pena L. First description of feline inflammatory mammary carcinoma: Clinicopathological and immunohistochemical characteristics of three casus. Breast Cancer Research 2004; 6: 300-307.
4. Tavassoli FA. Infiltrating carcinoma: special types. Inflammatory carcinoma. In Pathology of the Breast 2nd edition. New York: McGraw-Hill 1999; 538–541.
5. Giordano SH, Hortobagyi GN. Inflammatory breast cancer: clinical progress and the main problems that must be addressed. Breast Cancer Research 2003; 5:284–288.
6. Kleer CG, van Golen KL, Merajver SD. Molecular biology of breast cancer metastasis. Inflammatory breast cancer: clinical syndrome and molecular determinants. Breast Cancer Research 2000; 2: 423–429.
7. Susaneck SJ, Allen TA, Hoopes J, Withrow SJ, Macy DW. Inflammatory mammary carcinoma in the dog. Journal of the American Animal Hospital Association 1983; 9: 971–976.

8. Perez-Alenza MD, Tabanera E, Pena L. Inflammatory mammary carcinoma in dogs: 33 cases (1995–1999). Journal of the American Veterinary Medical Association 2001; 219: 1110–1114.

9. Clemente M, Rerez-Alenza MD, Illera JC, Pena L. Histological, Immunohistochemical, and Ultrastructural Description of Vasculogenic Mimicry in canine Mammary Cancer. Veterinary Pathology 2012; 47(2): 265-274.

10. Jaiyesimi IA, Buzdar AU, Hortobagyi G. Inflammatory breast cancer: a review. Journal Clinical Oncology 1992; 10: 1014-1024.

11. Illera JC, Perez-Alenza MD, Nieto A, Jimenez MA, Silvan G, Dunner S, Pena L. Steroids and receptors in canine mammary cancer. Steroids 2006; 71: 541-548.

12. Pena L, Perez-Alenza MD, Rodriguez-Bertos A, Nieto A. Canine inflammatory mammary carcinoma: histopathology, immunohistochemistry and clinical implications of 21 cases. Breast Cancer Research and Treatment 2003; 78: 141-148.

13. Pene L, Perez-Alenza MD, Silvan G, Lopes C, Nieto A. Steroid hormone profile of canine inflammatory mammary carcinoma: a preliminary study. Journal of Steroid Biochemistry&Molecular Biology 2003; 84: 211-216.

14. Marconato L, Romanelli G, Stefanello D, et al. Prognostic factors for dogs with mammary inflammatory carcinoma:43 cases (2003-2008). Journal of the American Veterinary Medical Association 2009; 235: 967-972.

15. Attia-Sobol J, Ferriere JP, Cure H, Kwiatkowski F, Achard JL, Verrelle P, Feillel V, De Latour M, Lafaye C, Deloche C. Treatment results, survival and prognostic factors in 109 inflammatory breast cancers: univariate and multivariate analysis. European Journal Cancer 1993; 29A: 1081-1088.

16. Resetkova E. Pathologic aspects of inflammatory breast carcinoma: part 1. Histomorphology and differential diagnosis. Seminars in Oncology 2008; 35: 25-32.

17. Taylor G, Meltzer A. Inflammatory carcinoma of the breast. American Journal of Cancer 1938; 33: 33049.

18. Kim T, Lau J, Erban J. Lack of uniform diagnostic criteria for inflammatory breast cancer limits interpretation of treatment outcomes: a systematic review. Clinical Breast Cancer 2006; 7: 386-395.

19. Kumar V, Abbas AK, Fausto N, ed.: Robbins and Cotran Pathologic Basis of Disease, 7th ed. Elsevier Saunders, Philadelphia, PA, 2005.

20. Allen SW, Prasse KW, Mahaffey EA. Cytologic differentiationn of bening from malignant canine mammary tumors. Veterinary Pathology 1986; 23: 649-655.

21. Ferguson RH. Canine mammary gland tumors. Veterinary Clinics of North America Small Animal Practice 1985; 15: 501-511.

22. Hellmen E. The pathogenesis of canine mammary tumors. Cancer Journal 1996; 9: 282-286.

23. Sarli G, Prezioso R, Benazzi C, Castellani G, Marcato PS. Prognostic value of histologic stage and proliferative activity in canine malignant mammary tumors. Journal of Veterinary Diagnostic Investigation 2002; 14: 25-34.

24. Alpaugh ML, Tomlinson JS, Shao ZM, Barsky SH. A novel human xenograft model of inflammatory breast cancer. Cancer Research 1999; 59: 5079-5084.

25. Ellis DL, Teitelbaum SL. Inflammatory carcinoma of the breast: a pathologic definition. Cancer 1974; 33: 1045-1047.

26. Amorim RL, Souza CHM, Bandarra EP, Sanches OC, Piza ET. Immunohistochemical study of estrogen and progesterone reptors and cell proliferative indexes in canine inflammatory mammary carcinoma: 9 cases. Brazilian Journal of Veterinary Pathology 2008; 1(1): 16-20.

Chapter 3

Indicators of Poor Welfare in Dairy Cows Within Smallholder Zero-Grazing Units in the Peri-Urban Areas of Nairobi, Kenya

1. Introduction

Animal welfare lacks a good universal definition and a satisfactory distinction from the term "well being". However, a consensual definition is essential for practical, legislative and scientific purposes. Without a clear definition, animal welfare cannot be effectively studied or conclusively assessed to provide remedial measures to its violation [1-3]. Animal welfare is therefore defined as the ability of an animal to interact or cope comfortably with its environment, resulting in satisfaction of both its physical and mental state [4-6]. This satisfaction enhances expression of normal behavioural patterns by the animal [7,8].

In the context of welfare, "environment" refers to internal factors (within the animal) and external factors (in the animal's physical environment) to which the animal responds with its physiological and psychological systems [6,9]. In contrast, animal "well being" is defined as the animal's perception of its state in trying to cope with its environment [1,5]. Concisely, animal "well-being" refers to the current state of the animal, but animal welfare is a more general term referring to past, present and future implications of the animal's state [10].

The assessment of animal welfare is base on the provisions of five freedoms, which include:

- Freedom from hunger and thirst, availed through provision of ready access to water and a diet to maintain health and vigour,
- Freedom from pain, injury and disease, availed through disease prevention and treatment,
- Freedom from fear and distress, availed through avoidance of conditions that cause mental suffering,
- Freedom to have normal behaviour patterns, availed through provision of sufficient space and appropriate physical structures,
- Freedom from thermal or physical discomfort, availed through provision of a comfortable environment.

Knowledge of animal physiology, animal behavior and animal needs based on the five freedoms is paramount in assessing as well as enforcing animal welfare. Animals need to be provided with amble comfort related to these five freedoms. They should be kept in housing or environments that will minimize adverse climatic variations or exposures to extremes of cold or heat, rain, strong continuous winds and direct solar exposures. Appropriate conditions minimizing trauma, development of lesions and disease outbreaks are essential. Continuous availability of water and provision of adequate wholesome feeds, which consist of balanced constituent rations supplying specific nutritional needs to the body, is required. Animals should be provided with housing conditions and environments that allow them to display natural behavior such as unhindered movement, free expression of oestrus or heat symptoms necessary for mating or insemination in order to have continued sustainable reproduction, social relationships that include animal-to-animal and animal-to-human cordial interactions; and finally minimizing or preventing any causes of suffering as much as possible [11].

Smallholder dairy farming occupies a vast proportion of agricultural production and the main livelihood of the people in most developing (third world) countries particularly in Africa, Asia and South America. In Kenya, smallholder zero-grazing dairy units contribute about 80% of the national commercial dairy herd [12] and over 70% of all the marketed milk [13-16]. Each of the Kenyan smallholder zero-grazing dairy units has 2 to 10 milking cows most of which are exotic breeds (Friesian, Ayrshire, Guernsey, Jersey or crosses of these exotic breeds). Some smallholder farmers, who have better financial resources, manage to have up to 20 or more cows. The cows are raised on small plots of land measuring between 0.25 to 2 acres. Only few smallholder farmers would have land measuring a maximum of 5 acres. The Kenyan smallholder zero-grazing dairy units are unique because they have varied designs and management practices. They vary in housing designs, nutritional and management protocol from unit to unit to the extent that they can correctly be referred to as zero-grazing "subunits" that are devoid of a consistent production system. The nutritional regimes and management practices not only vary from unit to unit, but also within the same unit from time to time [17]. The cows in these units are invariably zero-grazed [13,18] and have sub-optimal production [14,18,19], which is attributed to a number of constraints such as inadequate feeding, poor nutrition, substandard animal husbandry, lack of proper dairy farming facilities that include inadequate space to move and interact freely. All these factors predispose the cows to diseases and other stressful conditions [14,20,21].

A high number of smallholder zero-grazing dairy units are concentrated in the peri-urban areas owing to availability of ready market for milk and milk products among city and town residents [13,18]. The high and rapid population growth in developing countries has led to a reduction of agricultural lands that support the livelihood of the people. This has triggered a shift from fewer large-scale farms to numerous intensified smallholder production units in an endeavor to maximize economic profits [22]. The resulting low income following land subdivision to smallholder enterprises, affects the livelihood of majority of the citizens in the involved countries [16,21]. The low income poses financial challenges that make it difficult to afford adequate dairy farming facilities, hence the progressively deteriorating husbandry standards that precipitate stressful conditions, which further exacerbate poor welfare of the dairy cattle in these smallholder units. These interacting multiple factors, cause a vicious circle of events that eventually have negative effects on physiology, behavior, disease susceptibility and productivity of the dairy cows [23,24]. The welfare of food animals has become a major concern to consumers of animal products in many parts of the world. Consumers of products such as meat and meat products, milk and eggs are demanding to know how the animals from which these products have been obtained are handled with respect to animal welfare ethics [25,26].

Dairy cattle housing should provide the animal with protection from harsh environmental extremes [27]. Good housing systems are those that are well designed for ease of management and maintenance at all times [27-29]. It is proposed that all confinement for animals should be constructed and operated to meet the legal requirements for protection of the animal as well as maintain high quality animal products [30]. Good animal housing systems are those that enhance provision of all the five freedoms that an animal should have to satisfy its welfare [28,31]. If these basic needs cannot be met in the animal house, then health, welfare and production of the animal will be compromised. These concerns are particularly critical in the smallholder zero-grazing systems, in which dairy cows are confined throughout their growth and production life. Naturally, cattle are grazing animals and therefore pasture-grazing is a more welfare-friendly system because it allows free expression of normal animal behavior compared to the restricted indoor zero-grazing systems. Conversely, high yielding dairy cows may not get all their nutritional demands from grazing only, and this may compromise their welfare with regard to nutrition. This means that both zero-grazing and pasture-grazing systems have positive and negative effects on the welfare of dairy cattle [32]. However, zero-grazing systems demand more articulate precision in design, construction and management because they have a higher inclination to compromising welfare of the housed dairy cattle. Although pasture-grazing allows free expression of normal cattle behavior and provides sufficient comfortable lying space, the pasture forage has lower nutritional value than the high plane feeding of the zero-grazing units and therefore cattle in pastures may spent long hours grazing depending on the quality and amount of forage in the pasture, hence less time resting, which influences the resting aspect of welfare negatively [33]. In comparison, indoor housing systems provide high level feeding and increase intake rates, thus fulfilling nutritional requirements faster, reducing eating times, leaving more time for cattle to rest and ruminate [34]. However, indoor housing systems have limited space allowance, which increases competitive aggressive behavior within the herd [35], restriction of natural foraging behavior and opportunity to feed selectively [36], negative effects on the cow comfort [33], and high incidence of diseases such as lameness and mastitis [37,38]. All these factors in the indoor housing have adverse effects on the welfare of cattle. In Kenya, the practice of zero-grazing dairy production is inevitable owing to the reduced land sizes. Hence, the importance of drawing reliable direct indicators of poor welfare existing in these zero-grazing systems in order to introduce corrective remedial measures, particularly in relation to designing of the construction of welfare-acceptable and cow-comfortable zero-grazing units no matter how simple or cheap.

Improvements of animal welfare may be achieved through (a) assessment of animal welfare, (b) identification of risk factors potentially leading to welfare problems and (c), interventions in response to the risk factors. Improvements can be enhanced by directly dealing with the risk factors of animal welfare within the farming unit. Therefore, there must be good reliable way of measuring or assessing whether or not poor animal welfare exists within the practiced farming systems. In this process the animal based parameters help us to identify the animal's response to the system, and therefore indicating the negative impact of the potential risk factors existing within the farming system [39]. Traditionally, farm animal welfare assessment has focused on the measurement of resources provided to the animal such as housing-and-housing design criteria [40,41]. Although such indirect resource-based welfare assessment criteria are quick, easy and have some degree of reliability, basing the welfare verdict solely on their findings may not necessarily mean that the welfare of the animals is good or poor. Other husbandry aspects that affect animal welfare are management practices and the human-animal relationship, but their measurement may be more difficult. However, the provision of good management and environmental resources does not necessarily result in a high standard of animal welfare. Direct animal-level parameters such as health or behavior can be taken as indicators of the animals' feelings and a measure of bodily state of the animal. These are more reliable because they indicate how the animal has been affected by some factors existing within the proximate environment or housing system of the animal and how it has responded to these factors. Welfare assessment should therefore be based primarily on such animal-related parameters. In practice, resource or management-based parameters should also be included in an on-farm assessment protocol when closely correlated to animal-associated measurements and because they can form the basis for the identification of causes of welfare problems [39]. It is however challenging to select and develop reliable and at the same time feasible measurements for on-farm assessment protocols. Attempts to create an operational welfare assessment protocol primarily relying on animal-related parameters have mainly been made with regard to dairy cows [42-45].

Animal-level indices for on-farm welfare assessment can be divided into ethological or behavioural and pathological or health parameters; physiological indicators are mostly unavailable for feasibility reasons. Ethological parameters include individual animal behavior, animal-to-animal interaction, human-animal interaction, agonistic behavior and other abnormal behavior. The commonest animal health indicators of cattle welfare are lameness, external body injuries, disease incidence, body condition score and body cleanliness. The main welfare health problem in cattle is lameness, particularly caused by lesions resulting from disruptions of the horn of the claw predisposed by factors such as concrete floors, zero-grazing systems and uncomfortable stalls [45,46]. One of the main shortcomings that exacerbates welfare problems of lameness in cattle and this would even be more prevalent in zero-grazing systems in developing countries, is the lack of valid and reliable lameness diagnostic methods. There is generally lack of sensitive methods of recognizing early change in the gait of lame cattle [44,47,48]. The most reliable and sensitive way of detecting early changes in gait for diagnosis of lameness is the use of automated gait-scoring computer aided systems, which are very scarcely used all over the world [49]. Moreover, these automated facilities are expensively unaffordable to the poor smallholder farmers in developing countries such as Kenya. Claw disorders particularly those related to laminitis are highly prevalent in smallholder zero-grazing dairy units and subunits in the peri-urban areas of Nairobi, Kenya and probably in other parts of Kenya with similar production systems [50]. These have been found to be highly associated with housing and management factors within the zero-grazing units [17,50]. This high prevalence of claw lesions together with a high prevalence of injuries or signs of injuries in specific parts of the body as well as soiling and body condition scores of dairy cows in the smallholder zero-grazing units in the peri-urban areas of Nairobi, Kenya [51,52] was thought to be reliable indicators of the state of welfare of dairy cattle particularly when correlated with the prevailing zero-grazing conditions.

Parameters used to assess animal welfare should be able to inform us about the state of welfare. Three requirements are essential for parameters or indicators used to assess animal welfare. These include: "validity", which asks the question, "what does the parameter in consideration tell us about the animal's welfare state?"; "reliability", which considers inter-observer reliability and asks the question, "do different observers see the same thing?" and the third requirement is "feasibility", which considers the practical aspects of doing the recordings, asking the questions, "how easy is it to record the parameter?, how long does it take to assess the parameter?, and what equipment is needed for measuring the parameter?" [39].

There is a high likelihood among farmers with zero-grazed dairy cows to focus more on whatever it takes to cause their cows produce as much milk as possible at the expense of the health and welfare considerations of the animal. High milk yielding cows often develop a compromise of energy-balance deficits, which infringes on their welfare. As a result of energy deficit stress, these dairy cows become easily susceptible to metabolic and reproductive problems [53]. The uniqueness of the zero-grazing systems in Kenya which consists of subunits that are inconsistently varied in designs, in feeding regimes in relation to feed types, quality and quantity, as well as substandard management practices makes them a rich source of information on management of welfare of cattle. Information acquired from studies in these smallholder zero-grazing subunits will serve to demonstrate how animal-level parameters can be useful in indicating the welfare state of the dairy cattle and how these indicators are associated with the housing design, feeding and management practices in these varied and substandard zero-grazing units and generally suggest possible remedial welfare improvement measures.

The intent of this paper is to present the results from two studies carried out at different times with collection of data from some of the zero-grazing units in the same area but looking at separate objectives. These studies dealt with assessment of the state of welfare of dairy cattle in those units and the prevalent risk factors for poor welfare. In particular, it was planned 1) to determine the role of claw lesions in predicting the welfare of zero-grazed dairy cows with respect to housing designs, floor type, feeding and management practices in the peri-urban areas of Nairobi Kenya; 2) and to determine the role of body injuries, body soiling and body condition scores in predicting the welfare of zero-grazed dairy cows with respect to housing designs, floor type, feeding and management practices in the peri-urban areas of Nairobi Kenya.

2. Material and methods

2.1. Assessment of animal welfare

Assessment of animal welfare can be done using both animal-based and environmental-related parameters (which includes housing factors and management factors) [40,44,54].

These parameters can be evaluated using indicators that show the state of the animal such as production performance, physiological, pathological, ethological and integrated factors [3,55].

2.1.1. Production performance as an indicator of welfare

The production performance indicators of animal welfare are growth rate, productivity, reproductive output and duration of productive life of an animal [1,56]. Many researchers have stated that if the welfare of an animal is good, then production will be optimal [1,57,58]. However, high productivity may not necessarily be an indicator of good welfare, nor low productivity an indicator of poor welfare [46]. For example, dairy cows with high milk production are likely to be predisposed to increased lameness, mastitis, damaged udder ligaments, infertility and problems at parturition [59,60]. It has been suggested that milk yield can be used as an on-farm indicator of animal welfare [44].

2.1.2. Physiological indicators

The main physiological indicators of welfare are hormone levels from the pituitary and adrenal glands and the changes induced on target organs by these hormones such as tachycardia, blood pressure, hyperglycaemia, lymphocytosis and eosinopaenia [3]. The advantages of physiological indicators of animal welfare are that their measurements use reliable analytical methods [61,62] that are less invasive within the body [6]. Cortisol levels indicate the degree of stress experienced by an animal [63]. However, other normal activities such as mating, can lead to an increase in stress hormone levels. Moreover, results of different studies on stress hormones have been inconsistent and hence their reliability as indicators of animal welfare is doubtful [64]. In spite of these arguments, the use of stress hormone response as a welfare indicator has gained credibility because it can easily be measured [65].

Methods used as welfare indicators should not be generalized to all species but rather considered within species, and the search for more reliable methods should be intensified [66]. It has been shown that heart rate, adrenal function, brain biochemistry, regulatory responses and the suppression of functions are the main physiological responses to short-term welfare problems [5]. Adrenocorticotropic hormone (ACTH) challenge technique and the immune response provide measurement of long-term welfare problems. In bovines, the heart rate has been found to be a suitable parameter for studying dairy cow response to stress [67,68].

2.1.3. Pathological indicators

Pathologic signs are widely accepted as indicators of poor welfare because they are a manifestation of current suffering of the animal [3]. Reduction in health could be a reflection of compromised welfare; hence animal-level parameters are likely to be the best welfare indicators [42,44]. Clinical signs of disease and injuries are the animal-level parameters associated with reduced health that may be useful indicators of poor animal welfare [5,44]. Lameness, skin injuries and measurement of immune function are the most commonly used pathological indicators of poor welfare in dairy cattle [3,44]. However, absence of injury and disease is not sufficient proof of good animal welfare [69]. Therefore, pre-pathological state of the animal which includes suppressed immunity (hence increasing vulnerability to diseases), reduced ability to reproduce and cessation of normal growth, tend to suggest that the animal is already suffering and these factors could be used as indicators of poor welfare [70,71]. Assessment of pre-pathological immunity state is based on white cell counts in blood or milk [72]. However, results obtained from such studies have been inconsistent [63]. Some of the short comings of these studies are that pre-pathological conditions do not necessary lead to adverse effects on animals [3] and also animal welfare may be impaired at the time of pre-pathological assessment [66].

2.1.4. Ethological indicators

Behaviour is an important indicator of animal welfare. It can be measured and recorded with minimal animal disturbance [73]. However, the main difficulty is the understanding of animal's normal, natural or ideal behavior in order to quantify abnormal behaviour [74]. Behavioural indicators of poor welfare include the inability of the animal to carry out normal behaviour and the exhibition of a persistent undesirable action by a minority of the population that could be termed as abnormal behaviour [3,61]. Abnormal animal behaviour is classified into five categories which include: detrimental behaviour that causes injury, sham behaviours that are performed in the absence of adequate substrate or environmental stimuli, apathetic behaviour that is a reduced attentiveness towards external stimuli, escape behavior that manifests as a desire to leave the confined environment and redirected behaviour that may ritualize into stereotypes [75]. Abnormal behaviour is damaging to the animals [76]. Expression of abnormal behaviour is a sign that an animal has problems adapting to its environment [3]. It may be an expression of the level of distress that the animal is experiencing [6].

2.1.5. Bovine ethology

Cattle are referred to as group animals because they express synchronized behaviour within the herd [73]. On daily basis, cows confined and housed spend 5-6 hours eating, 4-9 hours ruminating and 11-11.5 hours lying down [3,77,78]. However, the behavioural patterns may vary according to the type of housing system in which they are [79,80]. Friesian cows under cubicle system were found to have lying time of 13.7 hours/day compared to 6.5 hours/day in open out-door systems [81]. Reduced lying time has been found to exacerbate the incidence of claw lesions [82]. Prolonged standing causes cows to expend more energy and exposes hooves to longer periods on slurry, which may increase incidence of lameness [17,83]. Eating behaviour is the most characteristic indication of the state of comfort in animals, that is, the degree to which the biological requirements of animals are met [84]. It has been observed that feeding cows with smooth quality fodder and high concentrates is very beneficial compared to rough fodder. The explanation here is that reduced eating time reduces standing time of the animals [84]. Increased milk yield has been observed in cows with longer lying times. This is thought to be due to increased blood supply to the udder through the milk vein, increasing nutrient supply to the udder [86,87].

2.2. Study procedures

2.2.1. Study area

The study was carried out in the peri-urban areas of Nairobi, Kenya. Nairobi is the capital city of Kenya with an area of 696 square kilometers and a population of over 2.1 million people. It is surrounded by a fertile peri-urban agricultural region lying between 01° 18′S and 36° 45′E, and 1798 meters above sea level. It has an annual rainfall estimated at 765 mm maximum and 36 mm minimum in two distinct seasons (March to June, and October to December). The rest of the months of the year are moderately dry. The cold months are beginning of July to the end of August with temperatures ranging from 18° C to 21°C at day time and 11°C to 15°C at night time. The North-Western side of Nairobi is the coolest with high humidity, while the Eastern side is the warmest with very low humidity. The region has a high concentration of zero-grazed smallholder dairy units owing to its ready market for milk and milk-related dairy products.

2.2.2. Study design

Study 1 – Can claw lesions be used for predicting welfare of zero-grazed dairy cows?

The study consisted of a cross-sectional study in which each zero-grazing unit was visited once and each cow included in the study was examined only once. Even when a zero-grazing unit was visited more than once, no cow was examined twice. Thirty-two smallholder zero-grazing dairy units were purposively selected from those with median cow number of 10 (ranging from 5 to 20 adult cows). It was difficult to get enough farmers allowing their cows to be used for the study, hence another major criteria for inclusion of the zero-grazing dairy units was the willing smallholder farmers. Selection of the zero-grazing dairy units was facilitated by local veterinarians and animal health technicians with whom the farmers were more acquainted. A total of 300 dairy cows that included Friesians 76% (n=228), Ayrshires 20% (n=60) and 4% (n=12) being Guernsey and Jersey crosses were recruited from the 32 smallholder zero-grazing units. Cows that were included in the study had calved at least once, from which 40% were in their first and second parities and 60% in their third and fourth parities. Both lame and non-lame cows of any of the breeds were included in the study group. Selection of the cows meeting the inclusion criteria was performed as previously described [50]. Briefly, in each smallholder unit, cows that met the selection criteria were isolated from the rest and serially numbered as 1, 2, 3, to S, where S was the last serial number depending on the total number of cows isolated in that unit. To avoid biased sampling, a farm worker numbered the isolated cows. From the serially numbered cows, the investigator, starting with either serial number 1 or 2, systematically selected every second cow in the series. For example in the series S1, S2, S3, S4, S5, S6, S7, S8, S9, and S10, if the first cow selected was S1 the next one selected serially would be S3, S5, S7 and S9 respectively, thus all odd serial numbers. But if the first cow selected was S2, then the next ones selected serially would be S4, S6, S8 and S10 respectively, thus all even serial numbers. If the first cow selected in one smallholder unit was serial number S1, then in the next smallholder unit, the first cow selected would be serial number S2. This selection of the first cow was alternated between odd and even numbers from one smallholder unit to the other until investigation in all the 32 units was completed. Therefore, the cows selected in any individual smallholder unit were either all with odd or all with even serial numbers.

Data on claw disorders were collected by examining only the hind claws of each cow, due to poor restraint facilities that make it difficult to examine the fore limbs. General observation of gait for signs of lameness was done first. The floor state and small sizes of the units made the examination for lameness quite restrictive, and it needed an experienced veterinarian to conclude on whether a cow was lame or not, particularly when mildly lame. Each cow was restrained in a standing posture in the crush or the sleeping cubicle. Lifting of one hind limb at a time was done using a rope tied to an overhead pole or cross-bar. After washing with soap and water, claws were examined for any lesions, particularly on the weight-bearing surface. About 1-2 mm thickness of the horn of the sole was trimmed-off using a sharp quittor knife to expose any underlying lesions. Trimming did not reach the level of the corium and therefore was non-invasive and non-painful to the cows. In case of painful claw condition, local analgesia using 2% lignocaine hydrochloride and a tourniquet at mid-metatarsus was applied. The lesions found on each cow were recorded.

Data on cow-level factors were collected by the first author (as interviewer) administering questionnaires either to farmers, or the stockmen managing the cows in the zero-grazing units (as respondent interviewees) before examination of the cows. The data which included breed, parity, milk yield per day, and lactation stage were pre-coded and recorded in the questionnaires. The questionnaires were structured simple "Yes" and "No" and "I do not know" responses to minimize variations and information bias from the respondents. Data on farm-level factors were collected during visitation to each of the 32 farms. Some data (housing and stall design, presence and number of cubicles, type of cubicle bedding and floor, presence or absence of a curb, and lunging space, and adequacy of feeding space) were collected through observation. Other data such as kerb height were collected through measurements, while the rest (frequency of concentrate feeding, mineral supplementation, type of fodder, and frequency of slurry removal from the walk-alleys were collected by the first author interviewing the farmer, or stockmen. All the information collected from the zero-grazing units by measurements and by interview on the questionnaires was recorded in data collection sheets in codes allocated for each parameter.

Study 2 - Are body injuries, body soiling or body condition scores useful in predicting the welfare of zero-grazed dairy cows?

In this cross-sectional study each zero-grazing smallholder unit (defined as one with a minimum of 3 and a maximum of 16 adult dairy cows) was visited once for the whole study period. A total of 80 smallholder zero-grazing dairy units were included in the study (It is important to note that apart from these zero-grazing units being in the same area as those in study 1, none of them was included in both studies). Selection of the 80 zero-grazing units to include in study 2 was performed as for study 1. Furthermore, for logistical reasons units were also chosen based on the farmers' willingness to co-operate and to allow their dairy units to be used in the study.

The animals included for examination were adult dairy cows, whether in milk or dry. In any smallholder unit that had 5 or less adult cows, all the adult females were selected for examination. In those having more than 5 adult cows, only 5 were selected for examination. The five were selected using a simple systematic sampling method, similar to the one used in study 1. In all the 80 smallholder units, a total of 306 dairy cows were selected for examination.

In each unit, the selected cows were closely examined for signs of external body injuries. Injuries were recorded according the body regions on which they occurred. These body regions were mainly those that were prone to injury from housing structures and they included the neck, brisket, carpal joint area, rib-cage area, area over the tuber coxae, ischial area, hock joint area, teats and udder. The main signs that were considered as indicators of body injuries included external presence of raw wounds, ulcerations, swellings, scars, localized hair loss and skin hyperkeratosis/callus-like formation.

2.2.3. Evaluation of housing and animal management

Some of the factors of housing design and the quality of construction finishes were evaluated only by visual observation while others were assessed by taking actual measurement of the dimensions. Those factors that were evaluated only by visual observation included types and state of roofing, walls, and floor (mainly at the walk alleys and cubicles), as well as types and adequacy of feed bunks/troughs, presence or absence of neck-bars over the feed bunks and presence or absence of cubicles. Presence and type of cubicle bedding was also observed. Those housing factors that were evaluated by measuring actual dimensions included height of neck-bar from the upper edge of the feed bunk, width of the walk alleys from the rear edge of the cubicles to the front (near edge) of the feed bunk as well as width and length of the cubicles. Besides the physical aspects of the facilities, other animal-related aspects were also evaluated. The stocking density was evaluated by calculating cows to cubicle ratios. Presence of slurry on the walk alleys and gross body soiling of the cows was noted. Frequency of slurry removal was obtained through questionnaires. The individual body condition score (BCS) was evaluated on a simple scale of 1 to 5, which included half points that separated between the unit body condition scores. BCS 1 meant poor body condition, BCS 2 represented moderate body condition, BCS 3 represented good body condition, BCS 4 meant a fat cow, and BCS 5 represented a very fat cow. The farmers' and stockmen's perspective or knowledge on animal welfare was evaluated through interviewing them as respondents. All the data were recorded in data collection sheets.

2.2.4. Data management and analysis

The data representing each parameter information was coded with a specific numerical code for each parameter for the purposes of entry into Microsoft Office Excel sheets. The data were imported into SAS© 2002-2003 (SAS Institute Inc., Cary, NC, USA). Descriptive statistics were computed for cow-level and farm-level factors. From study 1, the prevalence rate of each claw disorder was calculated independent of other claw disorders. The prevalence of each claw disorder was calculated as the number of cows (CL) affected by the specific claw disorder divided by the total number of cows (300) examined, then multiplied by 100 to make it a percentage.

$$\text{Prevalence } (\%) = \frac{CL \times 100}{300}$$

Chi-square (χ^2) statistics were used to determine unconditional associations between all risk factors and the claw lesions. An association was considered significant at the level of $P<0.05$. Multiple logistic regressions were done through a step-down regression in which the risk factors that made the least variation to the occurrence of the claw lesions were eliminated one at a time through consideration of their odds ratios. Only the factors that were found to influence the occurrence of claw lesions significantly were retained in the model. The effects of confounding the risk factors were dealt with in the analysis but they were minimal because of some similarities of the management in the smallholder farms.

From study 2, prevalence of body injuries were calculated as simple percentages of occurrences of lesions, injuries and the risk factors. By use of SAS (Statistical Analytical

System) descriptive statistics were generated and tests of simple associations between zero-grazing unit-level and animal-level factors were done using Chi Square (χ^2) statistics at $p<0.05$ significance level. Chi Square values were determined using 2x2 contingency tables. In these associations, the Chi Square calculations were determined by evaluating each risk factor (variable) against each welfare predictor (outcome) on the animal. The degrees of freedom (df) in each case was standard, being calculated by [(rows-1) (columns-1), hence [(2-1) x (2-1) = 1]. Therefore df was 1 for each association test.

3. Results and discussion

3.1. Lameness and claw disorders as indicators of welfare

A high prevalence of acquired claw disorders was encountered in the cows from both studies, but higher in the first than the second study. The difference can be attributed to the fact that in study 1 the claws were trimmed during evaluation, while in study 2 only observation for lameness was done without trimming for specific examination of the claws. In study 1, out of 300 cows the prevalence was 88% (n=264) of which 69% (n=182) were subclinical (the affected cows were not lame), the diagnoses being made through trimming of the claws; and 31% (n=82) were clinical (the affected cows were lame), with animals showing evidence of lameness. About 70% (n=211) of the cows had laminitis, which was either sublinical laminitis in 49% (n=148) diagnosed by presence of sole haemorrhages seen after trimming a thin layer of the horn of the sole, or chronic laminitis in 21% (n=63) diagnosed by presence of extensive diffuse sole haemorrhages coupled with various degrees of claw deformities. The Pictorial description of the claw lesions and the associated predisposing causes was detailed in a previous publication [50]. In study 2, lame cows were encountered in 73% (n=58) of the 80 zero-grazing units, for which the total prevalence was 35% (n=107) among the 306 cows examined. The lameness was caused by different claw disorders, which included various degrees of claw deformities ranging from moderate claw overgrowth to severe twisting of the claws. Lameness caused by lesions in proximal parts of the limbs (proximal to the claws) had very low prevalence of less than 2% in both studies; most of these lesions did not cause any lameness.

3.2. Body injuries as indicators of welfare

Injuries on body surface were found distributed in various body regions among the 306 cows that were examined from the 80 smallholder zero-grazed dairy units in study 2 (Table 1). These body regions included the neck, brisket, hock joint area, carpal joint area, tuber coxae, ischial and rib cage areas, teats and udder. These areas being protuberant were prone to be easily injuried by house structures. The protuberant areas of the body are the parts on which pressure is exerted the most when lying down, and therefore injuries in these areas indicate the comfort state of the lying places of the animal house, hence reflecting good or poor animal welfare with respect to lying comfort. Injuries on the mentioned body protuberances also serve as indicators of the traumatic tendencies of certain structural parts of the animal housing unit, and this in turn reflects good or poor animal welfare state of the housing unit.

In 65% (n=52) of the zero-grazed units, cows showed injuries in the dorsal part of the neck between the middle area and over the shoulders, which presented various signs such as hyperkeratosis and callus-like skin tissue, large patched hair loss, raw wounds, and scars (Figure 1). These affected 60.8% (n=186) of the 306 cows examined. Hyperkeratosis and callus-like skin tissue were the predominant lesions indicating chronic injuries to the skin and constituted 70% (n=130) of the cows with signs of neck injuries. Prevalence of hair loss and raw wounds or scars on the dorsal aspect of the neck as signs of injury was low, being 20% (n=37) and 10% (n=19) of the cows with signs of neck injuries respectively. Evaluation of the housing structures showed that only in 35% (n=28) of the zero-grazing units they were not the cause for trauma to the neck areas of the cows. The low level of neck-bars over the feed bunks was the main risk factor for injuries on the dorsal surface of the neck. Hyperkeratosis and callus-like skin in the dorsal surface of the neck are caused by constant friction against the neck-bar during the many hours of feeding at the feed bunks. A neck-bar is fixed over the feed bunk to prevent cattle from wasting feeds and placing their forelimbs into the feed bunks (Figure 2). Similar effects of neck-bars have been previously described [88]. The neck-bars over the feed bunks were present in 60% (n=48) of the zero-grazing units, and in 77.1% (n=37) of these units the neck-bars were fixed at less or up to 50cm of the top edge of the feed bunk, while in 22.9% (n=11) of the units they were more than 50 cm from the top edge of the feed bunk. When the level is too low, the dorsal surface of the neck would always scrap against the neck-bar as long as the animal is at the feed bunk feeding, and injuries are exacerbated by animals pushing one another and fighting at the feed bunks due to inadequate feeding space or social dominance molestation. All the neck-bars in these zero-grazing units were made of timber, some of which had side-facing sharp edges that contact the dorsal surface of the neck, precipitating the occurrence of injuries (Figure 2). Also, the width of some feed bunks was excessive that cows struggled to reach the feed on the far end and this predisposed them to more of the neck injuries.

Table 1. Distribution of injuries on various parts of the body surface as found among 306 cows examined in the 80 smallholder zero-grazed dairy units evaluated for welfare of dairy cattle in the peri-urban areas of Nairobi, Kenya.

	Zero-grazing units with cows showing surface body injuries		Cows with surface body injuries	
Body region	**n**	**%**	**n**	**%**
Carpal joint	77	96	230	75.16
Hock joint	76	95	260	85.00
Rib cage area	76	95	228	74.51
Tuber coxae	72	91	204	66.70
Ischial area	61	76	124	40.52
Neck	52	65	186	60.78
Brisket	51	64	134	43.79
Teats / udder	50	63	89	29.10

Inadequate feeding space per animal at the feed bunk was a common finding in these smallholder zero-grazing dairy cattle units. This led to increased competitiveness and aggressive behavior of the cows toward each other and particularly toward the subordinate cattle during feeding times. Such behavior is likely to result in physical injuries not only in the neck area but also in other regions of the body, and to reduce feeding time as well, a fact that also infringes partly on freedom from hunger (one of the five freedoms of animal welfare).

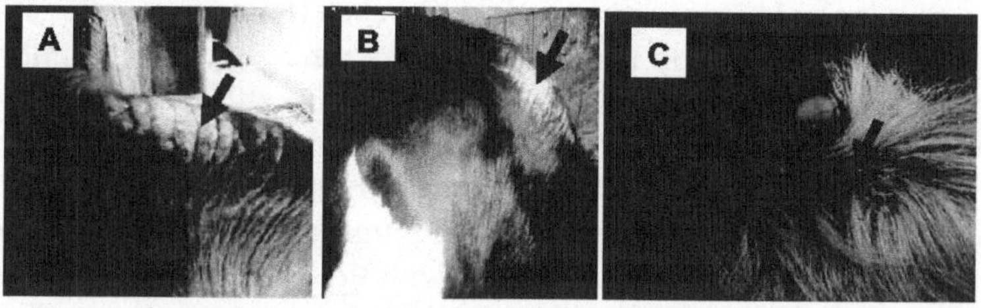

Figure 1. Signs of injuries on the dorsal surface of the neck in some of the cows among the 80 farms evaluated for welfare of dairy cattle in the smallholder zero-grazing units in the peri-urban areas of Nairobi, Kenya. Picture A shows severe hyperkeratosis, callus-like skin with complete hair loss (arrow), Picture B shows moderate hyperkeratosis and a patch of hair loss (arrow), and Picture C shows beginning of hair loss with skin crust (arrow).

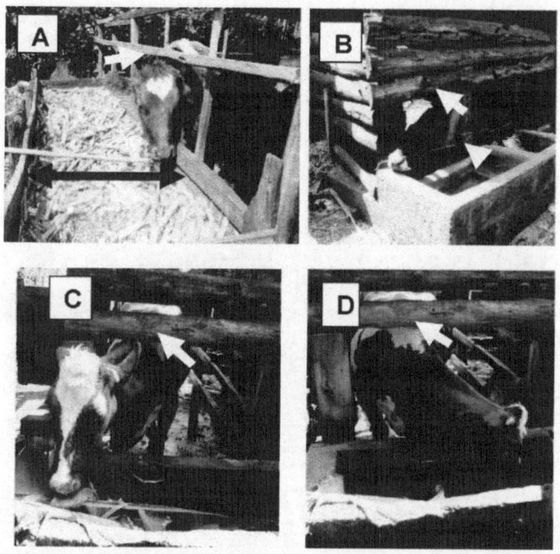

Figure 2. Position of the neck-bars in some of the zero-grazing units evaluated for dairy cattle welfare in the peri-urban areas of Nairobi, Kenya. Pictures A, C and D show low-level positioned neck-bars (arrow) that always rubs the dorsal surface of the cow neck whenever she feeds from the feed bunk; Picture A also shows excessively wide feed bunk (double-headed arrow) from which a cow struggles to reach feed in the far wide-end; Picture B shows a cow attempting to squeeze the head and the neck between a very low sharp-edged neck-bar (arrow) and a broken sharp-edged under-bar (arrow head).

Signs of injuries on the cranial surface of carpal joint area of the cows were observed in 96% (n=77) of the 80 units evaluated. These included healing wounds and scars, soft tissue swellings, hardening of skin in callus-like appearance and various degrees of hair loss. Out of the 306 cows examined, 75.2% (n=230) had signs of injuries in the carpal joint area. The main signs of injury in this area of the body were healing wounds and scars found in 75% (n=173) of the 230 cows with carpal area injuries, but soft tissue swellings and hair loss alone were found in 15% (n=34) and 10% (n=23) of the cows respectively. The high prevalence of signs of injuries on the cranial surface of the carpal joint area served as indicators of the rough and abrasive state of the floors where the cows lie on. It also meant that the cubicles in which the cows lay had inadequate or no bedding at all (Figure 3). Cattle get up from the lying posture by first kneeling on the carpus before extending the hind limbs to support their weight and finally stand up. This behavior predisposes cattle to likelihood of injuries to the carpal area every time the animal kneels on bare abrasive floor or bare concrete cubicle surfaces. Concrete or loose stone floors of the walk alley and cubicle lying surfaces were the commonest abrasive surfaces in these zero-grazing units. Repeated friction and contusion on such floors may cause injuries that will heal with time, leaving scars and hair loss. The repeated prolonged friction on the cranial surface of the carpus might eventually extend deep and lead to contusion of the underlying subcutaneous connective tissue with subsequent development of false pre-carpal bursa that consequently results into carpal hygroma (Figure 4). Inadequate lunge space and bob zone in the animal cubicle may exacerbate occurrence of injuries on the cranial surface of the carpus. All these traumatic signs indicate existence of poor animal welfare in the evaluated zero-grazing units.

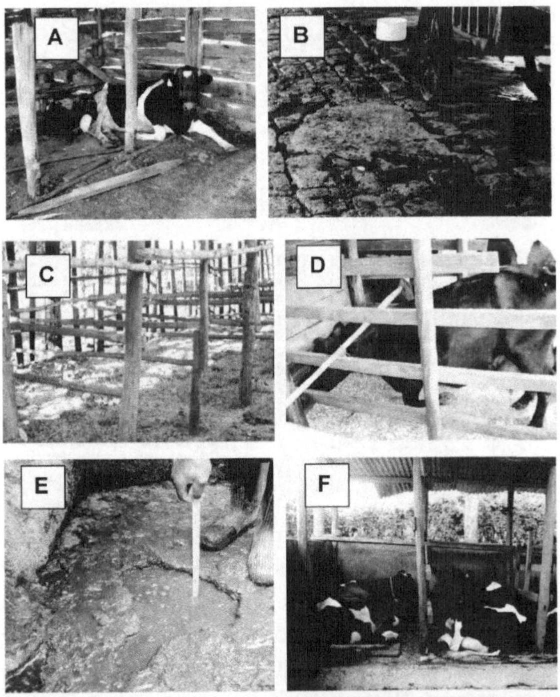

Figure 3. Bare or damaged floors and cubicles without bedding, which predisposed the cows to injuries and poor welfare. Picture A shows a cow lying on bare floor of a cubicle that is fallen apart with wooden planks on the floor. Picture B shows a floor made of blocks of stone with gaps between them. Picture C shows cubicles with loose stones in them. Picture D shows a cow attempting to stand by kneeling, which injures the carpus if the cubicle or concrete floor is bare and lunge space small, note the neck is under a wooden cross-bar. Picture E is a damaged pot-holed concrete floor. Picture F shows cows lying on rubber mats.

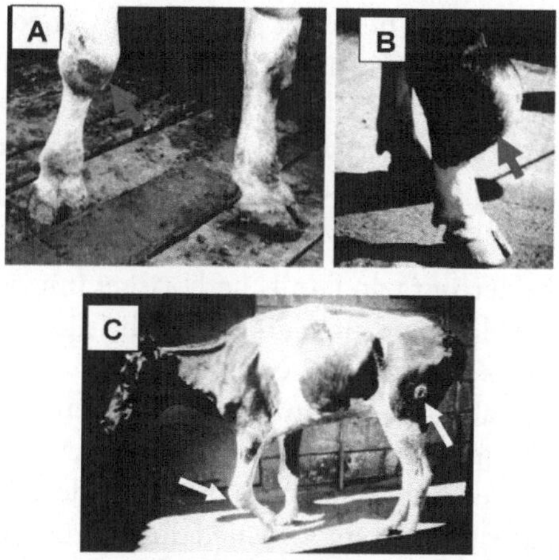

Figure 4.Signs of injuries on the cranial surface of the carpus. Picture A shows early swelling developing on the carpus (arrow); Picture B shows massively swollen carpal hygroma (arrow) as a result of prolonged repeated contusion of soft tissues cranial to the carpal joint subsequently forming a subcutaneous pre-carpal bursa. This swelling was full of viscous straw-coloured sterile fluid. Sometimes the carpal hygroma lesion could become infected and progress to joint ankylosis as in Picture C (arrow), which impairs the animal ability to move and feed, hence originating loss of body condition, which is also a sign of poor welfare. Frequent lying down from standing discomfort in a lame cow may result to development of decubital wounds as seen on the caudo-lateral aspect of the thigh in Picture C (arrow) and these aggravate poor animal welfare.

In this study, floors were evaluated in the walk alleys where the cows spent most of their time standing during feeding times. In total, 28.8% (n=23) of the 80 studied units were earthen floors in the walk alleys, while the remainder 71.3% (n=57) had concrete or stoned floors. The concrete floors were grossly worn-out and pot-holed in 41.3% (n=24) of the 57 units with concrete walk alleys, while 26.2% (n=15) were smooth and slippery and 32.5% (n=18) were good and non-slippery (32.50%). In 53.75% (n=43) of the units there was no bedding material in the cubicles or animal resting areas, these areas were bare earth in 53.5% (n=23) and bare concrete in 46.5% (n=20). The bedding materials used in the rest of the zero-grazing units were wheat straw, saw-dust, wood-shavings, plastic mats or bare wooden slabs. The grossly worn-out or pot-holed concrete floors and bare concreted cubicles were the main causes of injuries and discomfort on the cranial surface of the carpal joint area whenever the cows rose up from the lying position. Slippery concrete on the walk alley poses a risk by increasing chances of slipping and falling, particularly in the presence of slurry on the floor, making of it an increased risk for poor animal welfare [28]. Considering that cows spend an average of about 12 hours per day standing even when provided with soft lying area [77,89], it makes it necessary to have soft, non-slip, smooth washable floor systems with adequate slope for drainage in order to enhance claw hygiene and health [28,31]. Such materials on floors would promote good animal welfare. The types and conditions of the floors in these studies predisposed the cows to poor claw health, hence the high prevalence of claw lesions subsequently precipitating to lameness [90,91]. Provision of comfortable bedding in the cubicles and resting areas of the cow housing unit influences cow resting behavior positively, by encouraging them to lie down frequently. Hence, by reducing the long hours of standing, which subsequently minimizes the risk of lameness from claw lesions [17,92], the cow welfare is enhanced. However, some of the bedding such as sawdust, which are used in these zero-grazing units owing to ease of their availability and cost, could be incriminated as risk factor for mastitis [93], but in the current studies, mastitis was not a problem.

Cows in 64% (n=51) of the zero-grazing units had brisket injuries, which were evidenced by extensive patches of hair loss and/or scars on the brisket (Figure 5). Brisket injuries were found in 43.8% (n=134) of the 306 cows examined in this study. Injuries at the brisket area were caused by abrasive action of bare concrete in the cubicles and by high and sharp upper edge of the feed bunk on which the brisket rubbed continuously during feeding (Figure 6). A good feed bunk that takes into consideration animal welfare should be made of concrete, because it can be smoothened during construction to eliminate sharp edges that would injure cattle as they feed [28,31,89]. The feed bunk front side should not be too high but low enough for cattle to reach feeds without the brisket rubbing against the upper edge of the bunk. The few concrete feed bunks that were worn-out, and a high number of others made of iron sheets and timber, had sharpened edges that predisposed the cows to injuries of the mouth, head and neck regions. Nails and iron sheet pieces are likely to break from the iron sheet-lined feed bunks with time, and if ingested by the cows can lead to hardware disease apart from causing direct wounds on the body surface in the head, neck and brisket regions. Therefore, the state of feed bunks as found in this study, exposed cows to poor welfare.

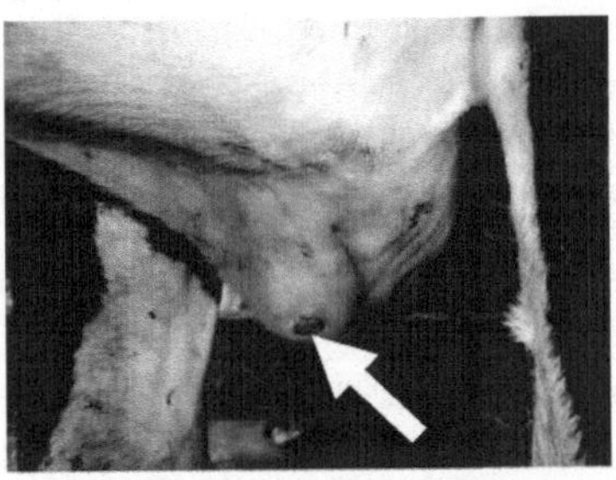

Figure 5. Brisket injury consisting of swelling, scar tissue and hair loss (arrow) in one of the examined cows.

Signs of injuries at the hock joint area were observed in 95% (n=76) of all the 80 zero-grazing units. These included healing wounds and scars, soft tissue swellings and hair loss (Figure 7). The lesions were found in 87% (n= 260) of the 306 cows examined. The high prevalence of injuries at the hock area was a good indicator of the uncomfortable state of the concrete floor and the bare concrete cubicles, which in turn were a definite reflection of the existing poor welfare of cattle in these zero-grazing units. Another region of the body with signs of injuries related to concrete floor and bare concrete cubicles was the ischial area. Injuries in this area were found in 76% (n=61) of the zero-grazing units and affected 41% (n=124) of the 306 cows examined. Cows tend to lie leaning more toward one side than the other, with the lateral aspect of the hock pressed against the floor (Figure 8). This explains the high prevalence of these injuries.

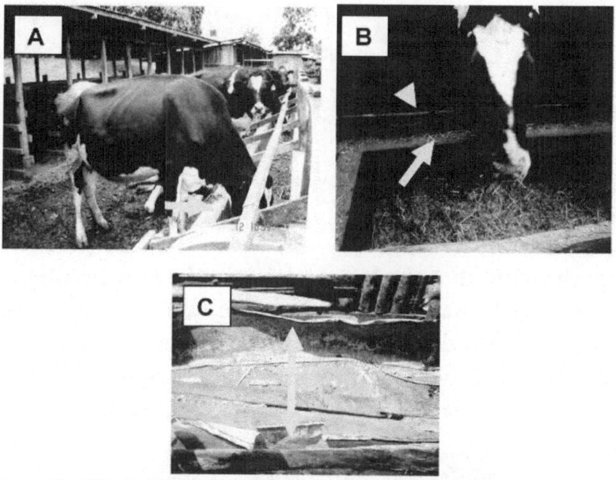

Figure 6.Various feed bunks with different designs and state of the upper front edge. Picture A shows concrete feed bunk with smooth upper front edge, which is at an acceptable low level off the brisket (arrow). Picture B shows low smooth-edged concrete feed bunk (arrow), but addition of wooden bars above the upper front edge (arrow head) on which the brisket could rub and be injured with time. Picture C shows the edges and main part of feed bunk lined with sharp broken iron sheet pieces (arrow), which could injure not only the brisket but also the tongue as it scoops the feed.

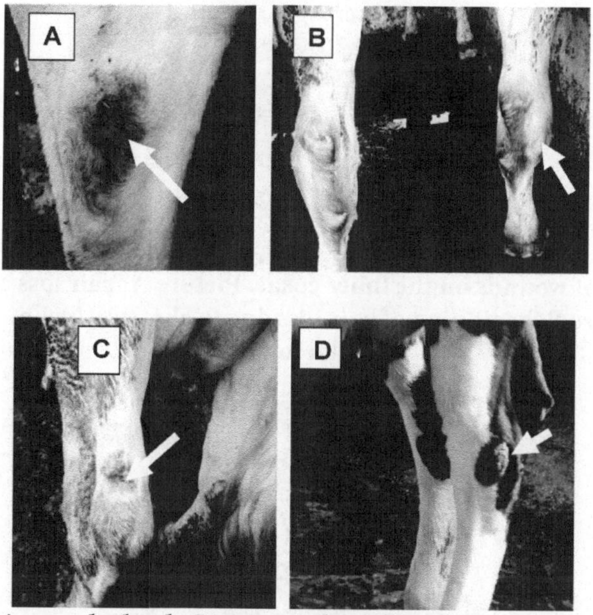

Figure 7.Injuries on the hock. Picture A shows hyperaemic skin with hair loss (arrow), Picture B shows hygroma swelling at the initial developing stage (arrow), Picture C shows healing wound caudal on the hock area (arrow). Picture D shows nodular scarring tumour-like swelling on the lateral aspect of the hock (arrow).

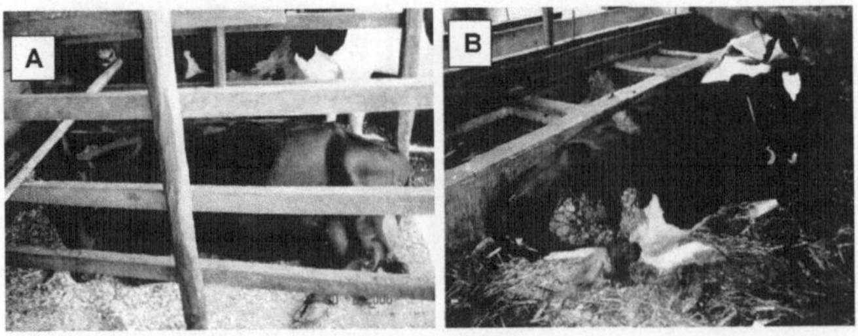

Figure 8.Pictures showing that the lying position of a cow presses on lateral aspect of one hock joint area such that if there is no adequate bedding material or padding, the hock area is easily injured by repeated pressure on hard floor particularly bare concrete floor. Picture A shows a cow lying on lateral aspect of the right hock, and Picture B the cow is lying on lateral aspect of the left hock.

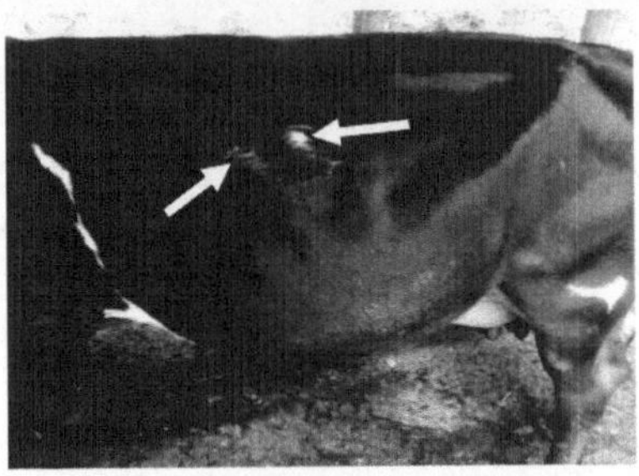

Figure 9.Scars sustained at the rib cage area (arrows) in one of the cows examined in the 80 zero-grazing units.

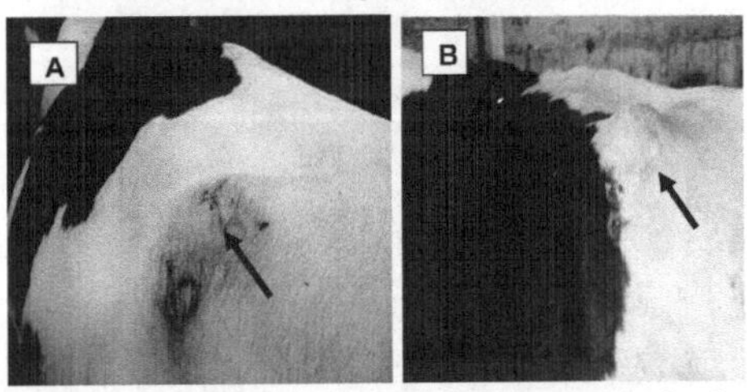

Figure 10.Signs of wounds on the tuber coxae. Picture A: hair loss and skin abrasion (arrow). Picture B: beginning of hair loss due to abrasion by housing structures (arrow)

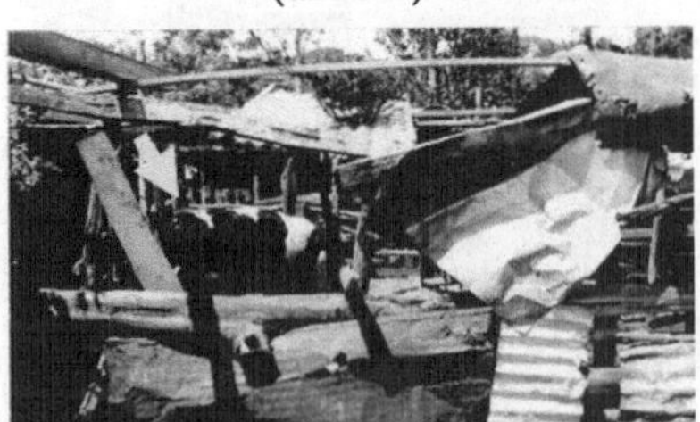

Figure 11.Collapsed iron sheet roof and sides in one of the zero-grazing units evaluated. Both the roof and side timber are broken and collapsing. Yet cows are still housed inside (arrow).

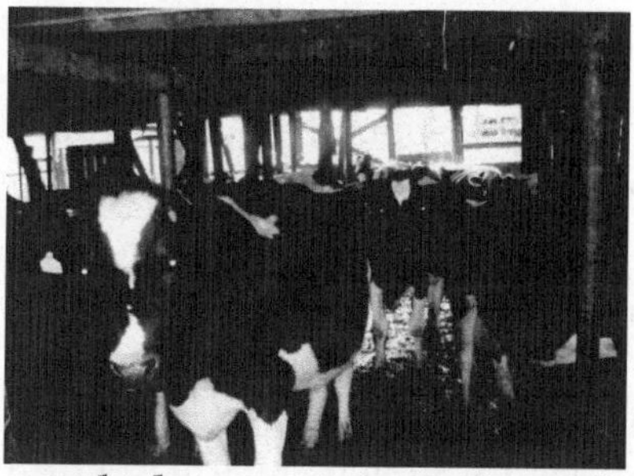

Figure 12.One of the overstocked zero-grazing units with narrowed walk alley and the cows hardly having any room to turn or move. Animal interactions here and scrambling for space can cause them to press each other against the sharp wooden structures leading to injuries on the rib cage, tuber coxae and other protuberances.

Other signs of injuries found on the cows in some of the units evaluated were located on the rib cage area (Figure 9) and the tuber coxae (Figure 10). On the rib cage area they were found in 95% (n=76) of the units and they affected 75% (n=228) of the 306 cows examined; lesions on tuber coxae were found in 91% (n=72) of the units and they affected 67% (n= 204) of the 306 cows examined. In both areas the signs of injuries were mainly healing wounds or scars. Tuber coxae and rib cage injuries were associated with small cubicle space and protruding traumatic parts of the cattle housing structures, such as side dividing timber or wooden pieces, nails and iron sheets on the side walls. Some of the studied units had broken wooden sidewalls and collapsing roofing material that easily injure the animals (Figure 11). Small-sized cubicles, measuring 1.80 meters by 0.95 meters or less, were found in 74.6% (n=50) of the units evaluated in this study. Overstocking was found in more than half of the zero-grazing units. It caused squeezing and competition for space and feed among the animals, which facilitates injury from the protruding traumatic objects and collapsed roofing material in the cattle housing units. Overstocking meant that there were more cows than the number of cubicles available to rest (Figure 12) and in some cases the feeding space was inadequate for all the cows present. All these factors contributed to poor welfare of the cattle.

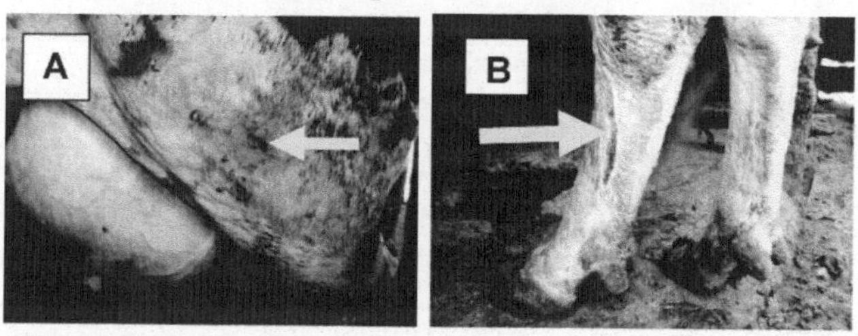

Figure 13.Pictures showing lateral limb injuries. Picture A shows a scarring bruised skin on the lateral side of the thigh (arrow); Picture B shows a healing longitudinal skin cut on the lateral aspect of the lower part of the limb (arrow).

Additional areas with lesions, but showing lower prevalence of injuries include the teats, udder, thighs and other areas of the limbs (Figure 13). These were mainly abrasions with hyperaemia of skin and hair loss. Injuries in these regions were mainly associated with roughness and bareness of the concrete floor and the cubicles. Occasionally, the skin in the thigh areas can also be injured by protruding sharp edges or objects in the housing unit. There were also pin-point nodular lesions on the teats of some of the cows, which resembled pox-like lesions. Although these lesions could have been caused by microorganisms such as viruses, poor environmental conditions would facilitate the entrance of such agents and persistence of infection.

The skin injuries observed in the current study were a reflection of the housing type and size, as well as the structures used to construct cattle houses. Similar injuries have been described in other studies [44]. Skin injuries in any part of the body of an animal are indicators of the welfare status of the animal particularly in relation to its environment. These lesions are associated with pain and suffering [43]. An environment that allows free movement of the animal without risk of disease or injury is paramount [28,31]. The key predisposing factors to external body injuries are the restrictiveness of housing types and structures that affect the cows' behavioral patterns [94]. The external injuries observed in the cows in this study were mainly located on body protuberances such as the hock and the tuber coxae. Others were in the areas of the body subjected to pressure during recumbency and feeding times such as the brisket, ischial region, udder, rib cage, and neck. These findings are in agreement with previous reports [94,95]. In this study, although injuries at different parts of the body were attributed to different risk factors, they still related to the nature of the housing environment.

Statistical analysis of simple associations between injuries and disease was carried out and several factors were associated. Injuries in the various body regions reported in the foregone pages were found to be associated with various factors within the zero-grazing units. The factors with strong association are presented in table 2.

Table 2.Risk factors associated with the occurrence of body injuries in the 306 cows examined in the 80 smallholder zero-grazing units evaluated for the welfare of dairy cattle in the peri-urban areas of Nairobi, Kenya.

Injured body region	Risk factor	Chi-square value (χ^2)	P value
Dorsal surface of the neck	Presence of neck bar	20.25	<0.0001
	Height of neck bar	22.93	<0.0001
Brisket area	Presence of neck bar	8.14	0.0043
	Height of neck bar	7.37	0.025
Teat /udder/thighs	Bare concrete floor	12.57	0.014
	Quality of bedding	5.15	0.023
Hock joint area	Narrow walk alley	10.68	<0.0011
Ischial region	Concrete floor	8.86	0.012

The presence of neck-bar over the feed bunk had a strong association with injuries on the dorsal surface of the neck (χ^2=20.25; p<0.0001) and the surface of the brisket (χ^2= 8.14; p=0.0043). The position of the height of the neck-bar from the top edge of the feed bunk was also found to influence presence or absence of injuries at the dorsal surface of the neck (χ^2=22.93; p<0.0001) and the surface of the brisket (χ^2=7.37; p=0.025. Injuries in the hock joint area were significantly influenced by narrow walk alleys (χ^2=10.68; p<0.001), whilst injuries at the ischial area were significantly associated with poor quality (excessively rough and pot-holed) concrete floors (χ^2=8.86; p=0.012). Teat, udder and thigh injuries were found to have a significant association with bare concrete-floored cubicles (χ^2 =12.57; p=0.014) and also with presence or absence of bedding and the quality of bedding (χ^2=5.15; p=0.023). Lameness was found to be associated with excess slurry in the walk alley (χ^2=29.58; p=0.042).

The housing systems in the smallholder zero-grazing units in this study greatly restricted the cows from freely expressing their normal behavior and enjoying free movement. The restricting sizes of these animal units are normally due to the small pieces of land owned and the financial constraints of these smallholder farmers, which makes it difficult for them to build cattle housing units with the recommended dimensions [29]. This means that it may be difficult to guarantee the freedom of expression of normal behavior and movement for the cows in such smallholder zero-grazing units. The restriction of movement is likely to predispose the cows to lameness [96]. The particularly small size of cubicles found in these units were contrary to what is recommended [97] and was incriminated as one of the factors that predisposed the cows to frequent injuries on the rib-cage, tuber coxae and ischial area, thus supporting previous findings [98]. All these housing factors predisposing the cows to body injuries and lameness are associated with causing pain and suffering, hence poor welfare.

3.3. Body condition score as indicators of welfare

Body condition score (BCS) was also found to be a good indicator of the dairy cow welfare for these zero-grazing units. It reflects mainly on the feeding regime, nutritional value of the diet and the feed quantities supplied to the cows. The average body condition score of the cows evaluated in these 80 units was 2.20. Out of the 306 cows examined, the distribution of the body condition score was found to be as is presented in table 3.

Table 3.Distribution of the body condition scores among the 306 cows examined in the 80 smallholder zero-grazing units evaluated for welfare of dairy cattle in the peri-urabn areas of Nairobi, Kenya.

BCS	Number of cows	Percentage of cows (%)
1 – 1.5	19	6
2 – 2.5	177	58
3 – 3.5	100	33
4 – 4.5	10	3
5	0	0
Total	306	100

From the results, about 91% (n=277) of the 306 cows examined had fair body condition (BCS between 2 and 3.5), which indicated that the feeding practiced in these zero-grazing units was moderate. Only a few cows had poor body condition below 1.5 (6%; n=19). Similarly, good body condition above 3.5 was found in only 3% (n=10) of the cows examined, which shows that nutritional quality and feed quantity or feeding regime in these zero-grazing units falls below the optimal expectations of good feeding practices for dairy cows. The body condition score (BCS) was influenced by the presence, amount and frequency of concentrate feeding, mineral supplementation and protein supplementation, as shown in Table 4. Body condition score 1 had significant association with occasional (irregular) feeding of concentrates (χ^2=14.77; p=0.022), absence of concentrate feeding (χ^2=7.90;

p=0.048), occasional mineral supplementation (χ^2=49.87; p<0.0001) as well as absence of mineral supplements (χ^2=8.23; p=0.042). Body condition score 2 was found to have a significant association with variation (number of times) in the frequency of concentrate feeding (χ^2= 22.69; p=0.012), regular (daily) concentrate feeding (χ^2=13.29; p=0.021) and regular mineral supplementation (χ^2=12.02; p=0.035). Body condition score 3 was found to have a significant association with high levels of concentrate feeding (χ^2=35.65; p=0.017), regular (daily) concentrate feeding (χ^2=13.29; p=0.021), variations in amounts of mineral supplementation (χ^2=29.08; p=0.016) and regular mineral supplementation (χ^2=15.03; p<0.01). Body condition score 4 was found to have a significant association with regular protein supplementation (χ^2=14.46; p=0.023).

Table 4. Factors associated with the body condition score (BCS) for the cows examined in 80 smallholder zero-grazing units evaluated for the welfare of dairy cattle in the peri-urban areas of Nairobi, Kenya.

BCS	Associated factor	Chi-square value (χ^2)	P value
1	Occasional concentrate feeding	14.77	0.022
	Absence of concentrate feeding	7.90	0.048
	Occasional mineral supplementation	49.87	<0.0001
	Absence of mineral supplementation	8.23	0.0415
2	Variation in frequency of concentrate feeding	22.69	0.012
	Regular concentrate feeding	13.29	0.021
	Regular mineral supplementation	12.02	0.035
3	High levels of concentrate feeding	35.65	0.017
	Variations in amounts of mineral supplementation	29.08	0.016
	Regular mineral supplementation	15.03	<0.01
	Regular concentrate feeding	13.19	0.022
4	Regular protein supplementation	14.46	0.0023

Generally, the feeding of forages to cows in these zero-grazing units was more consistent than the feeding of concentrates. Forages included mainly grasses such as napier grass (Pennisetum purpurem), Kikuyu grass (pennisetum clandestum), Rhodes grass [Chloris gayana], maize stover, and in few occasions banana plant stems. Forages were fed to all the cows in all the 80 zero-grazing units. Moreover, main variations in dairy cow feeding practices in these zero-grazing units were found on concentrate feeding. Concentrates were fed to cows only in 85% (n= 68) of the zero-grazing units evaluated in this study. In the remaining 15% (n=12) of the units, cows were not fed on concentrates at all. Of the zero-grazing units that provided concentrates, 98.5% (n=67) used commercially available concentrates, while 1.5% (n=1) used farm-made concentrate mixtures. The farm-made concentrate mixtures consisted of pollard, maize germ, wheat bran, yeast, cotton seed cake and minerals. The formulation ratios of the ingredients in the farm-made mixtures were not revealed to the investigator. In the farms that provided concentrates, 83.8% (n=57) fed it only to lactating cows while 16.2% (n=11) fed it to all cows. Concentrates were provided 2-3 times per day, intentionally coinciding with milking times. In the farms that provided concentrates, 32.4% (n=22) fed each cow on an average of 2-4 kilograms of concentrates per day, 29.4% (n=20) on an average of 5-7 kilograms per day, 23.5% (n=16) on an average of 8-10 kilograms per day and in 14.7% (n=10) on more than 10 kilograms per day (Table 5).

Table 5. Amount of concentrates fed to cows per day in 68 of the 80 smallholder zero-grazing units evaluated for welfare of dairy cattle in the peri-urban areas of Nairobi, Kenya.

Daily concentrate amount(Kilograms / cow)	Number ofZero-grazing units	Percentage ofZero-grazing units
2 – 4	22	32.4
5 – 7	20	29.4
8 – 10	16	23.5
> 10	10	14.7
Total	68	100

According to data in table 5, concentrate feeding in most zero-grazing units was minimal in quantity, and particularly when considering that in many of these units it was partial since the cows were fed only when lactating.

Cows in 88.75% (n=71) of the zero-grazing units were given mineral supplements. In the remaining 11.25% (n=9) of the units, no minerals were provided for the cows. In the zero-grazing units that provided minerals, 77.5% (n=55) of them provided minerals ad libitum, 19.7% (n=14) at 200g to 500g per cow per day, and 2.8% (n=2) of them only occasionally during the lactation period. The mineral supplements were commercially bought and they included: "Unga high phosphorus"-SuperPHOS® (Danthil Enterprises) and "Maclick Super®" (Coopers Limited). The latter was available either in powder form or as a mineral lick block. The constituents of the mineral supplements included higher concentrations of the major elements such as calcium, phosphorus, sodium, chloride and magnesium and lower concentrates of trace elements such as iron, copper, manganese, zinc, sulphur, cobalt, iodine, selenium and molybdenum. Regular mineral supplementation has been shown to be protective on occurrence of some claw conditions such as sole bruising and white line separation [17].

Additional protein supplements such as cotton seed cake, sorghum, fish-meal and high protein forage (Alfafa/Lucerne-*Medicago sativa*) were provided in 36% (n=29) of the zero-grazing units. These protein supplements were added to concentrates, but the high protein forages such as Lucerne were mixed with fodder feeds. Protein supplements were added and fed to cattle only during early lactation. Protein supplementation had no influence on occurrence of claw lesions, but on body condition score, which is discussed in the paragraphs below.

Concentrates are rich in proteins and carbohydrates and have some levels of minerals and vitamins, hence their usefulness in supplementing forages that generally have less of these nutrients. Apart from being essential for growth and for improved milk production [6,99], concentrates also make the diet of dairy cows more complete, thus contributing to their good welfare [99]. However, if fed in large quantities, carbohydrate feeds could lead to ruminal tympany, sub-acute ruminal acidosis and subsequent laminitis [100], which consequently results in lameness that negatively impacts on the welfare of the cow [31,44]. The inconsistencies of concentrate feeding observed in this study including total failure to feed the cows on any concentrate, irregular feeding frequencies and feeding irregular amounts, demonstrated the farmers' ignorance concerning the need and the importance of concentrate feeding. Discriminatory feeding of concentrates only to lactating cows but denying it to the young, non-pregnant, as well as dry cows further supports evidences to this ignorance.

The farmers' perception of the need for concentrate feeding was only associated with the benefits of increased milk production. All these inconsistencies and irregularities of concentrate feeding deny the cow access to a balanced feed type that promotes health, growth and energy [99,101]. Such varied irregularity in concentrate feeding of dairy cattle from one zero-grazing unit to the next has not been reported elsewhere, and is in sharp contrast to the more standardized dairy cattle feeding regimes in intensively managed dairy production systems in the developed countries [102]. The association observed in this study between body condition status and the level of concentrate feeding demonstrates the benefit of concentrate inclusion in the diet. It further points out to the fact that lack of, and irregular concentrate feeding has a direct negative effect on the welfare of the cows. The stronger influence of occasional (irregular) concentrate feeding than its total absence on body condition score, can be attributed to the fact that when the cow's body is denied concentrates completely, it probably adjusts through compensatory mechanisms. Conversely, occasional inconsistent feeding does not allow the cow physiological adjustment to one consistent system, but rather destabilizes it, hence negatively affecting the general welfare of the animal.

The study also indicated that good body condition of the cows was enhanced when additional protein supplements were mixed with the concentrate feeds. These observations could be attributed to the fact that concentrates supply the primary nutrient requirements to the cow as well as sufficient reserves needed for secondary processes such as normal lactation [99,101], and increased milk production [18]. Therefore, concentrates are pertinent constituents of the dairy cow diet if the stress of both body maintenance and milk production has to be avoided.

Regular mineral supplementation supplied in a majority of the zero-grazing units in this study is a reflection of good animal welfare practice, since minerals enhance animal growth, reproduction and health [99,101]. In this study, the importance of mineral supplementation was evidenced by the association between regular supplementation and fair body condition, while occasional or absence of mineral supplementation was associated with poor body condition. Irregular mineral supplementation like was found with irregular concentrate feeding destabilizes the body more than complete absence of minerals, hence affecting body condition score that impacts negatively on the welfare of the cows. Findings from previous studies indicate that absence or insufficient mineral supplementation impacts negatively on growth rate and reproduction, leading to anoestrus [101,103], and hence inevitably affecting animal welfare.

3.4. Other parameters indicating poor welfare

Gross soiling with slurry on various areas of the bodies of the cows was observed in all the zero-grazing units evaluated in this study. In all the cows examined, all their limbs were soiled. The flanks and udder were soiled in 97% (n=297) and 90% (n=28) of the cows, respectively (Figure14). Soiling was an indicator of the management of the slurry in the zero-grazing unit, which means if the body is grossly dirty with raw or dried slurry, then possibly slurry is left to accumulate for long on the floor before being scrapped or washed off. Removal of slurry and cleaning of the cow housing floors was done at least once per day in 55% (n=44) of the units. For the remaining 45% (n=36) of the units, it was done only occasionally, either once a week or once every two weeks (Figure 15). The frequency of cleaning the slurry from the floor was significantly associated with soiling of flanks (χ^2=80; p<0.0001), limbs (χ^2=16.06; p<0.0011) and udder (χ^2=13.58; p=0.0035) (Table 6).

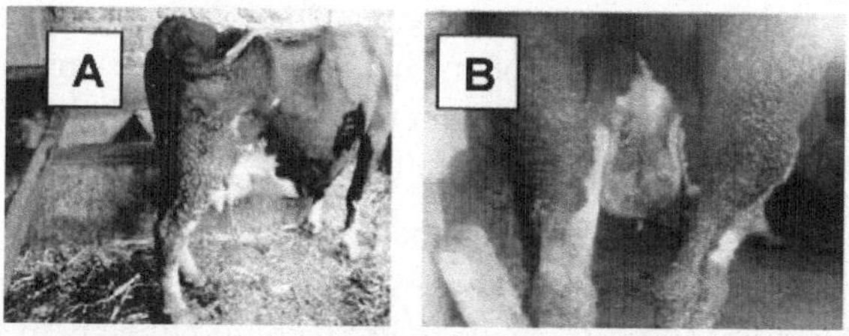

Figure 14. Gross soiling of the whole limb area in Picture A, and the udder plus whole hind quarters in Picture B, with slurry accumulated in the unit facilities.

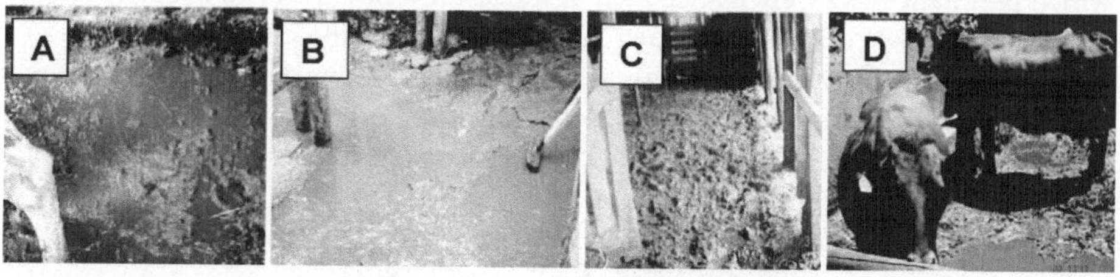

Figure 15. Slurry accumulated in animal facilities. Picture A shows slurry in an earthen floor. Picture B shows slurry in concrete floor. Picture C shows slurry and narrow walk alley. Picture D-Despite slurry accumulation on parks, the cows in this unit were clean because the cubicles had good clean bedding of sawdust, which meant the cows never lay on the slurry.

Table 6. Factors associated with soiling in various body parts of cows examined among the 80 smallholder zero-grazing units evaluated for welfare of dairy cattle in the peri-urban areas of Nairobi, Kenya.

Soiled body region	Associated factor	Chi-square value (χ^2)	P value
Flanks	Excess slurry in cow house	80	<0.0001
Limbs	Excess slurry in cow house	13.58	0.0035
Udder	Excess slurry in cow house	16.06	<0.0011

Although more than half of the smallholder units in the current study had slurry removed frequently, the excessive slurry found in the rest of the units is likely to affect health of the claws and the udders of the cows. The holding of slurry in cow housing units for long without cleaning it out, exposes the claws to continuous wet environment which softens the horny parts of the claws, predisposing them to development of lesions as previously reported [17,44]. Accumulated slurry also exposes udders to unhygienic conditions that predispose them to mastitis, particularly when the cows lie on it most of the time as observed previously [17,44]. The subsequent development of claw lameness and mastitis will cause pain and inevitably lead to poor welfare. Furthermore, this study was able to show that accumulation of slurry caused excessive soiling of the skin in some parts of the body mainly because most of the time the cows were found lying on it. This is supported by the strong statistical association between the presence of slurry and soiling of the hind quarters as well as the udder region. This may probably be exacerbated by poor housing designs, which were reported previously as the main predisposing factor for soiling of these body regions [104] due to likelihood of these designs forcing the cows to lie on the walk alleys where slurry accumulates. Moreover, prolonged soiling of the skin is not only likely to cause loss of hair especially when the matting is being removed after slurry dries on the skin, but it also interferes with normal health of the epidermis of the involved areas [54]. It is therefore important that slurry is removed from cattle houses at least once per day in order to promote good animal welfare [28].

None of the 80 zero-grazing units evaluated had proper milking parlour; instead the cows were milked in unsuitable improvised cubicles with protruding traumatic pieces of wood or nails in 76% (n=61) of the units, or in their sleeping cubicles in the remaining 24% (n=19) units (Figure 16). Only 12% (n=10) of the zero-grazing units had maternity stalls into which pregnant cows were transferred in the last few days prior to parturition. In the remaining 88% (n=70) of the units, cows calved in their resting cubicles (Figure 17) and in the walk alleys. Lack of maternity areas constituted a poor welfare risk factor, which exposed the cow and her newborn calf to trauma by the rest of the cows in the unit. Moreover, the level of hygiene within the cattle unit is reduced due to spread of bloody fetal fluids and placental remnants [28].

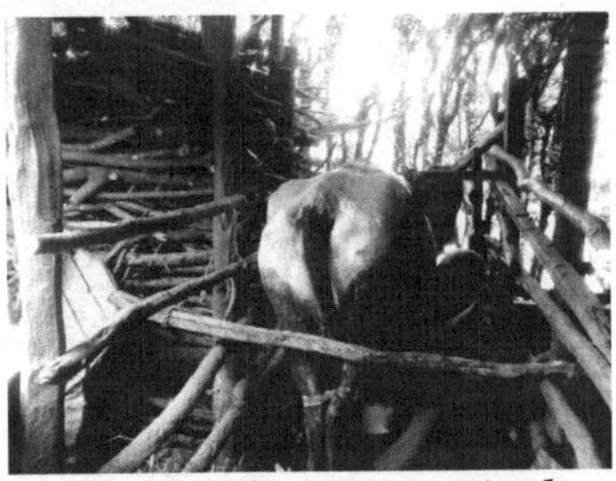

Figure 16.A cow being milked inside an improvised enclosure with a stack of firewood on the left, which poses a risk of injury to the cow when the animal struggles. The firewood can also slide off toward the cow from the top.

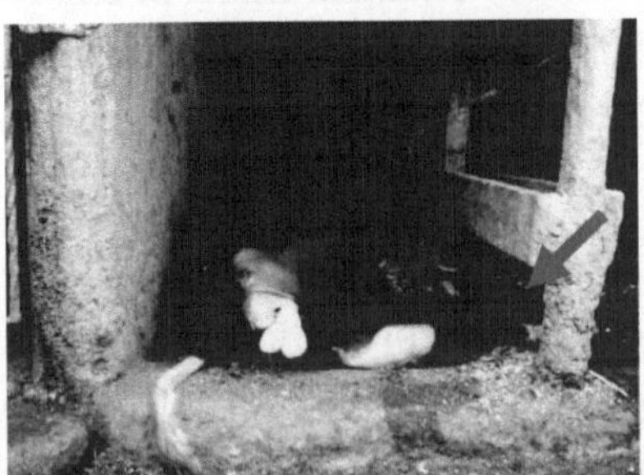

Figure 17. A cow calving in a lying position inside the sleeping cubicle. The cow is stuck in this position with her hind limbs having slipped under the lower side-bar (arrow), which further predisposed them to risk of injury. The head was also at risk of injury from being squeezed toward the inside wall.

3.5. Farmers and stockmen perspective on animal welfare

Farmers and stockmen acknowledged the need for cattle to have ready access to feed and to water in 98.75% (n=79) and 88.75% (n=71) of the zero-grazing units, respectively. In 47.5% (n=38) of the units evaluated, farmers and stockmen supported the need for alleviating unnecessary pain and suffering of the cattle as well as providing prompt medical attention when needed. In 31.25% (n=25) of the units, they also shared the opinion that animals suffer when mistreated and that there was the need to protect them from conditions that expose them to distress. The need for provision of a shelter and good housing systems to avoid animal discomfort and physical stress was acknowledged by farmers in 28.75% (n=23) of the units evaluated. The need to provide sufficient housing space with adequate facilities so as to allow for expression of normal behavioral patterns of animals was acknowledged by the farmers and stockmen in 5% (n=4) of the zero-grazing units evaluated in this study (Table 7).

Table 7. Percentages of responses from farmers and stockmen on their perspective of animal welfare issues in the 80 smallholder zero-grazing dairy units evaluated for the welfare of dairy cattle in peri-urban areas of Nairobi, Kenya.

Welfare input	Positive response (%)	Negative response (%)
Feed at all times	98.75	1.25
Water at all times	88.75	11.25
Medical attention when required	47.50	52.50
Appropriate treatment / handling	31.25	68.75
Comfortable housing	28.75	71.25
Adequate space for movement	5.00	95.00

The farmers and stockmen were found to have poor human-animal interaction, as exemplified by shouting and whipping of the cows particularly during milking times. Such interactions caused fear that made the cattle aggressive, leading to agonistic behavior towards making them difficult to handle contrary to good animal welfare recommendations [28]. Nevertheless, the few farmers who supported the need for alleviation of animal pain and suffering as well as provision for animal comfort were found to be better informed on other factors that also contribute to the improvement of production. Generally, the farmers and stockmen interviewed in the current study seemed to have the attitude that animal suffering and its alleviation were not important and that animal comfort was absolutely unnecessary. In spite of these attitudes, the farmers' and stockmen's perspective of animal welfare matters tend to agree with the understanding that animal welfare is affected by a hierarchy of needs whose importance is classified in priority order as life sustaining, health sustaining and comfort sustaining needs [6,105].

3.6. Mixing cattle of different age groups and with other species

In 74% (n=59) of the zero-grazing units evaluated in this study, cattle were housed separately according to their age groups, while for 26% (n=21) of the units the different groups were non-existent, with animals indiscriminately mixed irrespective of their age and lactation stage. Only male calves were separated from the rest of the cattle in all farms. In only 18% (n=14) of the studied units other species of animals such as poultry, pigs, sheep and goats were reared separately, although their houses were attached to the cattle housing facilities. However, in some of the units, chicken house was on top of the cattle house (Table 8).

Table 8.Animal mixing practices in the 80 smallholder zero-grazing units evaluated for welfare of dairy cattle in the peri-urban areas of Nairobi, Kenya.

Mixing practice	Number of zero-grazing units	Percentage of zero-grazing units
Separate age groups	59	74
Mixing of age groups	21	26
Only cattle reared	66	82
Cattle and other species	14	18

Although only a small percentage (26%; n= 21) of the smallholder units in this study housed cattle of different age groups together, it still creates conditions that would enhance development of negative social interactions. Such interactions create fear and disrupt feeding for the subordinate cattle. Eventually, this will inevitably affect health and productivity of the animals negatively [3,101], and subsequently lead to increased stress and poor animal welfare. In the units that had poultry production in rooms on an upper floor above cow houses, particularly separated by timber from the cows below, the cow houses are likely to have accumulations of ammonia from the chicken waste (faeces). This will exacerbate effects of poor ventilation. In the rest of the cattle units that were the majority (74%; n=59), cattle were housed according to their appropriate age groups according to the universal recommendations [28,31].

4. Conclusions and recommendations

The studies presented herein conclude that poor cattle welfare exist in the Kenyan smallholder zero-grazing units, and were able to identify some of the factors responsible for it, through direct indicators in the animals such as lameness lesions, body surface injuries, body condition scores and soiling of the body with slurry. The main factors resulting in poor welfare of dairy cows in the zero-grazing units within the peripheral areas of Nairobi include substandard housing designs, cattle housing in poor state, suboptimal feeding and poor husbandry practices. In this work, physical and environmental parameters that can be used to assess the welfare level in these zero-grazing units were discussed. The farmer perceptions and ignorance on animal welfare issues additionally precipitates cattle poor welfare.

References

1. Broom D M. Definition of animal welfare. Journal of Agricultural and Environmental Ethics 1993; 6 15-25.

2. Hemsworth P H., Coleman, G.J. Human Livestock Interactions. The stockperson and productivity and welfare of intensively farmed animals. In: CAB International, Wallingford, UK 1998; p 152.

3. Fregonesi J A.. Production and behaviour of dairy cattle in different housing systems. PhD Thesis. Wye College, University of London; 1999.

4. Broom D M. Indicators of poor welfare. British Veterinary Journal 1986; 142 524 – 526.
5. Fraser D., Broom D M. Farm animal behaviour and welfare. 3rd edition. In: CAB International, Oxon 1997; p437.
6. Duncan I J H. Science-based assessment of animal welfare. Farm animals. Scientific and Technical Review of Office International Epizooties 2005; 24 483-492.
7. Hewson C J. What is animal welfare? Common definitions and their practical consequences. Canadian Veterinary Journal 2003; 44 496-499.
8. Carenzi C., Verga M. Animal welfare review of the scientific concept and definition. Italian Journal of Animal Science 2009; 8 21-30.
9. Broom D M. Animal welfare defined in terms of attempt to cope with the environment. Acta Agriculturae Scandinavica 1996; 27 22-28.
10. Gonyou H W. Animal welfare: Definitions and assessment. Journal of Agricultural and Environmental Ethics 1993; 6 37-43.
11. Abeni F., Bertoni G. Main causes of poor welfare in intensively reared dairy cows. Italian.Journal of.Animal Science 2009; 8 (Suppl. 1) 45-66.
12. Wanyoike M M., Wahome R G. Small-Scale farming systems. In: Workshop Proceedings on Cattle Production in Kenya-Strategies for Research Planning and Implementation. December 2003 KARI HQ. Published 2004; p 87-133
13. Wakhungu J W. Dairy cattle breeding policy for Kenyan smallholders: An evaluation based on a demographic stationery state productivity model. PhD. Thesis University of Nairobi, Kenya; 2001.
14. Owen E., Kitalyi A., Jayasuriya N., Smith T. Livestock and Wealth creation: Improving the husbandry of animals kept by resource poor people in developing countries. 1st Edition. Nottingham University press. 2005.
15. Muriuki H., Omore A., Hooston N., Waithaka M., Ouma R., Staal S J., Odhiambo P. The policy environment in the Kenya dairy sub-sector: A review. Smallholder Dairy Project Research and Development Report 2. 2003.
16. Small-holder Dairy Project (SDP). The uncertainity of cattle numbers in Kenya. Policy brief number 10. Small holder dairy project Nairobi, Kenya. 2005.
17. Nguhiu-Mwangi J., Mbithi P M F., Wabacha J K., Mbuthia P G. Factors associated with the occurence of claw disorders in dairy cows under smallholder production systems in urban and peri-urban areas of Nairobi, Kenya. Veterinarski Arhiv 2008; 78(4) 345-355.
18. Musalia L., Wangia S., Shivairo R., Okutu P., Vugutsa V. Dairy production practices among smallholder dairy farmers in Butere/Mumias and Kakemega Districts in Western Kenya. Tropical Animal Health and Production 2007; 39 199-205.
19. Ministry of Livestock and Fisheries Development (MOLFD). Towards a competitive and sustainable dairy industry for economic growth in 21st century and beyond. Draft Dairy Policy. 2006.

20. Gitau J K., McDermott J J., Walner-Toews D., Lissemore K D., Osumo J M., Muriuki D. Factors influencing calf morbidity and mortality in smallholder dairy farms in Kiambu District of Kenya. Preventive Veterinary Medicine 1994; 21(2) 167-178.

21. Mutugi J J. Various livestock productions systems. In: Workshop Proceedings; on Cattle Production in Kenya. Strategies for research planning and Implementation. December 2003 KARI HQ, published 2004; p 3-35.

22. Bebe B O., Udo H M J., Rowlands G.J., Thorpe, W. Smallholder dairy systems in Kenya highlands: Cattle population dynamics under increasing intensification. Livestock Production Science 2003; 82 211-221.

23. Broom D W. Effects of Dairy cattle breeding and production methods on Animal welfare. In: Proceedings of the 21st World, Buiatrics Congress, Montevideo, Uruguay Sociedad de Medicina Veterinaria del Uruguay. 2001.

24. OIE Terrestrial Animal Code. Animal welfare issues. (OIE) World Organization for Animal Health, Rome. 2005. Chapter 7.

25. Wechsler B., Schaub J., Friedli K., Hauser R. Behaviour and leg injuries in dairy cows kept in cubicle systems with straw bedding or soft lying mats. Applied Animal Behavior Science 2000; 69 189-197.

26. Horgan R. European Union welfare legislation: Current position and future perspectives. Electrònica de Veterinaria REDVET®, volume VII, number 12. 2006; p 1-8.

27. Hristov S., Stankovic B., Zlatanovic Z., Joksimoviv, M T., Davidovic V. Rearing conditions, health and welfare of dairy cows. Biotechnology in Animal Husbandry 2008; 24 (1-2) 25-35.

28. Department of the Environment, Food and Rural Affairs (DEFRA). Code of Recommendations for the Welfare of Livestock: Cattle. Defra Publications, London. 2003.

29. Webster A J. Animal welfare. Limping towards Eden. Blackwell Publishing. Oxford UK. 2005

30. Leaver J D. Dairy cattle. In: Ewbank R., Kim-Madslien F., hart C B. (eds.), Management and Welfare of Farm Animals, 4th edition. The UFAW Handbook. Universities Federation for Animal Welfare, Wheathampstead, UK 1999;p 17-47.

31. Farm Animal Welfare Council (FAWC). Second Report on Priorities for Research and Development in Farm Animal Welfare. DEFRA, London. 1993.

32. Charlton G L., Rutter S M., East M., Sinclair L A. Preference of dairy cows: Indoor cubicle housing with access to a total mixed ration vs. access to pasture. Applied Animal Behaviour Science 2011; 130 (1) 1-9.

33. Krohn C C., Munksgaard L. Behaviour of dairy cows kept in extensive (loose housing/pasture) or intensive (tie stall) environments, II. Lying and lying down behaviour. Applied Animal Behavior Science 1993; 37 1-16.

34. Delaby L., Peyraud J L., Delagarde R.. Effect of the level of concentrate supplementation, herbage allowance and milk yield at turn-out on the performance of dairy cows in mid lactation at grazing. Animal Science 2001; 73 171-181.

35. Devries T J., von Keyserlingk M A G., Weary D M. Effect of feeding space on the inter-cow distance, aggression and feeding behaviour of free-stall housed lactating dairy cows. Journal of Dairy Science 2004; 87 1432-1438.

36. Rutter S M. Review: Grazing preferences in sheep and cattle: Implications for production, the environment and animal welfare Canadian Journal of Animal Science 201; 90 (3) 285-293

37. Fregonesi J A., Leaver J D. Behaviour, performance and health indicators of welfare for diary cows housed in strawyard or cubicle systems. Livestock Production Science 2001; 68 205-216.

38. Haskell M J., Rennie L J., Bowell V A., Bell M J., Lawrence A B. Housing systems, milk production and zero-grazing effects on lameness and leg injuries in dairy cows. Journal of Dairy Science 2006; 89 4259-4266.

39. Waiblinger S., Menke C. The relationship between attitudes, personal characteristics and behaviour of stockpeople and subsequent behaviour and production of dairy cows. Applied Animal Behavioral Science,. 2002; 79 195-219.

40. Bartussek H. (2001). A historical account of the development of the Animal Needs Index ANI-35L as part of the attempt to promote and regulate farm animal. 2001.

41. Bracke M. B. M., Metz J H M., Spruijt B M., Schouten W G P. Decision support system for overall welfare assessment in pregnant sows B: Validation by expert opinion. Journal of Animal Science 2002; 80 1835-1845

42. Capdeville, J., Veissier I. A method of assessing welfare in loose housed dairy cows at farm level, focussing on animal observations. Acta Agriculturae Scandinavica 2001; 30 62-68.

43. Main D C., Whay H R., Green L E., Webster A J. Effect of the RSPCA (Royal Society for the Prevention of Cruelty to Animals) freedom food scheme on the welfare of dairy cattle. Veterinary Record 2003; 153 227-231.

44. Whay H R., Main D C J., Green L E., Webster A J F. Assessment of the welfare of dairy cattle using animal–based measurements: Direct observations and investigation of farm records. Veterinary Record 2003; 153 197 – 202.

45. Cook, N B., Nordlund K V. Review: The influence of the environment on dairy cow behaviour, claw health and herd health lameness dynamics. Veterinary Journal 2009; 179: 360-369.

46. von Keyserlingk M A G., Rushen A M., Weary D M. Invited review: The welfare of dairy cattle and the role of science. Journal of Dairy Science 2009; 92: 4101 – 4111.

47. Channon A J., Walker A M., Pfau T., Sheldon I M., Wilson A M. Variability of Manson and Leaver locomotion scores assigned to dairy cows by different observers. Veterinary Record 2009; 164 388-392.

48. Tadich N., Flor E., Green L. Association between hoof lesions and locomotion score in 1098 unsound dairy cows. The Veterinary Journal 2010; 184 60-65

49. Flower F C., Sanderson D J., Weary D M. Hoof pathologies influence kinematic measures of dairy cow gait. Journal of Dairy Science 2005; 88 3166-3175.

50. Nguhiu-Mwangi J., Mbithi P M F., Wabacha J K., Mbuthia P G. Risk (Predisposing) Factors for Non-InfectiousClaw Disorders in Dairy Cows UnderVarying Zero-Grazing Systems. In: A Bird's-Eye View of Veterinary Medicine. Carlos C. Perez-Marin (ed). InTech, Janeza Trdine, Rijeka, Croatia. 2012. p393-422

51. Aleri J W., Nguhiu-Mwangi J., Mogoa E M. Housing-design as a predisposing factor for injuries and poor welfare in cattle within smallholder units in periurban areas of Nairobi, Kenya. Livestock Research for Rural Development 2011; 23 (3) online edition. http://www.lrrd.org/lrrd23/lrrd23.htm

52. Aleri J W. Welfare of Dairy Cattle in the Smallholder (Zero-grazing) Production Systems in Nairobi and its Environs. MSc thesis. University of Nairobi, Nairobi, Kenya. 2011.

53. Bertoni G., Calamari, L., Trevisi E., How to define and evaluate welfare in modern dairy farms. In: Proceedings of the 13th International Conference on Production Diseases in Farm Animals. Leipzig, Germany. 2007; p 590-606

54. Winckler C. On-farm welfare assessment in cattle: From basic concepts to feasible assessment systems. World Biuatrics Congress 2006 in Nice, France. 2006.

55. Smidt D. Advantages and problems of using integrated systems of indicators as compared to single traits. In: Indicators Relevant to Farm Animal Welfare (D.Smidt (ed.), Vol 23,. Martinus Nijhoff Publishers, The Hague, Netherlands. 1983; p 201-207.

56. Gröhn Y T., Rajala-Schultz P J., Allore, H G., DeLorenzo M A., Hertl J A., Galligan D T. Optimizing replacement of dairy cows: Modelling effects of diseases. Preventive Veterinary Medicine 2003; 61 27-43.

57. Hemsworth P H., Beveridge L., Matheus L R.. The welfare of extensively managed dairy cattle – A review. Applied Animal Behaviour Science 1995; 42 161-182.

58. Huzzey J M., Veira D M., Weary D M., von keyserlingk M A G. Prepartum behaviour and dry matter intake identify dairy cows at risk of metritis. Journal of Dairy Science 2007; 90 3220-3233.

59. Fleischner P M., Metzner M., Beyerbach M., Hoedemaker M., Klee W. The relationship between milk yield and the incidence of some diseases in dairy cows. Journal of Dairy Science 2001; 84 2025-2035.

60. Kelm S C., Freeman A E. and NC-2 Technical Committee Direct and correlated responses to selection for milkyield: Results and conclusions of Regional Project NC-2, Improvement of dairy cattle through breeding, with emphasis on selection. Journal of Dairy Science 2000; 83 2721-2732.

61. Duncan I H., Dawkins M S. The problem of assessing "well-being" and sufffering in farm animals. In: Indicators Relevant to Farm Animal Welfare. Vol 23, D.Smidt (ed.). Martinus Nijhoff Publishers, The Hague, Netherlands. 1983; p13-24.

62. Signoret J P. General conclusions. In: Indicators Relevant to Farm Animal Welfare. D. Smidt, (ed.),. MartinusPublishers, The Hague, Netherlands. 1983; p 245- 247.

63. Broom D M., Johnson K G. Stress and animal welfare. Chapman Hall, London. 1993. p 221.

64. Rushen J. Problems associated with the interpretation of physiological data in the assessment of animal welfare. Applied Animal Behaviour Science 1991; 28 381-386.
65. Dantzer R. Research perspectives in farm animal welfare: the concept of stress. Journal of Agricultural and Environmental Ethics 1993; 6 86-92.
66. Pederson B K. Animal welfare: A holistic approach. Acta Agriculturae Scandinavica 1996; 27 76-81
67. Hopster H. and Blokhuis H J. Validation of a heart-rate monitor for measuring a stress response in dairy cows. Canadian Journal of Animal Science 1994; 74 465-474.
68. Lindberg C. Animal behaviour and animal welfare. Journal of Biological Education. 1995; 29 16-22.
69. Duncan I J H., Poole T B. (Promoting the welfare of farm and captive animals. In: Managing the Behaviour of Animals. P. Monaghan and D. Wood-Gush (eds.),. Chapman and Hall, Cambridge, UK. 1990;.p193-232.
70. Moberg G P. A model for assesing the impact of behavioural stress on domestic animals. Journal of Animal Science. 1987; 65 1228-1235.
71. Moberg G P. Suffering from Stress: An approach for evaluating the welfare of an animal. Acta Agriculturae Scandinavica 1996;.27 46-49.
72. Smidt D., Schlichting M C., Ladewig J., Steinhardt M. Ethological and ethophysiological research for farm animal welfare. Archiv-fur-Tierzucht 1995; 38 7-19.
73. Kilgour R. Stress and behaviour: An operational approach to animal welfare. In: Farm Animal Housing and Welfare. S.H. Baxter, Baxter, M.R., and MacCormakck, J.A.C. (eds.),. Martinus Nijhoff Publishers, The Hague, Netherlands. 1983; p 36-44.
74. Duncan I J H. Welfare is to do with what animals feel. Journal of Agricultural and Environmental Ethics 1983; 6 8-14.
75. Wiepkema P R. On the significance of ethological criteria for assessment of animal welfare. In: Indicator Relevent to Farm Animal Welfare. (D.Smidt (ed.), Vol 23,. Martinus Nijhoff Publishers, The Hague, Netherlands. 1983; p71-79.
76. Fraser A F. Behaviour disorders in domestic animals. In: Abnormal Behaviour in Animals. M.W. Fox. (ed.),.Saunders, Philadelphia, USA. 1968; p179-187.
77. Phillips C J C. Cattle behaviour. Farming Press Books, Ipwich, UK. 1993; p 212.
78. Albright J L., Arave C W. The behaviour of cattle. CAB International Wallingford, UK. 1997; p 306.
79. Jensen P., Recen B.,Ekesbo, I. Methods of sampling and analysis of data in farm animal ethology. Birkhauser verlag, Basel. 1986; pp 86..
80. Herlin, A H., Nichelmann M., Wierenga, H K., Braun, S. Some effects of housing systems on social and abnormal behaviour of dairy cows. In: Proceedings of the International Congress on Applied Ethology held in Berlin. M. Nichelmann and H.K. Wierenga, (eds.), Berlin Germany 1993; p 389-391.
81. Miller K., Wood-Gush D G M. Some effects of housing on the social behaviour of dairy cows. Animal Production 1991; 53 271-278.

82. Leonard F C., O'Connell J., O'Farell K. Effect of different housing conditions on behaviour and foot lesions in Friesian heifers. The Veterinary Record 1994; 134 490-494.

83. Sumner J. Design of dairy cow housing in the United Kingdom. Dairy Food and Environmental Sanitation 1991; 2: 650-653.

84. Varlyakov I., Tossev A., Sivkova K., Dragneva R. Studies on the range of behaviour reactions of dairy cows. In: International Congress of the International Society for Applied Ethology. Rutter, S., Randle, H., and Eddison, J.(eds.), Universities Federation for Animal Welfare, UK. 1995; p 247-248.

85. Manson F J. A study of lameness in dairy cows with reference to nutrition and hoof shape. PhD Thesis. The West of Scotland Agricultural College, University of Glasgow, Dumfries, Scotland. 1986.

86. Metcalf J A., Roberts S J., Sutton J D. Variations in blood flow to and from the bovine mammary gland measured using transit time ultrasound and dye dilution. Research in Veterinary Science 1992; 53 59-63.

87. Rulquin H., Caudal J P. Effect of lying or standing on mammary bloodflow and heart rate of dairy cows. Ann.zootech. (paris). 1992; 41 101

88. Kirkegaard P., Agger J F., Bjerg B. Association between dairy cow somatic cell count and four types of bedding in free stalls. 11th ICPD. Acta. Veterinaria Scandinavica Supplement 2003; 98.

89. Weary D M., Marina A G., von Keyserlingk M A G. Building better barns – seeing the freestall from cow's perspective. American Association of Bovine Practitoners Proceedings, Vancorver, BC, Canada 2006; 39 32-39.

90. Nguhiu-Mwangi J. Characteristics of laminitis and associated claw lesions in dairy cows in Nairobi and its environs. PhD Thesis. University of Nairobi, Nairobi, Kenya. 2007.

91. Nguhiu-Mwangi J., Mbithi P M F., Wabacha J K., Mbuthia P G. Prevalence of laminitis and the patterns of claw lesions in dairy cows in Nairobi and the peri-urban districts. Bulletin of Animal Health and Production in Africa. 2009; 57 199-208.

92. Rutherford K M D., Fritha M L., Mhairi C J., Sherwood L., Alistair B L., Marie J H. Lameness prevalence and risk factors in organic and non-organic dairy herds in the United Kingdom. The Veterinary Journal 2009; 180 95-105.

93. Radostitis O M., Gay C C., Blood D C., Hinchcliff K W. Veterinary Medicine, 9th Edition. W.B. Saunders Company Ltd, Philadelphia, Pennsylvania. 2003.

94. Kiellard C., Ruud L E., Zarella A J., Østeras O. Prevalence and risk factors for skin lesions on legs of dairy cattle housed in free stalls in Norway. American Journal of Dairy Science. 2009; 92 5487-5496.

95. Zurbrigg K., Kelton D., Anderson N., Millman S. Stall dimensions and prevalence of lameness, injury and cleanliness on tie-stall dairy farms In Ontario. Canadian Veterinary Journal 2005; 46 902-909.

96. Greenough, P R. Bovine Laminitis and Lameness: A Hands on Approach. Saunders Elsevier. London, UK. 2007; p 70 – 83.

97. Leaver J D. Milk production. Science and practice. Longman, London, UK. 1983; p 173.

98. Weary D M., Tucker C. The science of cow comfort. In: Proceedings of the Joint Meeting of the Ontario Agriculture Business Association and the Ontario Association of Bovine Practitioners, April 2003 Guelph, Ontario. 2003; p 1 -15.

99. Lukuyu M., Romney D., Ouma R., Keith S. Feeding dairy cattle. In: A manual for smallholder farmers and extension workers in East Africa. SDP / KDDP, Nairobi, Kenya. 2007; p 62.

100. Plaizier J C., Krause D O., Gozho G N., McBride B W. Sub acute ruminal acidosis in dairy cattle. The physiological causes, incidence and consequences. The Veterinary Journal 2008; 176 (1) 21-3

101. Kilgour R., Dalton D C. Livestock behaviour. A practical guide. Granada Publishing, London, UK. 1984; p 320.

102. Somers J G C., Frakena J K., Noordhuizen-Stassen E N., Metz J H M. Prevalence of claw disorders in Dutch dairy cows exposed to several floor systems. Journal of Dairy Science 2003; 86 2082-2093.

103. Roche J F. The effect of nutritional management of dairy cows on reproductive efficiency. Animal Reproduction Science 2006; 96 282-296.

104. Whistance L K., Arney D R., Sinclair L.A., Phillips C J C. Defaecation behaviour of dairy cows housed in Straw yards or cubicle systems. Applied Animal behaviour Science 2007; 105 14 – 25.

105. Hurnik J F., Lehman H. Ethics and farm animal welfare. Journal of Agriculture Ethics 1988; 1(4) 305-318.

Chapter 4

Mycobacterium avium Complex in Domestic and Wild Animals

1. Introduction

Mycobacteria from the *Mycobacterium avium* complex (MAC) cause a variety of diseases including tuberculosis-like disease in humans and birds, disseminated infections in AIDS patients and otherwise immunocompromised patients, lymphadenitis in humans and mammals and paratuberculosis in ruminants. *M. avium* subsp. *paratuberculosis* (*Map*) is the etiologic agent of Johne´s disease in cattle and it has been identified in human patients with Crohn's disease. The MAC comprises slow growing mycobacteria that are ubiquitous in the environment (soil and water), and have a wide source range, causing disease in various domestic and wild mammals and birds [1].

The aim of this study was to discuss the classification and biology, epidemiology, clinical signs, pathology, diagnostic techniques, and public health concerns in *Mycobacterium avium* complex in domestic and wild animals.

2. Classification and biology of *Mycobacterium avium* complex

The phylum Actinobacteria is large and very complex; it contains one class (Actinobacteria), five subclasses, six orders, 14 suborders, and 40 families. The orders, suborders, and families are defined based on 16S rRNA sequences and distinctive signature nucleotides. The suborder Corynebacterineae contains seven families with several well-known genera. Three of the most important genera are *Corynebacterium, Mycobacterium,* and *Nocardia* [2].

The species of *Mycobacterium*, sole genus of the family Mycobacteriaceae, is composed of a group of high genomic C+G content (~61 to 71%), facultative intracellular, Gram-positive microorganisms comprising more than 130 established and validated species and subspecies [3], with surprisingly diverse phenotypes related to growth rate, metabolic activity, colony appearance, environmental distribution, and pathogenic potential for eukaryotic hosts [4]. Although most of these species are saprophytic, important human and animal pathogens have been identified. Pathogenic members are usually characterized by their slow growth in culture, with generation times of 12 to 24 h, and must be incubated for 2 to 40 days after inoculation of a solidified complex medium to form a visible colony, whereas nonpathogenic members grow considerably faster [5]. Mycobacteria are acid-fast bacilli, acidophilic, small, slightly curved or straight rods that sometimes branch or form filaments. Mycobacterial filaments differ from those of actinomycetes in readily fragmenting into rods and coccoid bodies when distributed. They are aerobic, immobile, non-sporulated and catalase positive bacteria. Their cell wall is lipid-rich and contain waxes with 60 to 90 carbon mycolic acids, which are complex fatty acids with a hydroxyl group on the β-carbon and an aliphatic chain attached to the α-carbon. The presence of mycolic acids and other lipids, in high concentration outside the peptidoglycan, makes mycobacteria acid-fast dye resistant (basic fuchsin cannot be removed from the cell by acid alcohol treatment), as well as resistant to immune system defense mechanisms and disinfectants [2,6].

2.1. *Mycobacterium avium* complex (MAC)

Bacteria from the *Mycobacterium avium* complex (MAC) differ in virulence and ecology, and are the most frequently isolated non-tuberculous mycobacteria [7]. *Mycobacterium* members of MAC have the capacity to survive and multiply under a wide range of environmental conditions, including low pH, extreme temperatures, chlorine or ozone treatment and low oxygen level. Thus, plus their ability to utilize many substances as nutrients, enables them to grow successfully in many biotopes [1]. The environmental sources responsible for MAC infection in different populations, the specific routes of infection and transmission, the potential for latent infection and reactivation of disease are not yet well defined [4,8]. Ingestion of environmental organisms followed by invasion through the gastrointestinal tract has been suggested as the main route of infection because the organisms are frequently isolated from stools of different animals. There is also an important positive correlation between the presence of MAC in respiratory samples and the subsequent development of disseminated disease [9]. Traditionally, MAC includes two species, *Mycobacterium avium* and *Mycobacterium intracellulare* [3]. Recently, advances in molecular taxonomy have fuelled identification of novel species within the MAC, including the *Mycobacterium chimaera* incorporating sequevar MAC-A organisms isolated from humans with pulmonary cavitations, pulmonary abscess, chronic obstructive pulmonary disease and bronchiectasis [10]; the *Mycobacterium colombiense* incorporating sequevar MAC-X organisms isolated from the blood and sputum of HIV infected patients in Colombia [11], and from diseased lymph nodes in children [12,13]; the *Mycobacterium arosiense,* recently described in an immunocompromised child with disseminated osteomyelitic lesions [14]; the *Mycobacterium vulneris* [15], *Mycobacterium marseillense, Mycobacterium timonense* and *Mycobacterium bouchedurhonense* isolated from patients with pulmonary disease. On the basis of genotypic, phenotypic and growth characteristics, biochemical tests and historical reasons, multiple subspecies of *Mycobacterium avium* are recognized. These include the subsp. *avium*, subsp. *paratuberculosis*, subsp. *hominissuis* and subsp. *silvaticum* [3]. All four *Mycobacterium avium* subspecies and *Mycobacterium intracellulare* are capable of infecting a diverse range of host and possess a high degree of genetic similarity [17]. Contemporary methods for MAC identification, e.g., high performance liquid chromatography (HPLC) of cell wall mycolic acids and genetic probes based on rRNA targets, e.g. AccuProbe, cannot discriminate among *Mycobacterium avium* subspecies. Given the differences in pathogenicity among *Mycobacterium avium* subspecies and the implications regarding the infection source, a practical and accurate method of simply identifying *Mycobacterium avium* subspecies is needed [18].

2.2. *Mycobacterium avium* subsp. *avium*

Before establishing the *Mycobacterium avium* subsp. *avium (Maa)* designation, this bacterium was simply referred to as *Mycobacterium avium* and has long been recognized as a primary pathogen causing avian tuberculosis in wild and domestic birds as well as in a variety of fowl, game birds and water-fowl. The most common route of infection for susceptible animals is the alimentary tract. Respiratory tract is also suggested as a potential source of infection [19].

2.3. *Mycobacterium avium* subsp. *paratuberculosis*

Mycobacterium avium subsp. *paratuberculosis (Map)* is the etiologic agent of Johne's disease or paratuberculosis, a chronic granulomatous enteritis of ruminant livestock and wildlife, with worldwide distribution having a significant impact on the world economy [5]. For veterinary medicine, *Map* is the MAC member of greatest importance, and is capable of infecting and causing disease in a wide array of animal species, including nonhuman primates, without the need for co-existent immunosuppressive infections [18]. *Map* is one of the slowest growing mycobacterial species, hence primary isolation from specimen, requires prolonged culture incubation and can take several months. Unlike most other *Mycobacterium avium* subspecies, isolation of *Map* requires the addition of the siderophore mycobactin to culture media [20]. From phenotypic analysis, the *Map* group has been subdivided into two main types, bovine and ovine, that vary in hosts, diseases caused, and growth phenotypes [21]. Genotypically, these findings were based primarily on comparisons of the integration *loci* of the IS*900* insertion sequence (IS) and used polymorphisms in IS*1311* to separate sheep and cattle isolates into separate populations [22].

2.4. *Mycobacterium avium* subsp. *hominissuis*

MAC isolates of genotypes IS*901*- and IS*1245*+ and serotypes 4 to 6, 8 to 11 and 21 are less virulent for birds and are designated *M. avium* subsp. *hominissuis* (*Mah*). *Mah* was proposed to distinguish organisms found in humans and pigs from those isolated from birds [3]. Those are genomically diverse, the more diverse group of strains, low-virulence, opportunistic pathogens for both animals and humans [18]. Considered ubiquitous in the environment (the most likely source of infection for humans), *Mah* can cause serious systemic infection in immunocompromised patients, such as those infected with HIV. Additionally, this opportunistic pathogen can cause cervical lymphadenitis in children with cystic fibrosis, and lung infections in patients with underlying lung disease [23]. Domestic water distribution systems have been reported as possible sources of *Mah* infections in hospitals, family houses, and commercial places [24]. In animals, *Mah* is found as a cause of lymphadenitis of the head and mesenteric lymph nodes of swine documented at slaughter [18], and can also lead to systemic infection of parenchymatous organs [23]. *Mah* were recovered from affected lymph nodes of red deer from Austria [25].

2.5. *Mycobacterium avium* subsp. *silvaticum*

Mycobacterium avium subsp. *silvaticum* applies to the previously named wood pigeon bacillus, an acid-fast organism causing tuberculosis-like lesions in these wood pigeons. The inability to grow on egg media, the stimulation of growth by pyruvate and at pH

5.5 and their mycobactin dependency upon primary isolation, gradually losing this phenotype upon subculture, have been described as characteristics of *Mycobacterium avium* subsp. *silvaticum* [17].

2.6. *Mycobacterium intracellulare*

Mycobacterium intracellulare, initially named *Nocardia intracellularis*, is an environmental organism and opportunistic pathogen, isolated from a variety of animal hosts and environmental sources. *Mycobacterium intracellulare* is a closely related pathogen of birds with a lower prevalence [26]. In general, it has been subject to less study than *Mycobacterium avium*, as the latter is more prevalent in clinical and environmental samples, has a wider apparent host range, and contributes almost exclusively to disseminated MAC disease in human immunodeficiency virus patients [3]. The type strain of *Mycobacterium intracellulare* (ATCC 13950) was isolated from a human, specifically responsible for enlarged lymph nodes in children, who died from disseminated disease [3], and progressive pulmonary disease in elderly women [27]. *Mycobacterium intracellulare* appears to have a distinct ecological niche, more prevalent in biofilms and at significantly higher CFU numbers than *Mycobacterium avium* [28].

3. Clinical signs and morphology in domestic and wild species

All ruminant species, captive or free-ranging, are susceptible to disease and death due to MAC infection [29], and a wide diversity of non-ruminant species can become infected with mycobateria belonging to MAC, especially with *Map* and *Maa*. Paratuberculosis has been described in cattle, small ruminants, deer, and in South American camelids (llamas and alpacas) [30,31]. This chronic disease is one of the most serious affecting dairy cattle worldwide showing symptoms of an insidious intestinal pathology responsible for significant economic losses [5]. The close relationship between wild, captive and domestic ruminants and other species like birds is, nowadays, clinically relevant as the wild population could act as reservoir for this agent [32].

In cattle this disease is scored in four stages according to its evolution and symptoms, two of them evolving sub-clinically. Stage I, or silent infection, is the most observed in young animals, without significant clinical signs and only in *post mortem* evaluation it is possible to identify the agent by culture or histopathology analysis [33].

Stage II remains a subclinical disease, being observed in adult animals. It may be detected by alterations in immunological serological and/or cellular parameters. Intermittently, fecal culture and histopathology analysis of these animals could be positive to *Map* [33].

In stage III the clinical signs can be observed, occurring after several years of incubation. The initial clinical signs are subtle with gradual weight loss despite normal appetite, intermittent diarrhea along several weeks, drop in milk production and roughness of hair coat. These symptoms are included in the differential diagnosis of multiple diseases, so it is often misdiagnosed [34]. Usually, animals in this stage are positive upon ELISA and other serological tests, as for histopathological analysis of lesions, which are common in the terminal ileum [35] (Figure 2A).

The last stage of the disease (stage IV) comprises animals that rapidly progress from the stage III with rapid condition deteriorated. They became increasingly lethargic, weak and emaciated and present intermandibular edema due to hypoproteinemia. In this stage, the culture of the agent, molecular biology techniques of PCR, ELISA, serology and histopathology (Figure 1), all are positive for the majority of animals tested. The gastrointestinal tract is the preferential local to sample in order to isolate the agent, but in some conditions it can even be present in extraintestinal lesions, with the liver and lymph nodes being the most common sites [33].

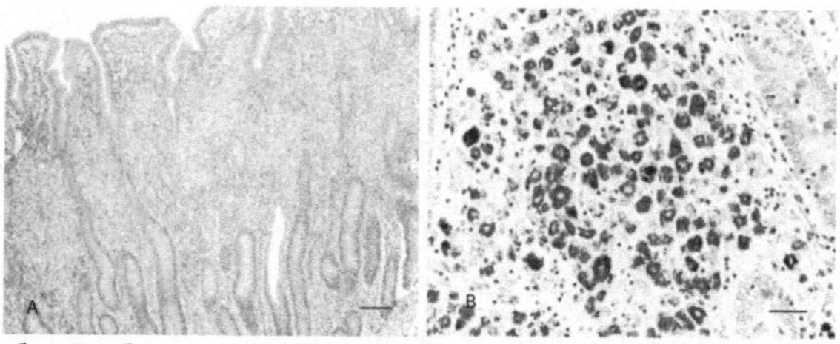

Figure 1. Morphological aspects of paratuberculosis lesions in the ileum of sheep. A- Thickening of the mucosa by an inflammatory infiltrate composed by epithelioid cells, macrophages and some multinucleated giant cells. (H&E stain, Bar=50μm) B- Acid-acohol resistant bacilli within the macrophages and epithelioid cells that infiltrate the mucosa. Notice the abundant number of mycobacteria that are visible at moderate amplification (Ziehl-Neelsen, Bar=30μm)

3.1. Clinical signs and lesions in wild species

Mycobacteria belonging to the MAC can affect a wide-range of wild animals, but little has been published on the clinical signs, which are rarely perceived or not documented. When present, the occurrence of clinical signs and lesions is highly variable in timing but often similar to those of their domesticated counterparts. The vast majority of reports on MAC species affecting wildlife mention the *Map* and the *Maa* as the mycobacteria most commonly isolated in these animals.

3.1.2. Wild ruminants

The lesions observed in wild species of sheep and goats are identical to those of their domestic counterparts, while in the South American camelids the lesional pattern is similar to that of cattle. However in llamas and alpacas, in contrast to what is generally described in cattle, lymph node necrosis and mineralization, along with multiorganic dissemination, have also been reported [30,31]. As in the previously mentioned species, the most significant MAC species capable of causing clinical disease in free-living, captive and farmed deer are *Map* and *Maa*. Although *Mah* has been also isolated from lesions in deer [25,26] and *Mycobacterium intracellulare* was also found in deer species but they are not so common and it's infection is usually subclinical. Despite the occurrence of paratuberculosis in adults, outbreaks of the disease frequently occur in young deer of 8-15 months of age, contrary to the clinical disease in sheep and cattle which usually affects adults of 3-5 years of age [36]. Clinical signs of paratuberculosis in deer are similar to those described in sheep and cattle, with diarrhea and loss of weight and body condition [37]. Accordingly, the intestinal lesions of paratuberculosis in deer primarily affect the jejunum and ileum, and are identical to the typical lesions observed in sheep and goats [30]; yet, necrosis and mineralization in lymph nodes draining the gastrointestinal tract, especially those draining the ileum and ileocecal valve, are a common feature (Figure 2B). The lymph nodes are often enlarged, and a range of changes from yellow watery areas to caseous necrosis is observed on cut surfaces. The histologic changes in these lesions are very similar to those caused by *Mycobacterium bovis* and other members of the MAC genus [38,39]. Balseiro et al., have proposed an histopathological classification of lesions observed in natural occurring cases of paratuberculosis in free-ranging fallow deer (*Dama dama*), according to which the lesions would be graded into four categories: focal, multifocal, diffuse multibacillary, and diffuse intermediate (multibacillary-lymphocytic) lesions. Focal lesions are composed of small granulomas, mainly in the jejunal and ileal lymph nodes, whereas multifocal lesions consist in well-demarcated granulomas in the intestinal lymphoid tissue and also in the intestinal lamina propria. Diffuse multibacillary lesions are characterized by a severe granulomatous enteritis and lymphadenitis. Macrophages and numerous Langhan's multinucleatd giant cells (L-MGC) containing many mycobacteria are present, resulting in macroscopic changes in the normal gut morphology. These changes are found from the proximal jejunum to the ileocaecal valve, but lesions are always particularly severe in the distal jejunum. In the diffuse intermediate (multibacillary-lymphocytic) lesions, there is a prominence of lymphocytes, macrophages and L-MGC, with small numbers of mycobacteria [40]. In deer with clinical signs of paratuberculosis, disseminated granulomatous lesions in the lung and liver can also be observed [38]. A recent report in free-ranging red deer (*Cervus elaphus*) supports the possibility of multiorganic dissemination of *Map* in deer, since the agent was isolated from kidneys with granulomatous lesions [41].

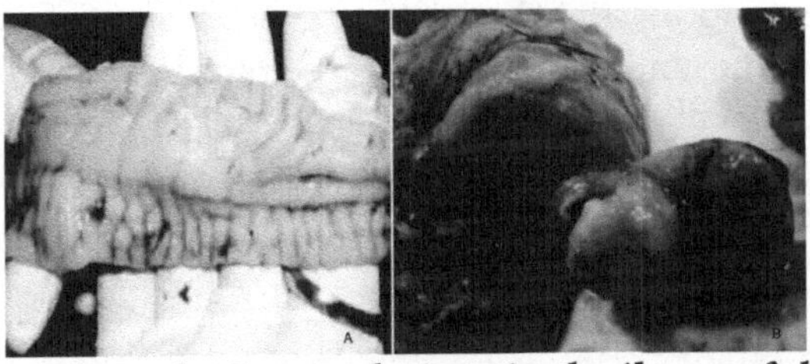

Figure 2.A – Paratuberculosis gross lesions in the ileum of sheep. Notice the increased thickness of the mucosa, with the characteristic folds and gyros B – Paratuberculosis lesions in the submandibularis lymph nodes of red deer (Cervus elaphus) with caseous necrosis.

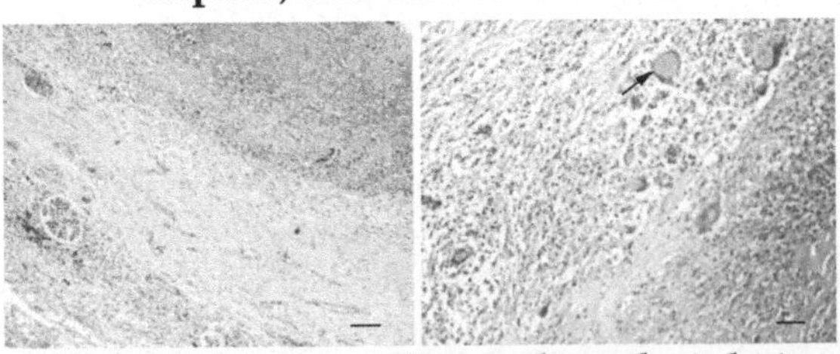

Figure 3. A - Morphological aspects of paratuberculosis lesions in the kidneys of deer (Cervus elaphus). A single granuloma with central caseous necrosis, surrounded by a thick fibrous capsule (H&E 100μm). B – Higher magnification of the previous image. Notice the presence of Langhan's MGC (Arrow. H&E 50μm).

In deer, the infection by *Maa* is self-limiting as in other mammalian species [36,42]. The lesions may be purulent, caseous, or granulomatous [26], and are mainly present in the retropharyngeal lymph nodes and lymph nodes draining the intestinal tract (mesenteric and ileocaecal), consistent with the feco-oral route of infection. The granulomatous lesions are grossly and histologically identical to the lesions caused by *Mycobacterium bovis* [42].

Mah lesions in deer are similar to those observed in animals with *Maa* infection, and although rare, both mycobacteria can cause systemic disease [26] with hematogenous spread to the liver and lungs to produce miliary lesions and a terminal septicemia [43]. Despite of these findings, *Map* and *Maa* infections can be present in apparently asymptomatic deer herds [44,45]. Furthermore, a study of wild Tule elks (*Cervus elaphus nannodes*) from California revealed no significant associations between MAC infection and microscopic lesions, such as presence of macrophages and/or multinucleate giant cells (MGC) in tissue sections [45] (Figure 3).

3.1.3. Non-ruminant species

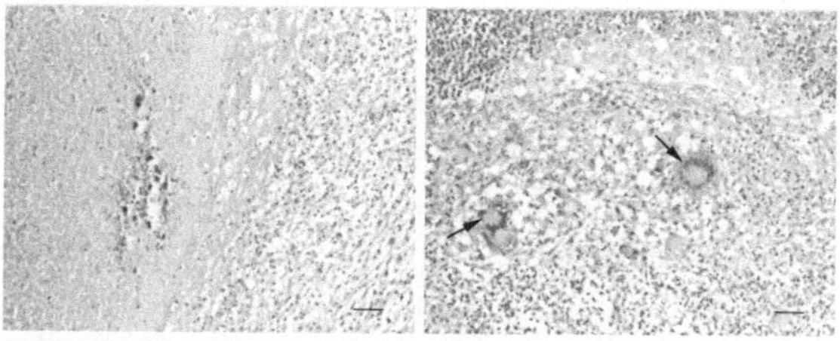

Figure 4. Morphological aspects of paratuberculosis lesions in wild boar (Sus scrofa). Presence of of multiple granulomas in the mesenteric lymph nodes (H&E 50µm). A – Notice the caseous necrosis surrounded by inflammatory cells predominantly macrophages and some fibroblasts. B – Higher magnification of the former image. Note the Langhan's MGC (Arrows. H&E 50µm).

Map has been isolated in a wide range of wild mammals, from rodents, badgers, racoons, nine-banded armadillos, opossums, northern short-tailed shrew, striped skunks [46-48], wild boars [32,49] and rhinoceros [50] to bears [51], but not all of them present the same susceptibility and develop clinical signs or lesions when infected. The lesions produced by *Map*, representative or not of paratuberculosis, as well as the clinical signs seen in non-ruminant wild animals are more subtle than those observed in wild-ruminant species. Monkeys (*Macaca arctoides* and *Papio sphinx*) have demonstrated susceptibility to *Map* infection and develop lesions that are confined to the intestine and abdominal lymph nodes, resembling the lesions of paratuberculosis in cattle and in humans Crohn's disease [52,53]. When infected by *Map* lagomorphs produce an intestinal disease similar to paratuberculosis in ruminants, and severe infection can occur naturally, in which extensive granulomas with numerous giants' cells carrying multiple acid-fast bacilli can be observed in the small intestine [54]. In foxes and stoats, *Map* affects the intestines and mesenteric lymph nodes with microscopic changes similar to those described in ruminants with subclinical paratuberculosis. The lesions are composed of single macrophage-like cells or discrete granulomas consisting of small numbers of macrophages, in the cortex and paracortex of the mesenteric lymph nodes. In the small intestine, only few numbers of intracellular acid-fast bacteria are present within the macrophages, and Langhan's-type MGC, irregularly scattered in the granulomas, in all layers of affected intestine [46,54,55]. The typical pathology of paratuberculosis has also been noted in wood mice, weasels, badgers [46], and rats infected with the predominant ruminant strains [56]. When present, in brushtail possum and hedgehogs infected with *Map*, the lesions observed are in the grastrointestinal tract [57]. A recent report revealed that wild Eurasian otters (*Lutra lutra* L.) could be infected with *Map*. In that study, no gross lesions were found, but the retropharyngeal and mesenteric lymph nodes presented disrupted architecture, lymphoid depletion and diffuse inflammatory infiltrate composed mainly of macrophages and, to a lesser extent, neutrophils. *Map* was identified by direct PCR in several organs, including the intestine and lymph nodes [58]. Reports in which *Map* was isolated from Eurasian wild boars (*Sus scrofa*) revealed that the infection can occur with or without lesions, the later being the most frequent. If present, lesions generally consist of granulomatous enteritis and mesenteric lymphadenitis [32,49]. In mesenteric lymph nodes, lymphadenitis with multifocal lesions ranging from less than 1 cm to large areas of more than 1 cm in diameter, of either necrotic or necrotic calcified granulomas are observed (Figure 4). The presence of lymphocytes and caseous necrosis are the most common findings in these lesions [59].

Despite *Maa* being widely reported in wild boar, data on clinical infection or mortality are scarce [49]. Apparently, natural infection with this mycobateria causes barely detectable clinical signs or lesions [49]. However, there are reports of *Maa* isolated from free-ranging Eurasian wild boars with tuberculous lesions in intestinal lymph nodes [60], and the experimental infection with high doses of *Maa* results in gross and histopathological lesions of tuberculosis in tracheobronchial and mandibular lymph nodes. All visible lesions are less than 10 mm in diameter and consist of typical tuberculous granulomas with a central caseous necrosis, variably mineralized, surrounded by macrophages, lymphocytes, neutrophils, eosinophils and occasional MGC surrounded by fibrous tissue. Acid-fast bacilli are rarely detected in the necrotic debris of these lesions [61]. Another study also showed that in wild boars with mesenteric and submaxillar lymphadenitis, *Mycobacterium avium* subspecies type 1 and *M. avium* subspecies type 2 were the most frequently isolated mycobacteria [62].

Regarding *Mah* in wild boar, recent reports suggest that this animal species may act as a reservoir for these mycobacteria, since it was detected in lymph nodes without gross lesions or microscopic lesions [60,63].

3.2. Bird species

Bird species, either domestic or free-living can be infected with MAC mycobacteria, but they are more susceptible to *Maa*, the causative agent of avian tuberculosis [19]. Infection by *M. avium* subsp. *paratuberculosis* has been also documented in birds, with and without clinical and pathological findings [46,57].

Maa belonging to serotypes 1, 2, 3, and 6 is the most common agent of avian tuberculosis, but other species belonging to MAC, such as *M. intracellulare*, are also sporadic causes of disease [19]. Tuberculosis affects a wide-range of bird species, and it has been documented in waterfowl, galliformes, columbiformes, passerines, psittacines, raptors, and ratites [64-67]. According to their susceptibility to the disease, it has been proposed the classification of bird species into four groups, from highly susceptible to highly resistant: (1) domestic fowl, sparrows, pheasants, and partridges; (2) guinea fowl and domestic turkeys; (3) domestic goose and duck; (4) domestic pigeon [19]. The clinical signs of avian tuberculosis are well established but are not pathognomonic, and are different according to the phase of infection and the predominant form of the disease in the bird species, which in turn is related to the species susceptibility to the agent. Avian tuberculosis usually presents three stages or phases: latency, lesion development, and period of cachexia [68,69]. In most reports on the initial phase of avian tuberculosis the absence of clinical signs is a common feature. On the contrary, in advanced cases, progressive weight loss, depression, white diarrhea with soiled feathers, increased thirst, respiratory distress, fatigue, and decreased egg production may be observed [68]. Generally, avian tuberculosis is an intestinal and hepatic disease that can disseminate to other organs including the lungs, air sacs, spleen, bone marrow, and skin [69]. This is considered as the classical form of infection, and it's marked by the presence of tubercles or granulomas in multiple organs. Lesions in the intestinal tract characterize a second form of infection, and a third type of infection, especially reported finches, canaries, and psittacines occurs without the development of tuberculous lesions [19,68,69]. The clinical signs of the intestinal form of tuberculosis are characterized by chronic wasting disease. In severe cases and as disease progresses, feathers are often dull or ruffled and comb, wattle, and earlobes are paler, thinner and dry. Birds become lethargic and emaciated with marked atrophy of breast muscles, displaying the typical "knife edged" keel. In extreme cases, the body fat disappears, and the bird's face looks smaller than normal. The body temperature of the affected birds remains normal, even in severe cases [68,69]. Sudden death may also occur, as well as dyspnea, granulomatous ocular lesions [70] and skin lesions, which are less frequent [68,69]. Sudden death may be the result of massive hemorrhage secondary to liver or spleen rupture. In such cases, the birds may exhibit good body condition but frequently show advanced lesions of tuberculosis. Lameness can be the result of bone dissemination, in particular to the bone marrow of long bones. Joints can also be affected, and as consequence, some birds may adapt a sitting position or even show paralysis. There are also reports of neurological signs, due to the involvement of vertebral or central nervous system [68]. The lesions of avian tuberculosis are mainly composed by epithelioid cells containing large numbers of bacterium, that may either diffusely infiltrate the organ or form discrete tubercles or granulomas [68]. In the classical and intestinal forms of the disease, studded greyish-white to greyish-yellow nodules are frequently observed. The nodules, which appear as tumour-like masses, bulge from the serosal surface of the intestine and can be palpable. These nodules may suffer ulceration, and the caseous material within may be discharge into the intestinal lumen leading to the excretion of mycobacteria in droppings. During dissemination, typical caseous lesions, without calcification, are always found in the liver and spleen, with considerable enlargement of the organs. Nodules are firm but can be incised easily since mineralization is rare in avian tuberculosis. Due to this, spleen takes irregular and "knobbly" appearance. With the disease progression, tubercular nodules in the bone marrow, ovaries and testes, are often seen. Pulmonary lesions, which are a striking feature of tuberculosis in other species, are rarely observed in birds [68,69]. Pulmonary avian tuberculosis is not common, but it has been reported occasionally in pigeons and water-fowl [19,65,69]. In the cachexia stage of avian tuberculosis, massive tubercles with large numbers of bacilli are observed [68,69].

In accordance to the clinical signs and lesional patterns of tuberculosis in domestic species, captive, exotic and wild birds, including raptors, generally develop the disseminated form of avian tuberculosis, involving the digestive tract, liver and spleen [66,71,72]. However, some studies reveal that exotic bird species may have lesions in the liver and spleen without intestinal involvement. These lesions are typical granulomas with a caseous or coagulative necrotic centre and MGC. Acid-fast bacilli are numerous in the central zone of the tubercle [69].

Infection of birds by *Map* has been reported, but it often occurs without clinical signs or lesions, despite the typical lesions of paratuberculosis being described in jackdaws (*Corvus monedula*), rooks (*Corvus frugilegus*), and crows (*Corvus corone*) [46,57]. A study also reported the occurrence of diarrhea, respiratory signs, hepatomegaly and splenomegaly in a diamond sparrow (*Emblema guttata*) with liver granuloma lesions, predominantly composed of lymphocytes and mononuclear cells [73].

4. Diagnostic techniques

The diagnosis of Mac is based on the clinical signs, post mortem gross lesions, and by demonstrating the presence of acid-fast bacilli using Ziehl-Neelsen staining. This is normally sufficient to establish the diagnosis [68,69,74,75]. *Ante mortem* diagnosis is based on clinical signs, leukograme, serology, culture and also acid-fast stain or biopsy samples of fluids or organs [76-80]. Radiography and ultrasonography are also useful in the medical evaluation of birds [79].

4.1. Isolation and identification

The golden standard test for mycobacterium diagnosis is the microbiological culture. Tissue culture seems to be slightly more sensitive than faecal culture and it allows the infection to be detected in some animals that had no specific lesions. The culture of bacteria requires weeks or months of incubation before colony growth occurs. This means that a significant amount of time is needed before a diagnosis can be made. It is also difficult to isolate bacteria in culture due to intermittent shedding and a low number of bacilli in faeces and tissues [81]. *M. genavense* is extremely difficult to isolate by culture [82,83]. *M. avium* complex grows best in media containing eggs or egg yolk and the incubation temperature should be set at 37ºC-40ºC. Culture can be performed in Dorset´s, Herrold´s egg yolk medium, Middlebrook 7H10 and 7H11 or Coletsos medium supplemented with 1% sodium piruvate [68,74,75]. For the isolation of *Map* or *M. silvaticum* addition of mycobactin is required in all media. *Map* is the slowest growing of the culturable mycobacteria [84]. Cultures should be incubated for at least 8 weeks. Typically, *M. avium* produces smooth colonies within 2-4 weeks and rough variants can occur [74]. Culture of *Map* from faeces or tissues of other animals such as sheep and goats is less successful due to the "S" strains that usually infect these animals [84]. The best organs to use for culture are usually liver and spleen but bone marrow can be used if carcass is decomposed, as it could be less contaminated [74]. Non-sterile specimens need to be processed with detergent alkali or acid to eliminate rapidly growing microorganisms before culture decontamination in order to remove faster growing microbial species. Incubation with various decontamination agents such as 0.6-0.75% hexadecylpryridinium chloride (HPC) or NaOH for 3 hours to overnight, have been used. It is important that decontamination does not remove too many viable mycobacterium cells [85,86]. Other methods like sedimentation and centrifugation can be employed if small numbers of mycobacteria are expected in the sample [85,87]. Shorter incubation times can be achieved using automated broth based systems, like liquid culture BACTEC system MGIT 960 [84]. These systems have been reported to be highly sensitive for culture [88]. For *M. genavense* the use of BACTEC system with no additives and pH 6.0 is recommended [89,90]. Middlebrook 7H11 with pH 6.0 supplemented with blood and charcoal is also recommended to promote growth of *M. genavense* [91]. In human AIDS patients, laboratory diagnosis of MAC infection is usually made by the BACTEC blood culture [92]. Conventional biochemical tests for species identification are lengthy and fail to distinguish between *M. avium* and *M. intracelullare* [74]. Identification of isolates by phenotypic characteristics of majority of clinically relevant mycobacteria can be based on growth rates, colony pigmentation and biochemical tests such as niacin production, nitrate reduction, tween 80 hydrolysis arylsulphatase, urease, tellurite reduction, thiophen-2-carboxylic acid hydrazide sensitivity catalase (qualitative and quantitative) growth on MacConkey and sodium chloride tolerance [88,93].

Classification of MAC organisms has been made by seroagglutination [19,74]. Seroagglutination is based on sugar residue specificity of surface glycopeptidolipids, and allows classification of MAC organisms into 28 serovars: 1 to 6, 8 to 11 and 21 are currently ascribed as *M. avium*, while serovars 7, 12 to 20 and 25 to *M. intracellulare*. However, no consensus was achieved on the other serovars [74]. MAC colonies can also be identified using high performance liquid chromatography (HPLC) for detecting mycolic acid [19]. HPLC and the use of monoclonal antibodies to major serovars in ELISA also facilitate typing of mycobacteria [19,75].

4.2. Immunological methods

The enzyme linked immunosorbent assay (ELISA) has been used for detecting antimycobacterial antibodies in the serum of ruminants [94]. However, serological assays for detecting *Mycobacterium* are problematic. The sensitivity of ELISA is dependent on the stage of the disease with a higher sensitivity of the test in case of higher bacterial load. The test can detect the most severe infections in multibacillar lesions but shows lower sensitivity in animals with paucibacillar lesions [84]. One important disadvantage is the inability to distinguish between different mycobacterial infections probably due to close antigenic relationship between *Maa* and *Map* [95].

Tuberculin test is the most widely used method in domestic fowl and the only for which an international standard for the reagent exists. Birds are tested by intradermal inoculation in the wattle with 0.05 ml or 0.1 ml of tuberculin (avian purified protein derivate – PPD) [74]. A positive reaction is identified as a hot and oedematous swelling at the site or by the presence of a small firm nodule of approximately 5 mm in diameter after 48 hours [19]. The tuberculin test and the haemagglutination test (stained antigen) are the immunological methods most frequently used for export testing [74]. In the stained antigen test an antigen stained with 1% malachite green is used for the rapid blood plate agglutination test [96].The diagnosis of *Mycobacterial* infections in live wild animals remains a challenge [95]. The comparative cervical tuberculin (CCT) skin test has been applied in wild animals such as in cervids [97], but the test presents two major limitations. It has been proved that CCT cannot detect some stages of infection [98], and wild ruminants must be captured twice increasing the stress and the risk of accidents for the animals and for handlers [95]. Alternative probes like the detection of interferon-γ (IFN- γ) assay and ELISA, which employ blood and serum respectively, could be an alternative in wild animals [95]. Advantages of ELISA and IFN-γ assay is that they enable testing without handling the animals twice and allow repeated testing, which are important advantages in case of wild ruminants [99]. ELISA detects humoral immune response whereas the CCT and IFN-γ assay detect cellular immune response [95]. The dominant response to mycobacterial infections in ruminants is cell-mediated. However, a recent study demonstrated that the IFN-γ assay may be of limited usefulness in some species of cervids [100].

4.3. Genetic methods

4.3.1. The contribution of molecular biology to MAC research

During the past several years, many molecular methods have been developed for direct detection, species identification, and drug susceptibility testing of mycobacteria. These methods can potentially reduce the diagnostic time from weeks to days with a higher sensibility. Molecular biology methods offer new opportunities to differentiate, identify and type bacterial species and strains. These methods use the variability of nucleic sequences of genes such as 16S rDNA, beta subunit RNA-ase (rpoB), gyrase (gyrB), rDNA internal transcribed spacer among other genes. Some of the methods available to differentiate and identify species of mycobacteria at the DNA sequence level are PCR, PCR-REA, sequencing analysis, spoligotyping and DNA fingerprinting. These methods have been applied to both the "universal" part of the genome and to specific mycobacterial genes.

Isolation of mycobacterial DNA can be done from living mycobacteria, not only from mycobacterial isolates but also directly from body fluids (sputum, bronchoalveolar lavages, and bronchial and tracheal aspirates, semen, milk, blood, cerebrospinal fluid), from tissues and from faeces and can be done using dead mycobacterial cells, namely from formalin-fixed and paraffin-embedded tissues and from forensic and archaeological samples [101]. One of the challenges with molecular detection of *Map* is to get the genomic DNA out of the bacteria, which is protected by its thick and waxy cell wall. One method commonly used is the mechanical disruption by the use of bead beating, a general term for using small beads mixed with the sample, usually in the presence of a proteolytic enzyme and lysis buffer, to break tissues or tough cell walls and spores by forceful shaking in a cell disrupter, or "bead beater". It is one of several suggested methods to lyse *Map* [102-105]. Others include homogenized (grinded) sample under liquid nitrogen in a mortar and pestle, combinations of enzymatic treatment, freeze-thaw/boiling and kits for plant DNA purification or for animal tissues DNA purification [103,105-109]. Commercially available kits, developed for DNA isolation from different matrices, are commonly used for the rapid isolation and detection of *Map* in milk.

4.3.2. Polymerase Chain Reaction (PCR)

The polymerase chain reaction (PCR) is an in vitro method for the amplification of DNA that was introduced in 1985 [110]. With the performance of a previous reverse transcription step, PCR can also be applied to RNA [111]. Reverse transcription PCR is a modification of this method used when the initial template is RNA rather than DNA, the reverse transcriptase enzyme first converts the RNA target into a complementary DNA copy (cDNA), that can be used to amplify the much higher numbers of copies of messenger or ribosomal RNA than the number of DNA copies present in bacteria, and it may detect specific expression of certain genes. Some modifications to single PCR were done to improve results and were used for MAC species detection, the multiplex PCR, the assay that include several primer pairs specific to different DNA targets to allow amplification and detection of several pathogens at the same time, and nested PCR, the product from one

PCR reaction serves as template in a second reaction with fresh reagents, thus diluting any PCR inhibiting substances and increasing the sensitivity. As example differentiation of *M. tuberculosis* complex, *M. avium* and other non-tuberculous mycobacteria (NTM) has been done by using hybridization probes [112]. Targeting the 16S rRNA gene, 3 different probes, specific for mycobacteria, *M. tuberculosis* complex and *M. avium,* were constructed and the thermal melting temperature (Tm) was different for *M. tuberculosis, M. kansasii, M. avium, M. intracellulare* and *M. marinum* allowing the differentiation. TaqMan PCR assay targeting 65 kD heat shock protein gene has been used for the detection of *M. genavense* and *M. avium* complex species in avian tissue samples [83].

Specific probes are available for the identification of *Mycobacterium avium* and *Mycobacterium intracellulare.* Amplification of the DT1 and DT6 fragments was considered equally sensitive for species identification [113]. Recently, numerous isolates suspected of be *Mycobacterium intracellulare* were reclassified as *Mycobacterium chimaera* sp. nov., as part of the MAC [114]. Strains of MAC can be identified by serological procedures, on the basis of differences in the C-mycoside glycopeptidolipids. To date, using 16S rRNA probes, 28 MAC serotypes have been identified from which the serotypes 1–6, 8–11, and 21 belong to *Maa.* Serovars 7, 12–20, and 25 have been ascribed to *Mycobacterium intracellulare.* Serovar-1 is the most common organism isolated from birds and from human. Serotypes 1 and 2 are most commonly isolated from domestic birds, and serovar 3 is recovered sporadically from wild birds. Serotypes 1, 2, and 3 are considered virulent for chickens. Serotypes 1, 4, and 8 have been reported to predominate among isolates from AIDS patients [19].

Other approach to the differentiation of MAC strains was obtained with the description of repetitive insertion sequence IS*900* in *Map* strains and IS*901* or IS*902* in *M. avium* subsp. *silvaticum* strains [115]. Examination of serotyped strains revealed IS*901* only in strains of serotypes 1, 2, and 3 [19].

The discovery of insertion sequences in mycobacterial genomes, e.g. IS*900* in *Map* [116], IS*901* [117], IS*1245* [118], IS*1311* [119] in the MAC strains was a major breakthrough in the study of mycobacterial infections. When characterized and used in the proper context, the species-specific IS (insertion sequences) elements can be useful classification tools to distinguish subsets of the MAC [18,120]. However, there are two problems described that can question their utility for this purpose. First, a number of IS elements have been uncovered in strains considered to be MAC organisms, but without adequate strain characterization, it is difficult to judge which organisms harbour such elements. Second, IS elements are by nature mobile elements, so there is a risk that similar elements are found in unrelated bacteria because of mobility to or from MAC organisms [3].

IS*900* was the first IS characterized within the *Mycobacterium* genus [116,121] and is the most widely used target sequence for detection of *Map* and presently considered specific for this agent. The *Map* genome is reported to have 15 to 20 copies of the insertion element, and the sequenced strain K-10 has 17 copies [122]. Cousins et al. recommended that restriction digestion should be used to confirm the profile of the IS of the amplified product [123]. However, Englund et al. identified a *Mycobacterium* sp. with an IS*900* like sequence in which the restriction sites after amplification with the original primers were identical to the restriction sites in amplified DNA of *Map* [124]. Therefore, restriction endonucleases analysis did not solve the problem of false positives. Englund et al. recommended that a positive IS*900* PCR should be confirmed by subsequent sequencing or by a PCR assay targeting another gene in *Map* [124]. In a study performed by Vansnick et al. two sets of newly developed PCR primers based on the insertion sequence IS*900* and the unique sequence f57 were developed and the combination of the two PCR assays has proven to be useful for the identification of *Map* [125]. *Map* genome has revealed the presence of 17 IS*900*, 7 IS*1311*, and 3 IS*1245* insertion elements. The IS*900* element seems unique to *Map* and has been widely used as a diagnostic tool to detect *Map* in clinical samples from both animals and humans [5].

The specific DNA sequence IS*900* was also used as the target for *Map* detection in Nested PCR. In 2002, IS*900*-nested PCR was used to determine the specificity and sensitivity of a commercial ELISA test [126]. However, the nested PCR method is now being replaced by Real-Time PCR [127].

RFLP analysis of the IS*900* element has been used a molecular tool to type *Map* isolates and allowed the division of *Map* into different groups, associated to different host species [3]. The IS*900* element is by far the most widely used target for the molecular detection of *Map* and has been used in the form of direct PCR [108,125], *in situ* PCR [128] nested PCR [126,129,130], and real-time PCR [131-133]. Sequencing of the amplified product for IS*900* is therefore necessary to confirm that the amplicon is truly IS*900*.

Additional gene loci specific for *Map* have been identified and suggested for use in diagnostics: ISMav2 [134], f57 [135], IS*Map*02 [136], and other *Map* specific coding sequences [137].

To identify the methods which are best suited for diagnostics, eight single-round and five nested PCR systems including twelve different primer pairs based on IS*900* (9x), 7 ISMav2 (1x), f57 (1x), and locus 255 (1x) sequences were compared by Möbius et al., which concluded that stringent selection of IS*900*-specific primers ensures that IS*900* remains a favourite target sequence for amplification of *Map* specific loci [138]. A PCR system targeting two different *Map* specific regions would have a still higher specificity. The following six single round PCR-systems were recommended by Möbius et al. [138]: IS*900* based PCRs of Englund et al. [139], and Doran et al. [140], the f57 based PCR assay [125], and the locus 255 based PCR assay [137]. However, despite their advantages, such as a hundredfold enhancement of sensitivity, nested PCR assays bear a high risk of contamination and crossing over and, therefore, cannot be recommended as a reliable method for routine diagnosis of *Map*.

The insertion sequence IS901 was discovered by Kunze et al. and shows around 60% sequence homology to IS*900* [117]. The stability of IS*901* in strains isolated primarily from clinical material from birds, domestic animals and from the environment is used for the rapid identification of IS*901*+ strains using the PCR method. Screening across a larger panel of isolates revealed that most isolates from birds and some animals contained the element, whereas isolates obtained from AIDS patients or the environment did not. Furthermore, it was found that most bird isolates had similar IS*901* patterns [3].

IS*1311* was first reported as a GenBank entry in 1994 (U16276) and was subsequently used for RFLP analyses [119,141]. This element is present in all members of the *M. avium* subspecies, including *Maa*, *Mah*, and *Map* [142], and is not present in *M. intracellulare*

[22,141]. The element itself has 85% sequence identity to IS*1245*. With the wide range of *M. avium* hosting for this element, it is possible that IS*1311* represents an "older" IS element which may have been present prior to subspecies divergence [3]. RFLP analysis of IS*1311* and the use of IS*1311* PCR-REA also revealed distinct pattern types, corresponding to different genotype species strains of *M. avium* subsp. *paratuberculosis* [22,142].

The IS*1245* was first described in 1995, is present in up to 27 copies in *Mycobacterium avium* [118], was presented as having a more restricted range than IS*1311*, and was found to be stable during in vivo and in vitro passage, making it a popular target for restriction fragment length polymorphism strain typing. It is described as limited to the subspecies of *M. avium*, i.e., *Maa* (that would include *Mah*), *Map* subsp. *paratuberculosis*, and *M. avium* subsp. *silvaticum*. By PCR analysis, this element was not found in *M. intracellulare* or in 17 other mycobacterium species [3]. Standardization of IS*1245* RFLP analysis was proposed in 1998 as a tool for MAC molecular epidemiology [143]. Some *M. avium* isolates have been documented as being IS*1245* negative, but only a few such reports have presented further documentation of strain identity by a sequence-based method [144]. Beggs et al. found IS*1245* in strains of *M. intracellulare*, demonstrating that the element is present in other species of the *M. avium* complex [144]. In some reports, IS*1245*-negative isolates have been described that contain an hsp65 sequence identical to that of *M. avium* but that differs from *M. avium* in other taxonomic targets, such as the 16S rRNA gene and the ITS sequence [3].

Other identification methods of *M. avium* species or its subspecies are based on 16S rDNA [145], PCR-REA (Restriction Endonuclease Analysis) [146], sequence analysis of hsp65 [8] or a strategy based on large sequence polymorphisms [147]. Semret et al. evaluating the distribution of genomic polymorphisms across a panel of strains, verified that it was possible to assign unique genomic signatures to host-associated variants and based on these polymorphisms proposed a simple PCR-based strategy that can rapidly type *M. avium* isolates into these subgroups [147].

The sequence of the 16S rDNA gene is specific at the species level and is also a stable property of microorganisms. Wilton and Cousins described a method for the simultaneous identification of genus, species and strains of *Mycobacterium* sp. using conserved and variable sequences of the 16S rDNA gene [145]. Comparing the 16S rDNA sequences of mycobacterial pathogens, they found variable regions specific for individual species and used the information to develop a duplex amplification system, which makes it possible to identify the genus *Mycobacterium*, and the species *M. a. avium* and *M. intracellulare*. If combining the primers for 16S rDNA with primers specific to the gene that encodes the secretion protein MPB70 (specific for *Mycobacterium tuberculosis* complex) this system permits the detection and identification of clinically important mycobacteria in one single PCR. The disadvantage of this method is that it does not distinguish between *M. a. avium* and *M. a. paratuberculosis*.

Combining PCR amplification of the 16S rDNA gene and subsequent restriction analysis we have the PCR-REA (or PRA) method. Using the 16S rDNA gene primers according to Thierry et al. and the resulting PCR products, 1 300 bp in size digested with *Rsa I* it is possible to distinguish species of MAC (*M. a. avium* serotypes 1–3, 8–11 and 21, *M. a. paratuberculosis*) and *M. intracellulare* (serotypes 7, 12–20, 22–28) [148].

Standard (housekeeping) genes offer a higher level of sequence variation than do ribosomal genes but are nonetheless useful for taxonomic purposes due to the relative sequence conservation imposed to maintain function. In this category, the stress protein gene hsp65 is a preferred target for mycobacterial identification to the species level, having been routinely used in diagnostics since the development of rapid PCR-restriction enzyme analysis (PRA) methods. The *dnaJ* gene encodes a stress chaperone protein and is highly conserved among the bacterial genera [149]. Morakova et al. designed primers specific for the *dnaJ* gene in the *M. avium* species that allow amplification of the *dnaJ* gene in all isolates of all *M. avium* subspecies and the authors suggest using them as an internal standard in the multiplex PCR to control inhibition of the amplification, and consequently false negatives, because are highly specific for at least *M. avium* [108]. The same team designed a fast and specific PCR strategy for the detection and differentiation of *M. avium* subspecies for use in routine veterinary diagnosis [108]. They have developed a multiplex PCR based on IS*900*, IS*901*, IS*1245* and the *dnaJ* gene. This method allows the detection of *M. a. paratuberculosis*, *M. a. hominissuis* and *M. a. avium*/*M. a. silvaticum* in one PCR reaction (PCR multiplex) and theoretically enables the detection of mixed infections of *M. a. paratuberculosis* and *M. a. avium* or M. *a. paratuberculosis* and *M. a. hominissuis*. The sensitivity of this multiplex PCR is 103 CFU for each bacterial strain in one PCR reaction, which also enabled the use of this test directly for DNA isolated from the tissue of the heavily infected sheep.

Shin et al. designed a five-target multiplex PCR to discriminate MAC organisms isolated. This MAC multiplex was designed to amplify a 16S rRNA gene target common to all *Mycobacterium species*, a chromosomal target called DT1 that is unique to *Maa* serotypes 2 and 3, to *M. avium* subsp. *silvaticum*, and to *M. intracellulare*, and three insertion sequences, IS*900*, IS*901*, and IS*1311*. The results for the pattern of amplification allowed to determine whether isolates were mycobacteria, or members of MAC, and to classify them into one of the three major MAC subspecies, *Map*, *Maa*, *Mah* [18].

5. Public health concerns

Zoonotic aspects of mycobacteria transmitted by the environment and wildlife highlights a major health problem. MAC causes a variety of disorders including tuberculosis-like diseases in animals and in human immunocompetent or immunocompromised patients. Susceptibility to mycobacterial infections depends of risk factors since they are ubiquous in the soil and water [150]. Human exposure to mycobacterium present in wildlife and in nature can occur by a variety of routes. Humans are continuously exposed at a low level (50 to 5000 bacilli per day). Contact with water, municipal or natural are also important routes for mycobacteria infection. Birds are major excretors of the agent in their faeces and the bacteria can persist in the soil and in water for long [1].

Healthy humans have a low susceptibility to MAC infection and only a very small percentage of mycobacteria progress trough to infection, but in immunocompromised individuals infected with HIV or leukaemia patients, treated with steroid therapy, chemotherapy or other immunosuppressive medication, should be carefully considered regarding their possibility to come in contact with birds with mycobacterial infection [1,151]. Prior to the introduction of highly active antiretroviral treatment more than 40% of patients developed *M. avium* complex bacteriemia two years after the AIDS diagnosis

[152] and a disseminated MAC infection was found in as much as 50% of autopsied AIDS patients [153,154]. This has predominantly been attributed to the impairment of the adaptative part of the immune systems in HIV-1 infected individuals due to the loss of CD4+ T cells, as the susceptibility to opportunistic infections including *M. avium* infection is correlated with a decline in this cell type [155]. MAC usually produces clinical disease only when CD4+ are very low (< 50 cells/ml), which is seen in 4 to 5 per cent of HIV infected patients [88]. A recent study showed that exposure of dendritic cells to HIV-1 promotes or facilitates the intracellular growth of *M. avium* [153]. Signs and symptoms associated with MAC disease in AIDS cases are persistent high grade fever, high sweats, anaemia and weight loss in addition to nonspecific symptoms of malaise, anorexia, diarrhea, myalgia and occasional painful adenophaty [88]. Epidemiology of MAC complex in patients without HIV infection remains somewhat difficult to determine since the disease is relatively uncommon, it is not a reportable health event and environmental exposure varies greatly according to the geographic region [156]. In an epidemiological survey in USA from 2000 to 2003 performed in [156] in patients without HIV infection the rate of positive non-tuberculous cultures was 17.7 per 100,000. Surveys conducted in Europe estimated the rate of disease anywhere in the human body to be 0.8-3.1 per 100,000 [157,158]. In a recent study, Bodle et al. estimated the incidence of non-tuberculous mycobacteria in the respiratory tract disease in 2.0 per 100,000 and the disease in anywhere in the human body in 2.7 per 100,000 [156]. Another recently published study showed that the patient′s lung disease was likely acquired by inhalation of aerosols while showering [159]. *M. avium* may reach the lungs by aspiration because a considerable percentage of patients with non-tuberculous mycobacteria (NMT) disease have been found to experience gastroesophageal reflux disease [160,161].

Disease patterns of MAC are different in immunocompromised patients. In adults, infection is mainly pulmonary [1,151]. MAC is the most common of the nontuberculous mycobacteria found in apparently healthy children [162] and it's infection is characterized by a chronic granulomatous lymphadenopathy in the neck region that preferably is treated by excision of the affected lymph node [162,163]. The main hypothesis of infection is that oral contact with *M. avium*-infected water courses causes lymphadenitis in the head and neck region in children [162,164]. Among the members of MAC, *Maa* is predominant (87-98%) in AIDS patients and induces disseminated mycobacteriemia rather than restrict the bacteria to the lungs [1]. Since the advent of AIDS, HIV has become the major risk factor for MAC infection. In AIDS patients the main route of infection is the gastrointestinal tract and *M. avium* is naturally tolerant to the low pH that exists in the stomach [19,165]. Regarding therapeutics, *M. avium* is of special concern because drugs commonly used from treating tuberculosis in humans are not effective [166] and MAC strains are resistant to isoniazid, the most popular anti-tuberculosis drug [19,167]. Preexisting pulmonary conditions, patients with current illness or immunosuppressive medication are the most important risk factors for MAC infection amongst patients without HIV infection. MAC was also reported as the most common pathogen causing post transplant non-tuberculous mycobacteria disease [156]. Other factors are local traumas and surgical procedures injuries [168]. Chronic obstructive pulmonary disease, emphysema, pneumoconiosis, aspiration due to oesophageal disease, previous gastrectomy and chronic alcoholism are some of the conditions which have been linked to disease [88,154]. Disseminated MAC infection is more frequent in caucasians compared with Hispanic or African-americans individuals. However, there are no differences related with age [169,170]. Infection is more frequent in men than in women, particularly in homosexual and bisexual men, when compared to other HIV risk categories.

The zoonotic potential of *Map* has been debated for almost a century because of similarities between Johne´s disease in cattle and Crohn´s disease in humans. A quarter century later since *Map* was first proposed as an etiologic agent in Crohn´s disease based on the isolation of the organism from several patients the association as a causative agent or in an incidental away remains unresolved. Milk and water are potential sources for acquiring *Map* infection [171]. However, only a few samples of milk, positive by PCR for the presence of *Map* have yielded positive results in culture, suggesting that *Map* remains undetectable probably because the low number of viable *Map* in samples [172]. Published reports indicate that *Map* may not be completely inactivated by pasteurization of milk [173]. Serological response to *Map* in humans is also not conclusive [172]. Traditional methods of detecting bacteria, culture and stain are largely ineffective in detecting *Map* in humans. Bacteria are very difficult to culture and *Map* is able to exist in a spheroplast (cell wall deficient form) in humans so it cannot be identified by Ziehl-Neelsen staining [174-176]. Polymerase chain reaction has identified *Map* in greater than 90% of biopsy specimens from Crohn´s patients [177] and viable *Map* was detected in peripheral blood and serum in a higher proportion of individuals with Crohn's disease [178,179]. However, culture of *Map* from human specimens is a controversial question since some authors pointed out the difficulty of culturing *Map* [180,181]. At this moment is not possible to know if *Map* is a primary etiological agent or secondary invader and further research is need to understand the possible links between this agent and Crohn disease [1].

There is a recent interest in *Map* as an immune trigger of several autoimmune diseases [182,183]. Environmental agents are postulated to trigger autism. Recently, a theory proposing a mechanism by which *Map* triggers autism through molecular mimicry to the heat shock protein HSP65, which stimulates antibodies that cross react with myelin basic protein, a common feature of autism [184]. Another recent study has associated the presence of *Map* with Blau syndrome, an autossomal dominant, and systemic inflammatory disease. The mutations of Blau syndrome are on the same gene on chromosome 16 (CARD 15) that confers susceptibility to Crohns´disease [185]. *Map* was also implicated in sarcoidosis [186,187], which is a multisystemic granulomatous disease with many features in common with mycobacterial infection, and that, like Crohn´s disease, can be mimicked by slow bacterial infections [188,189].

Map was also linked to ulcerative colitis, irritable bowel syndrome, autoimmune (type 1) diabetes, Hashimoto thyroiditis and multiple sclerosis [179,184]. Increasing evidence suggests a role for *Map* in autoimmune (type I) diabetes. It is postulated that this bacterium acts via molecular mimicry between its antigens (HSP65) and the pancreatic enzyme glutamic acid decarboxylase (GAD) [190-195].

6. Conclusion

MAC comprises slow growing mycobacteria that are ubiquitous in the environment (soil and water), and have a wide source range, causing disease in various domestic and wild mammals and birds. MAC can affect a wide-range of wild animals, but little has been published up to the moment on the clinical signs, which are rarely exhibited or not documented. When present, the occurrence of clinical signs and lesions is highly variable in timing, though often similar to those of their domesticated counterparts.

The evidence for the zoonotic potential should not be neglected particularly in immunocompromised patients, both humans and animals.

Recent reports, suggesting an association between MAC and autoimmune and other chronic human diseases, alert to the importance of developing new studies on MAC biology, molecular diagnosis and epidemiology.

Research to understand the impact of MAC in public health is needed as well as the determination of transmission routes between humans and wildlife, which requires interdisciplinary collaboration among medical, veterinary and other public health officials.

References

1. Biet F, Boschiroli ML, Thorel MF, Guilloteau LA. Zoonotic Aspects of Mycobacterium bovis and Mycobacterium avium-intracellulare Complex (MAC). Veterinary research. 2005;36(3) 411-436.
2. Prescott LM, Harley JP, Klein DA. Microbiology. New York: McGraw-Hill; 2002.
3. Turenne CY, Wallace R, Behr MA. Mycobacterium avium in the Postgenomic Era. Clinical Microbiology Reviews. 2007;20(2) 205-229.
4. Smole SC, McAleese F, Ngampasutadol J, von Reyn CF, Arbeit RD. Clinical and Epidemiological Correlates of Genotypes within the Mycobacterium avium Complex Defined by Restriction and Sequence Analysis of hsp65. Journal of Clinical Microbiology. 2002;40(9) 3374-3380.
5. Harris NB, Barletta RG. Mycobacterium avium subsp. paratuberculosis in Veterinary Medicine. Clinical Microbiology Reviews. 2001;14(3) 489-512.
6. Carter G, Wise D. Mycobacterium. In: Carter G, Wise D (ed.) Essentials of Veterinary Bacteriology and Mycology. Iowa: Iowa State Pres; 2004. p. 207-213.
7. Mackenzie N, Alexander DC, Turenne CY, Behr MA, De Buck JM. Genomic Comparison of PE and PPE Genes in the Mycobacterium avium Complex. Journal of Clinical Microbiology. 2009;47(4) 1002-1011.
8. Turenne CY, Semret M, Cousins DV, Collins DM, Behr MA. Sequencing of hsp65 Distinguishes among Subsets of the Mycobacterium avium Complex. Journal of Clinical Microbiology. 2006;44(2) 433-440.
9. Inderlied CB, Kemper CA, Bermudez LE. The Mycobacterium avium Complex. Clinical Microbiology Reviews. 1993;6(3) 266-310.
10. Tortoli E, Rindi L, Garcia MJ, Chiaradonna P, Dei R, Garzelli C, Kroppenstedt RM, Lari N, Mattei R, Mariottini A, Mazzarelli G, Murcia MI, Nanetti A, Piccoli P, Scarparo C. Proposal to Elevate the Genetic Variant MAC-A, Included in the Mycobacterium avium complex, to species rank as Mycobacterium chimaera sp. nov. International Journal of Systematic and Evolutionary Microbiology. 2004;54(4) 1277-1285.

11. Murcia MI, Tortoli E, Menendez MC, Palenque E, Garcia MJ. Mycobacterium colombiense sp. nov., a Novel Member of the Mycobacterium avium Complex and Description of MAC-X as a New ITS Genetic Variant. International Journal of Systematic and Evolutionary Microbiology. 2006;56(9) 2049-2054.
12. Esparcia Á, Navarro F, Quer M, Coll P. Lymphadenopathy Caused by Mycobacterium colombiense. Journal of Clinical Microbiology. 2008;46(5) 1885-1887.
13. Vuorenmaa K, Ben Salah I, Barlogis V, Chambost H, Drancourt M. Mycobacterium colombiense and Pseudotuberculous Lymphadenopathy.. Emerging Infectious Diseases. 2009;15(4) 619-620.
14. Bang D, Herlin T, Stegger M, Andersen AB, Torkko P, Tortoli E, Thomsen VO. Mycobacterium arosiense sp. nov., a Slowly Growing, Scotochromogenic Species Causing Osteomyelitis in an Immunocompromised Child. International Journal of Systematic and Evolutionary Microbiology. 2008;58(10) 2398-2402.
15. Van Ingen J, Boeree MJ, Kásters K, Wieland A, Tortoli E, Dekhuijzen PNR, van Soolingen D. Proposal to Elevate Mycobacterium avium Complex ITS Sequevar MAC-Q to Mycobacterium vulneris sp. nov. International Journal of Systematic and Evolutionary Microbiology. 2009;59(9) 2277-2282.
16. Ben Salah I, Cayrou C, Raoult D, Drancourt M. Mycobacterium marseillense sp. nov., Mycobacterium timonense sp. nov. and Mycobacterium bouchedurhonense sp. nov., Members of the Mycobacterium Avium Complex. International Journal of Systematic and Evolutionary Microbiology. 2009;59(11) 2803-2808.
17. Thorel M-F, Krichevsky M, Vincent Lévy-Frébault V. Numerical Taxonomy of Mycobactin-Dependent Mycobacteria, Emended Description of Mycobacterium avium, and Description of Mycobacterium avium subsp. avium subsp. nov., Mycobacterium avium subsp. paratuberculosis subsp. nov., and Mycobacterium avium subsp. silvaticum subsp. nov. International Journal of Systematic Bacteriology. 1990;40(3) 254-260.
18. Shin SJ, Lee BS, Koh W-J, Manning EJB, Anklam K, Sreevatsan S, Lambrecht RS, Collins MT. Efficient Differentiation of Mycobacterium avium Complex Species and Subspecies by Use of Five-Target Multiplex PCR. Journal of Clinical Microbiology. 2010;48(11) 4057-4062.
19. Dhama K, Mahendran M, Tiwari R, Dayal Singh S, Kumar D, Singh S, Sawant PM. Tuberculosis in Birds: Insights into the Mycobacterium avium Infections. Veterinary Medicine International. 2011; 2011:1-14. http://dx.doi.org/10.4061/2011/712369.
20. Wells SJ, Collins MT, Faaberg KS, Wees C, Tavornpanich S, Petrini KR, Collins JE, Cernicchiaro N, Whitlock RH. Evaluation of a Rapid Fecal PCR Test for Detection of Mycobacterium avium subsp. paratuberculosis in Dairy Cattle. Clinical and Vaccine Immunology. 2006;13(10) 1125-1130.
21. Whittington RJ, Marsh I, McAllister S, Turner MJ, Marshall DJ, Fraser CA. Evaluation of Modified BACTEC 12B Radiometric Medium and Solid Media for Culture of Mycobacterium avium subsp. paratuberculosis from Sheep. Journal of Clinical Microbiology. 1999;37(4) 1077-1083.

22. Whittington R, I., Marsh EC, Cousins D. Polymorphisms In IS1311, an Insertion Sequence Common to Mycobacterium avium and M. avium subsp. paratuberculosis, Can Be Used to Distinguish Between and within these Species. Molecular and Cellular Probes. 1998;12(6) 349-358.

23. Álvarez J, García IG, Aranaz A, Bezos J, Romero B, de Juan L, Mateos A, Gómez-Mampaso E, Domínguez L. Genetic Diversity of Mycobacterium avium Isolates Recovered from Clinical Samples and from the Environment: Molecular Characterization for Diagnostic Purposes. Journal of Clinical Microbiology. 2008;46(4) 1246-1251.

24. Matlova L, Dvorska L, Palecek K, Maurenc L, Bartos M, Pavlik I. Impact of Sawdust and Wood Shavings in Bedding on Pig Tuberculous Lesions in Lymph nodes, and IS1245 RFLP Analysis of Mycobacterium avium subsp. hominissuis of Serotypes 6 and 8 isolated from pigs and environment. Veterinary Microbiology. 2004;102(3-4) 227-236.

25. Glawischnig W, Steineck T, Spergser J. Infections Caused by Mycobacterium avium subspecies avium, Hominissuis, and paratuberculosis in Free-Ranging Red Deer (Cervus elaphus hippelaphus) in Austria, 2001-2004. Journal of Wildlife Diseases. 2006;42(4) 724-731.

26. Thorel MF, Huchzermeyer HF, Michel AL. Mycobacterium avium and Mycobacterium intracellulare Infection in Mammals. Revue scientifique et technique (International Office of Epizootics). 2001;20(1) 204-218.

27. Kyriakopoulos AM, Tassios PT, Matsiota-Bernard P, Marinis E, Tsaousidou S, Legakis NJ. Characterization to Species Level of Mycobacterium avium Complex Strains from Human Immunodeficiency Virus-Positive and -Negative Patients. Journal of Clinical Microbiology. 1997;35(11) 3001-3003.

28. Falkinham JO, Norton CD, LeChevallier MW. Factors Influencing Numbers of Mycobacterium avium, Mycobacterium intracellulare, and other Mycobacteria in Drinking Water Distribution Systems. Applied and Environmental Microbiology. 2001;67(3) 1225-1231.

29. Manning EJ. Paratuberculosis in Captive and Free-Ranging Wildlife. The Veterinary clinics of North America. Food animal practice. 2011;27(3) 621-630.

30. Stehman S. Paratuberculosis in Small Ruminants, Deer, and South American Camelids. Veterinary Clinics of North America-Food Animal Practice. 1996;12(2) 441-455.

31. Committee on Diagnosis and Control of Johne's Disease NRC. Diagnosis and Control of Johne's Disease. Washington The National Academies Press; 2003. Available from: http://www.nap.edu/openbook.php?record_id=10625.

32. Álvarez J, de Juan L, Briones V, Romero B, Aranaz A, Fernández-Garayzábal JF, Mateos A. Mycobacterium avium subspecies paratuberculosis in fallow deer and wild boar in Spain. Veterinary Record. 2005;156(7) 212-213.

33. Rideout A, Brown S, Davis W, Gay J, Giannella R, Hines II M, Hueston W, Hutchinson L. Diagnosis and Control of Johne's Disease. Washington: The National Academies Press Washington; 2003.

34. Whittington RJ, Sergeant ESG. Progress Towards Understanding the Spread, Detection and Control of Mycobacterium avium subsp para-tuberculosis in Animal Populations. Australian Veterinary Journal. 2001;79(4) 267-278.

35. Coelho A. Estudo Epidemiológico da Paratuberculose Ovina na Região de Trás-os-Montes e Alto Douro. Vila Real: University of Trás-os-Montes and Alto Douro; 2006.

36. Mackintosh C, de Lisle G, Collins D, Griffin J. Mycobacterial Diseases of Deer. New Zealand Veterinary Journal. 2004;52(4) 163-174.

37. Reyes-Garcia R, Pérez-de-la-Lastra JM, Vicente J, Ruiz-Fons F, Garrido JM, Gortázar C. Large-Scale ELISA Testing of Spanish Red Deer for Paratuberculosis. Veterinary Immunology and Immunopathology. 2008;124(1-2) 75-81.

38. de Lisle GW, Yates GF, Collins DM. Paratuberculosis in Farmed Deer: Case Reports and DNA Characterization of Isolates of Mycobacterium paratuberculosis. Journal of Veterinary Diagnostic Investigation. 1993;5(4) 567-571.

39. de Lisle G, Yates GF, Montgomery H. The Emergence of Mycobacterium paratuberculosis in Farmed Deer in New Zealand - a Review of 619 Cases. New Zealand Veterinary Journal. 2003;51(2) 58-62.

40. Balseiro A, García Marín JF, Solano P, Garrido JM, Prieto JM. Histopathological Classification of Lesions Observed in Natural Cases of Paratuberculosis in Free-ranging Fallow Deer (Dama dama). Journal of Comparative Pathology. 2008;138(4) 180-188.

41. Matos A, Figueira L, Martins M, Matos M, Andrade S, Álvares S, Mendes A, Sousa N, Coelho A, Pinto M, editors. Renal Lesions in Deer (Cervus elaphus) - Mycobacterium avium subsp. paratuberculosis Involvelment. 30th Meeting of the European Society of Veterinary Pathology; 2012 September 5th to 8th Léon,Spain.

42. de Lisle G, Joyce MA, Yates GF, Wards BJ, Hoyle FP. Mycobacterium avium Infection in a Farmed Deer Herd. New Zealand Veterinary Journal. 1995;43(1) 1-3.

43. Griffin J. The aetiology of tuberculosis and mycobacterial diseases in farmed deer. Irish Veterinary Journal. 1988;42(1) 23-26.

44. Machackova-Kopecna M, Bartos M, Straka M, Ludvik V, Svastova P, Alvarez J, Lamka J, Trcka I, Treml F, Parmova I, Pavlik I. Paratuberculosis and avian tuberculosis infections in one red deer farm studied by IS900 and IS901 RFLP analysis. Veterinary Microbiology. 2005;105(3-4) 261-268.

45. Crawford GC, Ziccardi MH, Gonzales BJ, Woods LM, Fischer JK, Manning EJB, Mazet JAK. Mycobacterium avium subspecies paratuberculosis and Mycobacterium avium subsp. avium Infections in a Tule Elk (Cervus elaphus nannodes) Herd. Journal of Wildlife Diseases. 2006;42(4) 715-723.

46. Beard PM, Daniels MJ, Henderson D, Pirie A, Rudge K, Buxton D, Rhind S, Greig A, Hutchings MR, McKendrick I, Stevenson K, Sharp JM. Paratuberculosis Infection of Nonruminant Wildlife in Scotland. Journal of Clinical Microbiology. 2001;39(4) 1517-1521.

47. Corn JL, Manning EJB, Sreevatsan S, Fischer JR. Isolation of Mycobacterium avium subsp. paratuberculosis from Free-Ranging Birds and Mammals on Livestock Premises. Applied and Environmental Microbiology. 2005;71(11) 6963-6967.

48. Deutz A, Spergser J, Wagner P, Rosengarten R, Köfer J. Mycobacterium avium subsp. paratuberculosis in wild animal species and cattle in Styria/Austria. Berliner und Munchener Tierarztliche Wochenschrift. 2005;118(7-8) 314-320.

49. Machackova M, Matlova L, Lamka J, Smolik J, Melicharek I, Hanzlikova M, Docekal J, Cvetnic Z, Nagy G, Lipiec M, Ocepec M, Pavlik I. Wild boar (Sus scrofa) as a Possible Vector of Mycobacterial Infections: Review of Literature and Critical Analysis of Data from Central Europe Between 1983 to 2001. Veterinarni Medicina. 2003;48(3) 51-65

50. Cousins DV, Williams SN, Hope A, Eamens GJ. DNA Fingerprinting of Australian Isolates of Mycobacterium avium subsp paratuberculosis using IS900 RFLP. Australian Veterinary Journal. 2000;78(3) 184-190.

51. Kopecna M, Ondrus S, Literak I, Klimes J, Horvathova A, Moravkova M, Bartos M, Trcka I, Pavlik I. Detection of Mycobacterium avium subsp. paratuberculosis in Two Brown Bears in the Central European Carpathians. Journal of Wildlife Diseases. 2006;42(3) 691-695.

52. McClure HM, Chiodini RJ, Anderson DC, Swenson RB, Thayer WR, Coutu JA. Mycobacterium paratuberculosis Infection in a Colony of Stumptail Macaques (Macaca arctoides). Journal of Infectious Diseases. 1987;155(5) 1011-1019.

53. Zwick LS, Walsh TF, Barbiers R, Collins MT, Kinsel MJ, Murnane RD. Paratuberculosis in a Mandrill (Papio sphinx). Journal of Veterinary Diagnostic Investigation. 2002;14(4) 326-328.

54. Beard PM, Rhind SM, Buxton D, Daniels MJ, Henderson D, Pirie A, Rudge K, Greig A, Hutchings MR, Stevenson K, Sharp JM. Natural Paratuberculosis Infection in Rabbits in Scotland. Journal of Comparative Pathology. 2001;124(4) 290-299.

55. Beard RM, Henderson D, Daniels MJ, Pirie A, Buxton D, Greig A, Hutchings MR, McKendrick I, Rhind S, Stevenson K, Sharp JM. Evidence of Paratuberculosis in Fox (Vulpes vulpes) and Stoat (Mustela erminea). Veterinary Record. 1999;145(21) 612-613.

56. Florou M, Leontides L, Kostoulas P, Billinis C, Sofia M, Kyriazakis I, Lykotrafitis F. Isolation of Mycobacterium avium subspecies paratuberculosis from Non-Ruminant Wildlife Living in the Sheds and on the Pastures of Greek Sheep and Goats. Epidemiology and Infection. 2008;136(5) 644-652.

57. Nugent G, Whitford EJ, Hunnam JC, Wilson PR, Cross ML, de Lisle GW. Mycobacterium avium subsp. paratuberculosis Infection in Wildlife on Three Deer Farms with a History of Johne's Disease. New Zealand Veterinary Journal. 2011;59(6) 293-298.

58. Matos A, Figueira L, Martins M, Matos M, Álvares S, Pinto M, Coelho A. Disseminated Mycobacterium avium subsp. paratuberculosis Infection in Two Wild Eurasian Otters (Lutra lutra L.) from Portugal. Journal of Zoo and Wildlife Medicine (in press). 2012.

59. Matos A, Figueira L, Martins M, Matos M, Andrade S, Álvares S, Mendes A, Sousa N, Coelho A, Pinto M, editors. Granulomatous Lesions and Mycobacterium avium subsp. paratuberculosis in Portuguese Wild Boars (Sus scrofa).. 30th Meeting of the European Society of Veterinary Pathology; 2012 September 5th to 8th Léon,Spain.

60. Trcka I, Lamka J, Kopecna M, Beran V, Parmova I, Pavlik I. Mycobacteria in Wild Boar (Sus scrofa) in the Czech Republic. VETERINARSKI ARHIV. 2006;76(Supplement) S27-S32.

61. Garrido JM, Vicente J, Carrasco-García R, Galindo RC, Minguijón E, Ballesteros C, Aranaz A, Romero B, Sevilla I, Juste R, de la Fuente J, Gortazar C. Experimental Infection of Eurasian Wild Boar with Mycobacterium avium subsp. avium. Veterinary Microbiology. 2010;144(1-2) 240-245.

62. Lara GHB, Ribeiro MrG, Leite CQF, Paes AC, Guazzelli A, Silva AVd, Santos ACB, Listoni FJP. Occurrence of Mycobacterium spp. and other Pathogens in Lymph nodes of Slaughtered Swine and Wild Boars (Sus scrofa). Research in Veterinary Science. 2011;90(2) 185-188.

63. Cvetnić Ž, Špičić S, Tončić J, Račić I, Duvnjak S, Zdelar-Tuk M. Mycobacterium avium subsp. hominissuis in Wild Boar (Sus scrofa) in the Republic of Croatia. Veterinarinarski Arhiv. 2011;81(1) 67-76.

64. Sah R, Singh S, Arya S. Tuberculosis in some captive zoo birds: case records. Indian Journal of Veterinary Pathology. 1985;9(1) 84-87.

65. Dvorska L, Matlova L, Ayele WY, Fischer OA, Amemori T, Weston RT, Alvarez J, Beran V, Moravkova M, Pavlik I. Avian Tuberculosis in Naturally Infected Captive Water Birds of the Ardeideae and Threskiornithidae Families Studied by Serotyping, IS901 RFLP Typing, and Virulence for Poultry. Veterinary Microbiology. 2007;119(2-4) 366-374.

66. Heatley JJ, Mitchell MM, Roy A, Cho DY, Williams DL, Tully TN. Disseminated Mycobacteriosis in a Bald Eagle (Haliaeetus leucocephalus). Journal of Avian Medicine and Surgery. 2007;21(3) 201-209.

67. Dhama K, Mahendran M, Tomar S. Pathogens Transmitted by Migratory Birds: Threat Perceptions to Poultry Health and Production International Journal of Poultry Science. 2008 7(6) 516-525.

68. Tell L, Woods L, Cromie R. Mycobacteriosis in Birds. Review Science and Technology Office Internationale des Epizooties. 2001;20(1) 180-203.

69. Fulton RM, Thoen CO. Tuberculosis In: Saif YM (ed.) Diseases of Poultry. Iowa: Iowa State University Press; 2003. p. 836-844.

70. Pocknell AM, Miller BJ, Neufeld JL, Grahn BH. Conjunctival Mycobacteriosis in Two Emus (Dromaius novaehollandiae). Veterinary Pathology. 1996;33(3) 346-348.

71. Lairmore M, Spraker T, Jones R. Two Cases of Tuberculosis in Raptors in Colorado. Journal of Wildlife Diseases. 1985;2154-57.

72. Millán J, Negre N, Castellanos E, Juan Ld, Mateos A, Parpal L, Aranaz A. Avian mycobacteriosis in free-living raptors in Majorca Island, Spain. 2010;39(1) 1-6.

73. Miranda C, Matos M, Pires I, Correia-Neves M, Ribeiro P, Ã⊠lvares S, Vieira-Pinto M, Coelho AC. Diagnosis of Mycobacterium avium Complex in Granulomatous Lymphadenitis in Slaughtered Domestic Pigs. Journal of Comparative Pathology. 2012; doi: 10.1016/j.jcpa.2012.05.005. http://www.sciencedirect.com/science/article/pii/S0021997512000849.

74. OIE. Avian tuberculosis 2010. Available from: http://www.oie.int/en/international-standard-setting/terrestrial-> manual/access-online.

75. Aranaz A, Liébana E, Mateos A, Dominguez L. Laboratory Diagnosis of Avian Mycobacteriosis. Seminars in Avian and Exotic Pet Medicine. 1997;6(1) 9-17.

76. Altman RB, Clubb SL, Dorrestein GM, Quesenberry K. Avian Medicine and Surgery1997.

77. Fowler M. Zoo and Wild Animal Medicine Current Therapy 3. Philadelphia: W.B Saunders Company; 1993.

78. Tell LA, Ferrell ST, Gibbons PM. Avian Mycobacteriosis in Free-Living Raptors in California: 6 Cases (1997-2001). Journal of Avian Medicine and Surgery. 2004;18(1) 30-40.

79. Chebez J, Aguilar R. Order Falconiformes (Hawks, Eagles, Falcons, Vultures): Infectious Diseases: Avian Mycobacteriosis. In: Fowler ME (ed.) Biology, Medicine, and Surgery of South American Wild Animals. Iowa: Iowa State University Press; 2001. p. 115-124.

80. Soler D, Brieva C, Ribón W. Mycobacteriosis in Wild Birds : the Potential risk of Disseminating a Little-known Infectious Disease. Revista de Salud Pública. 2009;11(1) 134-144.

81. Pavlik I, Matlova L, Bartl J, Svastova P, Dvorska L, Whitlock R. Parallel Faecal and Organ Mycobacterium avium subsp. paratuberculosis Culture of Different Productivity Types of Cattle. Veterinary Microbiology. 2000;77(3-4) 309-324.

82. Tell LA, Foley J, Needham ML, Walker RL. Diagnosis of Avian Mycobacteriosis: Comparison of Culture, Acid-Fast Stains, and Polymerase Chain Reaction for the Identification of Mycobacterium avium in Experimentally Inoculated Japanese Quail (Coturnix coturnix japonica). Avian Diseases. 2003;47(2) 444-452.

83. Tell LA, Leutenegger CM, Scott Larsen R, Agnew DW, Keener L, Needham ML, Rideout BA. Real-Time Polymerase Chain Reaction Testing for the Detection of Mycobacterium genavense and Mycobacterium avium Complex Species in Avian Samples. Avian Diseases. 2003;47(4) 1406-1415.

84. Timms VJ, Gehringer MM, Mitchell HM, Daskalopoulos G, Neilan BA. How Accurately can we Detect Mycobacterium avium subsp. paratuberculosis Infection? Journal of Microbiological Methods. 2011;85(1) 1-8.

85. Whipple DL, Callihan DR, Jarnagin JL. Cultivation of Mycobacterium Paratuberculosis from Bovine Fecal Specimens and a Suggested Standardized Procedure. Journal of Veterinary Diagnostic Investigation. 1991;3(4) 368-373.

86. Reddacliff LA, Marsh IB, Fell SA, Austin SL, Whittington RJ. Isolation of Mycobacterium avium subspecies paratuberculosis from Muscle and Peripheral Lymph nodes Using Acid-pepsin Digest Prior to BACTEC Culture. Veterinary Microbiology. 2010;145(1-2) 122-128.

87. Whitlock RH, Wells SJ, Sweeney RW, Van Tiem J. ELISA and Fecal Culture for Paratuberculosis (Johne's disease): Sensitivity and Specificity of Each Method. Veterinary Microbiology. 2000;77(3-4) 387-398.

88. Katoch VM. Infections Due to Non-Tuberculous Mycobacteria (NTM). Indian Journal of Medical Research. 2004;120(1) 290-304.

89. Realini L, De Ridder K, Palomino J-C, Hirschel B, Portaels F. Microaerophilic Conditions Promote Growth of Mycobacterium genavense. Journal of Clinical Microbiology. 1998;36(9) 2565-2570.

90. Realini L, Van Der Stuyft P, De Ridder K, Hirschel B, Portaels F. Inhibitory Effects of Polyoxyethylene Stearate, PANTA, and Neutral pH on Growth of Mycobacterium genavense in BACTEC Primary Cultures. Journal of Clinical Microbiology. 1997;35(11) 2791-2794.

91. Realini L, De Ridder K, Hirschel B, Portaels Fo. Blood and Charcoal Added to Acidified Agar Media Promote the Growth of Mycobacterium genavense. Diagnostic Microbiology and Infectious Disease. 1999;34(1) 45-50.

92. Kulski JK, Khinsoe C, Pryce T, Christiansen K. Use of a Multiplex PCR to Detect and Identify Mycobacterium avium and M. intracellulare in Blood Culture Fluids of AIDS Patients. Journal of Clinical Microbiology. 1995;33(3) 668-674.

93. Katoch V, Sharma V. Advances in the Diagnosis of Mycobacterial Diseases. Indian Journal of Medical Microbiology. 1997;15(2) 49-56.

94. Coelho AC, Pinto ML, Silva S, Coelho AM, Rodrigues J, Juste RA. Seroprevalence of Ovine Paratuberculosis Infection in the Northeast of Portugal. Small Ruminant Research. 2007;71(1-3) 298-303.

95. Fernández JG, Fernández-de-Mera I, Reyes LE, Ferreras MC, Pérez V, Gortazar C, Fernández M, García-Marín JF. Comparison of Three Immunological Diagnostic Tests for the Detection of Avian Tuberculosis in Naturally Infected Red Deer (Cervus elaphus). Journal of Veterinary Diagnostic Investigation. 2009;21(1) 102-107.

96. Rozanska M. Preparation of Antigen for Whole Blood Rapid Agglutination Test and its Specificity for Diagnosis of Avian Tuberculosis. Bulletin of Veterinary Institute Pulawy. 1965;9(1) 20-25.

97. Griffin A, Newton AL, Aronson LR, Brown DC, Hess RS. Disseminated Mycobacterium avium Complex Infection Following Renal Transplantation in a Cat. Journal of the American Veterinary Medical Association. 2003;222(8) 1097-1101.

98. Monaghan ML, Doherty ML, Collins JD, Kazda JF, Quinn PJ. The Tuberculin Test. Veterinary Microbiology. 1994;40(1-2) 111-124.

99. Palmer MV, Waters WR, Whipple DL, Slaughter RE, Jones SL. Evaluation of an in Vitro Blood-Based Assay to Detect Production of Interferon-Υ by Mycobacterium bovis—Infected White-Tailed Deer (Odocoileus Virginianus) Journal of Veterinary Diagnostic Investigation. 2004;16(1) 17-21.

100. Waters WR, Palmer MV, Thacker TC, Orloski K, Nol P, Harrington NP, Olsen SC, Nonnecke BJ. Blood Culture and Stimulation Conditions for the Diagnosis of Tuberculosis in Cervids by the Cervigam Assay. Veterinary Record. 2008;162(7) 203-208.

101. Hosek J, Svastova P, Moravkova M, Pavlik I, Bartos M. Methods of Mycobacterial DNA Isolation from Different Biological Material: A Review. Veterinarni Medicina. 2006;51(5) 180-192.

102. Hurley SS, Splitter GA, Welch RA. Rapid Lysis Technique for Mycobacterial Species. Journal of Clinical Microbiology. 1987;25(11) 2227-2229.

103. Odumeru J, Gao A, Chen S, Raymond M, Mutharia L. Use of the Bead Beater for Preparation of Mycobacterium paratuberculosis Template DNA in Milk. The Canadian Journal of Veterinary Research. 2001;65(4) 201-205.

104. Lanigan MD, Vaughan JA, Shiell BJ, Beddome GJ, Michalski WP. Mycobacterial Proteome Extraction: Comparison of Disruption Methods. PROTEOMICS. 2004;4(4) 1094-1100.

105. Logar K, Kopinc R, Bandelj P, Staric J, Lapanje A, Ocepek M. Evaluation of Combined High-Efficiency DNA Extraction and Real-Time PCR for Detection of Mycobacterium avium subsp. paratuberculosis in Subclinically Infected Dairy Cattle: Comparison with Faecal Culture, Milk Real-Time PCR and Milk ELISA. BMC Veterinary Research. 2012; 8(1):49. http://www.biomedcentral.com/1746-6148/8/49.

106. Zecconi A, A M, Piccinini R, Robbi C, editors. A Comparison of Six Different Protocols to Extract M. paratuberculosis DNA from Bovine Faeces. 7th International Colloquium on Paratuberculosis; 2003; Bilbao-Spain.

107. Chui LW, King R, Lu P, Manninen K, Sim J. Evaluation of Four DNA Extraction Methods for the Detection of Mycobacterium avium subsp. paratuberculosis by Polymerase Chain Reaction. Diagnostic Microbiology and Infectious Disease. 2004;48(1) 39-45.

108. Moravkova M, Hlozek P, Beran V, Pavlik I, Preziuso S, Cuteri V, Bartos M. Strategy for the Detection and Differentiation of Mycobacterium avium Species in Isolates and Heavily Infected Tissues. Research in Veterinary Science. 2008;85(2) 257-264.

109. Slana I, Pribylova R, Kralova A, Pavlik I. Persistence of Mycobacterium avium subsp. paratuberculosis at a Farm-Scale Biogas Plant Supplied with Manure from Paratuberculosis-Affected Dairy Cattle. Applied and Environmental Microbiology. 2011;77(9) 3115-3119.

110. Saiki R, Scharf S, Faloona F, Mullis K, Horn G, Erlich H, Arnheim N. Enzymatic Amplification of Beta-globin Genomic Sequences and Restriction Site Analysis for Diagnosis of Sickle Cell Anemia. Science. 1985;230(4732) 1350-1354.

111. Lo YMD, Chiu RWK, Chan KCA, editors. Clinical Applications of PCR. Second Edition ed. New Jersey: Humana Press; 2006.

112. Lachnik J, Ackermann B, Bohrssen A, Maass S, Diephaus C, Puncken A, Stermann M, Bange F-C. Rapid-Cycle PCR and Fluorimetry for Detection of Mycobacteria. Journal of Clinical Microbiology. 2002;40(9) 3364-3373.

113. Devallois A, Picardeau M, Goh KS, Sola C, Vincent V, Rastogi N. Comparative Evaluation of PCR and Commercial DNA Probes for Detection and Identification to Species Level of Mycobacterium avium and Mycobacterium intracellulare. Journal of Clinical Microbiology. 1996;34(11) 2756-2759.

114. Schweickert B, Goldenberg O, Richter E, Göbel UB, Petrich A, Buchholz P, Moter A. Occurrence and Clinical Relevance of Mycobacterium chimaera sp. nov., Germany. Emerging Infectious Diseases. 2008;14(9) 1443-1446.

115. Green EP, Tizard MLV, Moss MT, Thompson J, Winterbourne DJ, McFadden JJ, Hermon-Taylor J. Sequence and Characteristics or IS900, an Insertion Element Identified in a Human Crohn's Disease Isolate or Mycobacterium paratuberculosis. Nucleic Acids Research. 1989;17(22) 9063-9073.

116. Green E, Tizard M, Moss M, Thompson J, Winterbourne D, Mc Fadden J, Hermon-Taylor J. Sequence and Characteristics of IS900, an Insertion Element Identified in a Human Crohn's Disease Isolate of Mycobacterium paratuberculosis. Nucleic Acids Research. 1989;17(22) 9063 - 9073.

117. Kunze ZM, Wall S, Appelberg R, Silva MT, Portaels F, McFadden JJ. IS901, A New Member of a Widespread Class of Atypical Insertion Sequences, is Associated with Pathogenicity in Mycobacterium avium. Molecular Microbiology. 1991;5(9) 2265-2272.

118. Guerrero C, Bernasconi C, Burki D, Bodmer T, Telenti A. A Novel Insertion Element from Mycobacterium avium, IS1245, is a Specific Target for Analysis of Strain Relatedness. Journal of Clinical Microbiology. 1995;33(2) 304-307.

119. Roiz MP, Palenque E, Guerrero C, Garcia MJ. Use of Restriction Fragment Length Polymorphism as a Genetic Marker for Typing Mycobacterium avium strains. Journal of Clinical Microbiology. 1995;33(5) 1389-1391.

120. Bartos M, Hlozek P, Svastova P, Dvorska L, Bull T, Matlova L, Parmova I, Kuhn I, Stubbs J, Moravkova M, Kintr J, Beran V, Melicharek I, Ocepek M, Pavlik I. Identification of Members of Mycobacterium avium species by Accu-Probes, Serotyping, and Single IS900, IS901, IS1245 and IS901-Flanking Region PCR with Internal Standards. Journal of Microbiological Methods. 2006;64(3) 333-345.

121. Collins D, Gabric D, de Lisle G. Identification of a Repetitive DNA Sequence Specific to Mycobacterium paratuberculosis. FEMS Microbiology Letters. 1989;51(1) 175 - 178.

122. Li L, Bannantine JP, Zhang Q, Amonsin A, May BJ, Alt D, Banerji N, Kanjilal S, Kapur V. The Complete Genome Sequence of Mycobacterium avium subspecies paratuberculosis. Proceedings of the National Academy of Sciences of the United States of America. 2005;102(35) 12344-12349.

123. Cousins DV, Whittington R, Marsh I, Masters A, Evans RJ, Kluver P. Mycobacteria Distinct from Mycobacterium avium subsp. paratuberculosis Isolated from the Faeces of Ruminants Possess IS 900 -like Sequences Detectable by IS 900 Polymerase Chain Reaction: Implications for Diagnosis. Molecular and Cellular Probes. 1999;13(6) 431-442.

124. Englund S, Bölske G, Johansson K-E. An IS900-like Sequence Found in a Mycobacterium sp. Other Than Mycobacterium avium subsp. paratuberculosis. FEMS Microbiology Letters. 2002;209(2) 267-271.

125. Vansnick E, de Rijk P, Vercammen F, Geysen D, Rigouts L, Portaels F. Newly Developed Primers for the Detection of Mycobacterium avium subspecies paratuberculosis. Veterinary Microbiology. 2004;100(3-4) 197-204.

126. Stabel JR, Wells SJ, Wagner BA. Relationships Between Fecal Culture, ELISA, and Bulk Tank Milk Test Results for Johne's Disease in US Dairy Herds. Journal of Dairy Science. 2002;85(3) 525-531.

127. Slana I, Kralik P, Kralova A, Pavlik I. On-farm Spread of Mycobacterium avium subsp. paratuberculosis in Raw Milk Studied by IS900 and F57 Competitive Real Time Quantitative PCR and Culture Examination. International Journal of Food Microbiology. 2008;128(2) 250 - 257.

128. Sanna E, Woodall CJ, Watt NJ, Clarke CJ, Pittau M, Leoni A, Nieddu AM. In situ-PCR for the Detection of Mycobacterium paratuberculosis DNA in Paraffin-embedded Tissues. European Journal of Histochemistry. 2000;44(2) 179-184.

129. Corti S, Stephan R. Detection of Mycobacterium avium subspecies paratuberculosis Specific IS900 Insertion Sequences in Bulk-Tank Milk Samples Obtained from Different Regions throughout Switzerland. BMC Microbiology. 2002;2(1) 15.

130. Doosti A, Moshkelani S. Application of IS900 Nested-PCR for Detection of Mycobacterium avium subsp. paratuberculosis Directly from Faecal Specimens. Bulgarian Journal of Veterinary Medicine. 2010;13(2) 92-97.

131. Rajeev S, Zhang Y, Sreevatsan S, Motiwala AS, Byrum B. Evaluation of Multiple Genomic Targets for Identification and Confirmation of Mycobacterium avium subsp. paratuberculosis Isolates Using Real-Time PCR. Veterinary Microbiology. 2005;105(3-4) 215-221.

132. Pribylova R, Slana I, Lamka J, Babak V, Hruska K, Pavlik I. Mycobacterium avium subsp. paratuberculosis in a Mouflon Herd without Clinical Symptoms Monitored Using IS900 Real-Time PCR: A Case Report. Veterinarni Medicina. 2010;55(12) 625-630.

133. Salgado M, Herthnek D, Bölske G, Leiva S, Kruze J. First Isolation of Mycobacterium avium subsp. paratuberculosis from Wild Guanacos (Lama Guanicoe) on Tierra del Fuego Island. Journal of Wildlife Diseases. 2009;45(2) 295-301.

134. Strommenger B, Stevenson K, Gerlach G-F. Isolation and Diagnostic Potential of ISMav2, a Novel Insertion Sequence-like Element from Mycobacterium avium subspecies paratuberculosis. FEMS Microbiology Letters. 2001;196(1) 31-37.

135. Poupart P, Coene M, Van Heuverswyn H, Cocito C. Preparation of a Specific RNA Probe for Detection of Mycobacterium paratuberculosis and Diagnosis of Johne's Disease. Journal of Clinical Microbiology. 1993;31(6) 1601-1605.

136. Stabel JR, Bannantine JP. Development of a Nested PCR Method Targeting a Unique Multicopy Element, ISMap02, for Detection of Mycobacterium avium subsp. paratuberculosis in Fecal Samples. Journal of Clinical Microbiology. 2005;43(9) 4744-4750.

137. Bannantine JP, Baechler E, Zhang Q, Li L, Kapur V. Genome Scale Comparison of Mycobacterium avium subsp. paratuberculosis with Mycobacterium avium subsp. avium Reveals Potential Diagnostic Sequences. Journal of Clinical Microbiology. 2002;40(4) 1303-1310.

138. Möbius P, Hotzel H, Raßbach A, Köhler H. Comparison of 13 Single-Round and Nested PCR Assays Targeting IS900, ISMav2, f57 and locus 255 for Detection of Mycobacterium avium subsp. paratuberculosis. Veterinary Microbiology. 2008;126(4) 324-333.

139. Englund S, Ballagi-Pordány A, Bölske G, Johansson K-E. Single PCR and Nested PCR with a Mimic Molecule for Detection of Mycobacterium avium subsp. paratuberculosis. Diagnostic Microbiology and Infectious Disease. 1999;33(3) 163-171.

140. Doran TJ, Davies JK, Radford AJ, Hodgson ALM. Putative Functional Domain within ORF2 on the Mycobacterium Insertion Sequences IS900 and IS902. Immunology and Cell Biology. 1994;72(5) 427-434.

141. Devallois A, Rastogi N. Computer-Assisted Analysis of Mycobacterium avium Fingerprints Using Insertion Elements IS1245 and IS1311 in a Caribbean Setting. Research in Microbiology. 1997;148(8) 703-713.

142. Collins DM, Cavaignac S, de Lisle GW. Use of four DNA Insertion Sequences to Characterize Strains of the Mycobacterium avium complex isolated from animals. Molecular and Cellular Probes. 1997;11(5) 373-380.

143. van Soolingen D, Bauer J, Ritacco V, Leão SC, Pavlik I, Vincent V, Rastogi N, Gori A, Bodmer T, Garzelli C, Garcia MJ. IS1245 Restriction Fragment Length Polymorphism Typing of Mycobacterium avium Isolates: Proposal for Standardization. Journal of Clinical Microbiology. 1998;36(10) 3051-3054.

144. Beggs ML, Stevanova R, Eisenach KD. Species Identification of Mycobacterium avium Complex Isolates by a Variety of Molecular Techniques. Journal of Clinical Microbiology. 2000;38(2) 508-512.

145. Wilton S, Cousins D. Detection and Identification of Multiple Mycobacterial Pathogens by DNA Amplification in a Single Tube. Genome Research. 1992;1(4) 269-273.

146. Godfroid J, Delcorps C, Irenge LM, Walravens K, Marché S, Gala J-L. Definitive Differentiation between Single and Mixed Mycobacterial Infections in Red Deer (Cervus elaphus) by a Combination of Duplex Amplification of p34 and f57 Sequences and Hpy188I Enzymatic Restriction of Duplex Amplicons. Journal of Clinical Microbiology. 2005;43(9) 4640-4648.

147. Semret M, Turenne CY, de Haas P, Collins DM, Behr MA. Differentiating Host-Associated Variants of Mycobacterium avium by PCR for Detection of Large Sequence Polymorphisms. Journal of Clinical Microbiology. 2006;44(3) 881-887.

148. Dvorská L, Bartoš M, Martin G, Erler W, Pavlík I. Strategies for Differentiation, Identification and Typing of Medically Important Species of Mycobacteria by Molecular Methods. Veterinarni Medicina. 2001;46(11-12) 309-328.

149. Nagai R, Takewaki S, Wada A, Okuzumi K, Tobita A, Ohkubo A. Development of Rapid Detection Method for Mycobacteria using PCR. Journal of Medical Technology (In Japanese). 1990;38(1) 1247-1252.

150. Cirillo JD, Falkow S, Tompkins LS, Bermudez LE. Interaction of Mycobacterium avium with Environmental Amoebae Enhances Virulence. Infection and Immunity. 1997;65(9) 3759-3767.

151. Arasteh KN, Cordes C, Ewers M, Simon V, Dietz E, Futh UM, Brockmeyer NH, L'Age MP. HIV-Related Nontuberculous Mycobacterial Infection: Incidence, Survival Analysis and Associated Risk Factors. European journal of medical research. 2000;5(10) 424-430.

152. Nightingale SD, Byrd LT, Southern PM, Jockusch JD, Cal SX, Wynne BA. Incidence of Mycobacterium avium-intracellulare Complex Bacteremia in Human Immunodeficiency Virus-Positive Patients. Journal of Infectious Diseases. 1992;165(6) 1082-1085.

153. Salte T, Pathak S, Wentzel-Larsen T, Åsjö B. Increased Intracellular Growth of Mycobacterium avium in HIV-1 Exposed Monocyte-Derived Dendritic Cells. Microbes and Infection. 2011;13(3) 276-283.

154. Wallace JM, Hannah JB. Mycobacterium avium Complex Infection in Patients with the Acquired Immunodeficiency Syndrome. A Clinicopathologic Study. CHEST Journal. 1988;93(5) 926-932.

155. Crowe SM, Carlin JB, Stewart KI, Lucas CR, Hoy JF. Predictive Value of CD4 Lymphocyte Numbers for the Development of Opportunistic Infections and Malignancies in HIV-Infected Persons. Journal of acquired immune deficiency syndromes. 1991;4(8) 770-776.

156. Bodle E, Cunningham J, Della-Latta P, Schluger N, Saiman L. Epidemiology of Nontuberculous Mycobacteria in Patients without HIV Infection. Emerging Infectious Diseases. 2008;14(3) 390-396.

157. Henry MT, Inamdar L, O'Riordain D, Schweiger M, Watson JP. Nontuberculous Mycobacteria in non-HIV Patients: Epidemiology, Treatment and Response. European Respiratory Journal. 2004;23(5) 741-746.

158. Maugein J, Dailloux M, Carbonnelle B, Vincent V, Grosset J. Sentinel-site Surveillance of Mycobacterium avium Complex Pulmonary Disease. European Respiratory Journal. 2005;26(6) 1092-1096.

159. Falkinham JI. Nontuberculous mycobacteria from household plumbing of patients with nontuberculous mycobacteria disease. Emerging Infectious Diseases. 2011;17(3) 419-424.

160. Koh W-J, Lee JH, Kwon YS, Lee KS, Suh GY, Chung MP, Kim H, Kwon OJ. Prevalence of Gastroesophageal Reflux Disease in Patients with Nontuberculous Mycobacterial Lung Disease*. CHEST Journal. 2007;131(6) 1825-1830.

161. Hernández-Garduño E, Elwood K. Nontuberculous Mycobacteria in Tap Water. Emerging Infectious Diseases. 2012;18(2) 353.

162. Thegerström J, Romanus V, Friman V, Brudin L, Haemig P, Olsen B. Mycobacterium avium lymphadenopathy among children. Emerging Infectious Diseases. 2008;14(4) 661-663.

163. Jindal N, Devi B, Aggarwal A. Mycobacterial Cervical Lymphadenitis in Childhood. Indian Journal of Medical Sciences. 2003;57(1) 12-15.

164. Primm TP, Lucero CA, Falkinham JO. Health Impacts of Environmental Mycobacteria. Clinical Microbiology Reviews. 2004;17(1) 98-106.

165. Bodmer T, Miltner E, Bermudez LE. Mycobacterium avium Resists Exposure to the Acidic Conditions of the Stomach. FEMS Microbiology Letters. 2000;182(1) 45-49.

166. Hoop RK. Public Health Implications of Epet Mycobacteriosis. Seminars in Avian and Exotic Pet Medicine. 1997;6(1) 3-8.

167. Suzuki AE, Inamine JM. Genetic Aspects of Drug Resistance in Mycobacterium avium. Research in Microbiology. 1994;145(3) 210-213.

168. Hellinger WC, Smilack JD, Greider JL, Alvarez S, Trigg SD, Brewer NS, Edson RS. Localized Soft-Tissue Infections with Mycobacterium avium / Mycobacterium intracellulare Complex in Immunocompetent Patients: Granulomatous Tenosynovitis of the Hand or Wrist. Clinical Infectious Diseases. 1995;21(1) 65-69.

169. Horsburgh CR, Selik RM. The Epidemiology of Disseminated Nontuberculous Mycobacterial Infection in the Acquired Immunodeficiency Syndrome (AIDS). American Journal of Respiratory and Critical Care Medicine. 1989;139(1) 4-7.

170. Modilevsky T, Sattler FR, Barnes PF. Mycobacterial Disease in Patients with Human Immunodeficiency Virus Infection. Archives of Internal Medicine. 1989;149(10) 2201-2205.

171. Hermon-Taylor J, Bull TJ, Sheridan JM, Cheng J, Stellakis ML, Sumar N. Causation of Crohn's Disease by Mycobacterium avium subspecies paratuberculosis. Canadian Journal of Gastroenterology. 2000;14(6) 521-539.

172. Bernstein CN, Blanchard JF, Rawsthorne P, Collins MT. Population-Based Case Control Study of Seroprevalence of Mycobacterium paratuberculosis in Patients with Crohn's Disease and Ulcerative Colitis. Journal of Clinical Microbiology. 2004;42(3) 1129-1135.

173. Grant IR. Zoonotic Potential of Mycobacterium avium ssp. paratuberculosis: The Current Position. Journal of Applied Microbiology. 2005;98(6) 1282-1293.

174. Wall S, Kunze ZM, Saboor S, Soufleri I, Seechurn P, Chiodini R, McFadden JJ. Identification of Spheroplast-like Agents Isolated from Tissues of patients with Crohn's Disease and Control Tissues by Polymerase Chain Reaction. Journal of Clinical Microbiology. 1993;31(5) 1241-1245.

175. Hines II ME, Styer EL. Preliminary Characterization of Chemically Generated Mycobacterium avium subsp. paratuberculosis Cell Wall Deficient Forms (Spheroplasts). Veterinary Microbiology. 2003;95(4) 247-258.

176. Sechi LA, Mura M, Tanda E, Lissia A, Fadda G, Zanetti S. Mycobacterium avium sub. paratuberculosis in Tissue samples of Crohn's Disease Patients. The new microbiologica. 2004;27(1) 75-77.

177. Bull TJ, McMinn EJ, Sidi-Boumedine K, Skull A, Durkin D, Neild P, Rhodes G, Pickup R, Hermon-Taylor J. Detection and Verification of Mycobacterium avium subsp. paratuberculosis in Fresh Ileocolonic Mucosal Biopsy Specimens from Individuals with and without Crohn's Disease. Journal of Clinical Microbiology. 2003;41(7) 2915-2923.

178. Naser SA, Ghobrial G, Romero C, Valentine JF. Culture of Mycobacterium avium subspecies paratuberculosis from the Blood of Patients with Crohn's Disease. The Lancet. 2004;364(9439) 1039-1044.

179. Bitti MLM, Masala S, Capasso F, Rapini N, Piccinini S, Angelini F, Pierantozzi A, Lidano R, Pietrosanti S, Paccagnini D, Sechi LA. Mycobacterium avium subsp. paratuberculosis in an Italian Cohort of Type 1 Diabetes Pediatric Patients. Clinical and Developmental Immunology. 2012;20121-5.

180. Naser SA, Collins MT, Crawford JT, Valentine JF. Culture of Mycobacterium avium subspecies paratuberculosis (MAP) from the Blood of Patients with Crohn's disease: A Follow-Up Blind Multi Center Investigation. The Open Inflammation Journal. 2009;2(1) 22-23.

181. Parrish NM, Radcliff RP, Brey BJ, Anderson JL, Clark DL, Koziczkowski JJ, Ko CG, Goldberg ND, Brinker DA, Carlson RA, Dick JD, Ellingson JLE. Absence of Mycobacterium avium subsp. paratuberculosis in Crohn's Patients. Inflammatory Bowel Diseases. 2009;15(4) 558-565.

182. Dow CT. Paratuberculosis and Type I Diabetes Is this the Trigger? Medical Hypotheses. 2006;67(4) 782-785.

183. D'Amore M, Lisi S, Sisto M, Cucci L, Dow CT. Molecular Identification of Mycobacterium avium subspecies paratuberculosis in an Italian Patient with Hashimoto's Thyroiditis and Melkersson-Rosenthal Syndrome. Journal of Medical Microbiology. 2010;59(1) 137-139.

184. Dow CT. Mycobacterium paratuberculosis and autism: Is this a trigger? Medical Hypotheses. 2011;77(6) 977-981.

185. Dow CT, Ellingson JLE. Detection of Mycobacterium avium ss. paratuberculosis in Blau Syndrome Tissues. Autoimmune Diseases. 2010;2010.

186. el-Zaatari FA, Naser SA, Markesich DC, Kalter DC, Engstand L, Graham DY. Identification of Mycobacterium avium complex in sarcoidosis. Journal of Clinical Microbiology. 1996;34(9) 2240-2245.

187. Oliveira-Filho JP, Monteiro LN, Delfiol DJZ, Sequeira JL, Amorim RM, Fabris VE, Del Piero F, Borges AS. Mycobacterium DNA Detection in Liver and Skin of a Horse with Generalized Sarcoidosis. Journal of Veterinary Diagnostic Investigation. 2012;24(3) 596-600.

188. Rook G, McCulloch J. HLA-DR4, Mycobacteria, Heat-Shock Proteins, and Rheumatoid Arthritis. Arthritis & Rheumatism. 1992;35(12) 1409-1412.

189. Mangiapan G, Hance A. Mycobacteria and Sarcoidosis: An Overview and Summary of Recent Molecular Biological Data. Sarcoidosis. 1995;12(1) 20-37.

190. Rosu V, Ahmed N, Paccagnini D, Pacifico A, Zanetti S, Sechi L. Mycobacterium avium subspecies paratuberculosis Is not Associated with Type-2 Diabetes Mellitus. Annals of Clinical Microbiology and Antimicrobials. 2008;7(1) 9.

191. Sechi LA, Paccagnini D, Salza S, Pacifico A, Ahmed N, Zanetti S. Mycobacterium avium Subspecies paratuberculosis Bacteremia in Type 1 Diabetes Mellitus: An Infectious Trigger? Clinical Infectious Diseases. 2008;46(1) 148-149.

192. Sechi LA, Rosu V, Pacifico A, Fadda G, Ahmed N, Zanetti S. Humoral Immune Responses of Type 1 Diabetes Patients to Mycobacterium avium subsp. paratuberculosis Lend Support to the Infectious Trigger Hypothesis. Clinical and Vaccine Immunology. 2008;15(2) 320-326.

193. Paccagnini D, Sieswerda L, Rosu V, Masala S, Pacifico A, Gazouli M, Ikonomopoulos J, Ahmed N, Zanetti S, Sechi LA. Linking Chronic Infection and Autoimmune Diseases: Mycobacterium avium Subspecies paratuberculosis,SLC11A1 Polymorphisms and Type-1 Diabetes Mellitus. PLoS ONE. 2009; 4(9):e7109. http://dx.doi.org/10.1371%2Fjournal.pone.0007109.

194. Rosu V, Ahmed N, Paccagnini D, Gerlach G, Fadda G, Hasnain SE, Zanetti S, Sechi LA. Specific Immunoassays Confirm Association of Mycobacterium avium Subsp. paratuberculosis with Type-1 but Not Type-2 Diabetes Mellitus. PLoS ONE. 2009; 4(2):e4386. http://dx.doi.org/10.1371%2Fjournal.pone.0004386.

195. Cossu A, Rosu V, Paccagnini D, Cossu D, Pacifico A, Sechi LA. MAP3738c and MptD are specific tags of Mycobacterium avium subsp. paratuberculosis infection in type I diabetes mellitus. Clinical Immunology. 2011;141(1) 49-57.

Chapter 5

Psittacosis

1. Introduction

Chlamydophila psittaci (Bacteria kingdom, Chlamydiae phylum, Chlamydiae class, Chlamydiales order, Chlamydiaceae family) is part of the genus *Chlamydophila*, where *Cp. abortus*, *Cp. caviae*, *Cp. felis*, *Cp. pecorum* and *Cp. pneumoniae* are the other five species of bacteria [1].

Avian chlamydiosis induced by this Gram-negative obligate intracellular bacteria [2] is traditionally known as ornithosis or psittacosis [3-5]. It is an infectious disease capable of infecting domestic and wild birds [6,7], being the Psittacidae family where most occurrences are reported [8].

Chlamydophila psittaci infects primarily birds [9], but mammals, including humans, are also susceptible of infection [10-11]. In fact, zoonotic status of this organism is largely described and emphasizes the scientific reports worldwide [12-15].

Chlamydophila psittaci can be found in bird feathers, excrements and blood, whether or not these animals are showing clinical signs of disease [16,17].

Psittacosis can be transmitted by vertical and horizontal via [2]. The agent is excreted on faeces and ingested from the food or inhaled via aerosols [13]. At the lungs of newly infected animals, the organism gets an infecting status becoming capable to replicate and causing clinical signs of disease [18,19].

There are three morphologically distinct forms of *Chlamydophila*:

- The elementary body, which is small, spherical, of about 0.2-0.3 mm in diameter;
- The reticular body, wider, of about 0.5-2.0 mm, which is able to replicate by binary division;
- And the intermediate body, with 0.3-2.0 mm in diameter, seen in infected host cells [18,20].

Parrots are often infected animals but they show no signs of disease unless they are stressed out [21], and thus can be a source of contamination to other birds and mammals, so as the man [3,4,22]. Infections in turkeys have been described long ago, with a mortality range of 5-40% without any treatment [23], and more recently in ducks, with a mortality of 30%, which was highlighted as an economic problem and health impairment [24]. The mortality rate in humans is low if treatment is appropriate. Therefore, setting up a quick prognosis is essential [20,23].

Clinical symptoms are very extensive in number and vary depending on the serotype of the bacteria and the animal affected. General infections may cause fever, anorexia, lethargy, diarrhoea and sometimes shock or even death. Chlamydiosis in psittacines is mostly chronic and cause conjunctivitis, enteritis, sacculitis, pneumonitis, hepatomegaly and droppings can range from green to yellow-green in colour [20]. Clinical signs in humans range from unapparent to severe systemic disease with interstitial pneumonia and encephalitis [12,20]. Signs of disease are headache, chills, malaise and myalgia with possible respiratory involvement. Infection of pigeons by *Chlamydophila* is vast and well reported [15]. These animals are a major spreader of the disease, and present clinical signs such as conjunctivitis, blepharitis and rhinitis [20]. *Chlamydophila psittaci* antibodies can be detected by several laboratory methodologies. The complement fixation test (CFT) is the most frequently used test [25,26]. Other serological tests such as PCR (polymerase chain reaction) and ELISA are used as well for its diagnosis [8,22,27].

Psittacosis or "parrot fever" was documented for first time in 1879, when Jakob Ritter described an epidemic and unusual pneumonia, associated with exposure to tropical birds in seven Switch individuals causing flu-like symptoms and pneumonia [28]. The term "psittacosis" (from the Latin word for parrot - *psittacus*) was firstly used by Morange, in 1895, when transmission of an infectious agent to humans from parrots was notorious [29-30].

Investigations of chlamydiosis began in 1907 when microorganisms within intracytoplasmic vacuoles in conjunctival scraping cells from humans with trachoma were found. Trachoma is a chronic infectious disease of the conjunctiva and cornea [18] a disease well known since ancient civilizations [31]. These organisms were named *Chlamydozoa*, from the characteristic shape of the mantle or "*chlamys*" in Greek [32].

A psittacosis outbreak occurred during the winters of 1929 and 1930 in Europe and in the United States. The causative agent of psittacosis was isolated from birds and infected humans and the source of contamination traced to parrots of the genus *Amazona*, originated in South America [33]. At the same time, a microorganism causing lymphogranuloma venereum (LGV) was isolated in humans [34]. Until then, it was believed avian psittacosis was restricted to *Psittaciformes* birds [18]. However, a number of studies demonstrated a much higher number of species concerned or potentially infected by this microorganism. In fact, Meyer and Eddie, in 1932, described a case of transmission of human psittacosis from domestic fowl [35] and Haagen and Mauer, six years later, reported an infection in fulmar (*Fulmarus glacialis*). Pinkerton and Swank, in 1940, proved the existence of this agent in domestic pigeons, as Wolins, in 1948, described the same disease in ducks [33]. Later studies of this matter enhanced the idea that psittacosis was not restricted to parrots, reporting infections in humans by contact with other affected birds [18,36].

Later, Everett and collaborators (1999), proposed a new classification, where the *Chlamydophila* genus would contain six species: *Chlamydophila pneumoniae, Chlamydophila pecorum, Chlamydophila abortus, Chlamydophila felis, Chlamydophila caviae* and *Chlamydophila psittaci* [1]. This taxonomic classification was accepted and is still used worldwide [17].

The aim of this study was to discuss phylogeny, epidemiology, clinical signs, pathology, diagnostic techniques, treatment, prevention and public health concerns in psittacosis with special attention due to *Chlamydophila psittaci* infection.

2. Phylogeny and biology of Chlamydiacea family

Bacteria kingdom consists of different phyla, including the Chlamydiae, holding the class with the same name. The order Chlamydiales belongs to the class Chlamydiae and the family Chlamydiaceae to the order described. The genus *Chlamydophila* belongs to the family Chlamydiaceae and accordingly with the National Center For Biotechnology Information Taxonomy Browser (www.ncbi.nlm.nih.gov), it has six species of bacteria [1]. The Chlamydiae genus contains three species: *C. trachomatis, C. suis* and *C. muridarum* [1].

In the genus *Chlamydophila, Chlamydophila abortus* is a bacterium whose disease is severe, especially in small ruminants [37], but it is also described as an important zoonotic disease [38-40].

Chlamydophila pneumoniae has been primarily described as an infection in humans but later has been reported in other animals as well, such as mammals, marsupials, reptiles and amphibians [41-44]. The transmission of *Cp. pneumoniae* among animals and humans was not yet described; however, Myers and collaborators proved that human could be infected from animal isolated bacteria following adaptation to the new host [44].

Chlamydophila caviae was found in animals such as rabbits, guinea pigs, horses, cats and dogs [45-48]. In 2006, it was reported the identification of this bacteria in humans, raising the possibility that it has a zoonotic potential, which has not been yet clarified [45].

Chlamydophila felis affects cats mainly under one year old and is very often associated with conjunctivitis [49-52]. Although there is evidence that this bacterium can cause keratoconjunctivitis in humans, there is still little evidence that can create systemic disease or severe pneumonia in the man [53].

Chlamydophila pecorum affects several small and large mammals such as ruminants, swine and koalas [54-59], but little or no studies have been published to date that can prove human infection from this agent.

Chlamydophila psittaci is the causative agent of Psittacosis and is capable of infecting domestic and wild birds [6, 60], but also reptiles [61] and mammals such as man [10,11]. This bacterium is definitely an important zoonosis and such potential has been widely reported across the years [12-15].

All species of the genera *Chlamydophila* and Chlamydiae have one or more serotypes, whose sequence are known [62-63] or are still under intense study [64].

a. *Chlamydophila psittaci*

Chlamydophila psittaci is negative to Gram test bacterium [2, 49, 57], having a cytoplasmic membrane and an outer three-layer membrane [65-66], with a significant cell wall fraction insoluble to ionic detergents [67]. In bacteria of the genus *Chlamydophila*, this portion is referred to as COMC (*Chlamydia* outer membrane complex), which is composed of MOMP (major outer membrane protein) and other small proteins [68]. MOMP is composed of cysteine-rich proteins and takes approximately 60% of the total weight of the outer membrane [69]. This constituent is important to maintain the integrity and rigidity of the bacteria, and the main antigen to host immune system [70].

b. *Chlamydophila psittaci biology*

Chlamydophila bacteria have three distinct forms during its life cycle: elementary body (EB), reticular body (RB) and intermediate body (IB) [19,20, 71].

The EB is small, electro-dense, spherical and about 0.2 to 0.3 mm in diameter [18,20]. The outer membrane is composed of proteins, lipids, lipopolysaccharides and proteins. However, unlike the Gram-negative bacteria, this species is devoid of muramic acid [72]. This is an active form of the bacterium capable of binding with the host cell allowing to reach its inside [19]. This first form is characterized by a highly electro-dense nucleoid [71, 73], located in the periphery and clearly separated from the cytoplasm [19, 71]. The Hc1 histone maintains the chromatin highly condensed [74]. Within the cell, the elementary body increases in size to form the reticular body, which is the metabolic active intracellular form of the organism [19, 20]. At this stage, the chromatin is dispersed, since the bacteria begin a process of transcription [20, 75].

The RB is of about 0.5 to 2.0 mm in diameter and its inner and outer membranes are relatively nearby, thereby reducing the virtual space between them [18, 20]. This form of the bacterium has the ability to split by binary fission, resulting in new RB [19, 65]. During this process, intermediate bodies can be observed within the host cell, measuring between 0.3 and 1.0 mm in diameter [18, 20].

This third form of the bacterium (IB) has a very specific presentation with an electro-dense core nucleoid surrounded by fibres dispersed radially [65, 73]. In the periphery, there exists an agglomerate of cytoplasmic granules, separated from the core by a translucent area [71]. When the replication process is over, several elementary forms are observed, which can be somewhat condensed, depending on their conformations [20]. The less condensed are more immature form, have further fibrous elements in the granular cytoplasm, bearing for the electro-dense nucleoid, which will become progressively highly condensed [71]. The nucleoid is close to the inner membrane [20].

The mature elementary bodies are condensed, having a homogeneous oval shaped nucleoid, irregular or an elongated, separated from the cytoplasmic organisms by a well visible electro-transparent area [20, 75].

Some studies have shown the existence of hemispherical-shaped projections of the cytoplasm on the surface of the elementary bodies and ridge-shaped projections of the reticular forms for this bacterium [76-78]. These projections range from the bacteria to the surface of the membrane inclusion and it is speculated that can possess pores of type III secretion [32].

c. *Pathogenesis*

Infection of *Chlamydophila psittaci* begins with the attachment of the elementary body to the host cell and subsequent parasite-mediated endocytosis [79]. The bacterium binds to the cell membrane receptor of the host cell, often associated with a cytoplasm protein known as clathrin [20]. This connection stimulates the cell to emit pseudopods; these increase in size until all bacteria have been surrounded, forming a vacuole delimited by clathrin, referred to as inclusion [18, 80]. In the vacuole, the bacterium has a biphasic cycle (Figure 1), alternating between states of elementary body and reticular body [19].

Once inside the vacuole, the EB are redistributed from the periphery of the cell and join in the region of the Golgi apparatus, which corresponds to the MTOC (Microtubule

Organizing Centre) [19, 80]. The non-acid inclusions are firstly too small, allowing to avoid its fusion with lysosomes, and are formed by endocytic constituents of the plasma membrane of the host cell such as proteins and lipids [19, 80]. All of these conditions lead to a more efficient survival and infection by the bacterium [20].

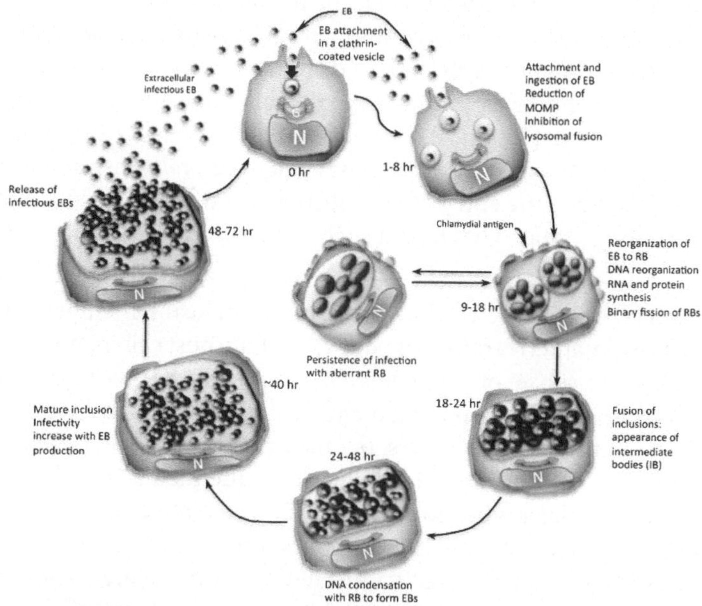

Figure 1.Chlamydia life cycle. Infection begins with the attachment of the elementary bodies (EB) to the surface of target epithelial cells. These cells promote a pseudopod formation to engulf the EB. Inside the cytoplasm this bacterium inhibits the fusion of the vesicle with the cell lysosomes. The nascent inclusion is accompanied by the transition from EBs to reticulate bodies (RB). Late in the cycle, RBs replicate by binary fission to generate both RBs and intermediate bodies (IB). At this stage, antigenic proteins are exposed into the cell surface. An elongated, aberrant RB could be formed at this time with an arrest on chlamydia cycle originating a persistent infection, or continuing the cycle. The various intracytoplasmic inclusions with bacterium inside, can also be fused in this phase, and the agent develop into intermediate bodies (IB), before DNA condensation and RB transformation into a newly EB. The mature inclusion increases in size with EB formation, until becoming infectious and released into the extracellular space to continue a new intracellular cycle. N – nucleus; G – Golgi apparatus: EB – elementary bodies; RB – reticulate bodies; IB – intermediate bodies.

On the first hours, the elementary bodies initiate to differentiate into reticular bodies. These forms of *Chlamydophila* are not infectious, have a non-condensed nucleoid and a greater size than EB [19, 65]. From eight to ten hours of cycle, the reticular bodies start to replicate by binary fission, remaining in contact with the inclusion membrane [20, 65]. In this moment, it's possible to see numerous mitochondria surrounding the inclusion [18, 20], possibly due to protein motors function as kinesins [81]. *Cp. psittaci* may not be able to generate as much energy in the form of ATP as other species of the genus, so a deeper association with the host cell mitochondria is necessary for the bacteria to recruit the necessary ATP by an alternative mechanism [20]. The migration of nutrients from the host cell into the inclusion is essential. Amino acids and nucleotides cross the inclusion membrane [20, 82]. Since the vacuole is not in the vicinity of lysosomes leads to the assumption that the releasing of nutrients by fusion with endocytic vesicles is unlikely [20]. It is known that exocytic vesicles containing sphingomyelin fuse with the membrane of the inclusion, delivering nutrients and lipids to the bacteria [80]. It was demonstrated that the inclusion membrane is permeable to small molecules of a molecular weight ranging from 100-520 Da [83,84]. After releasing the nutrients into the lumen of the bacterium by passive diffusion, membrane-specific carriers/transporters located in the membrane would facilitate the entry of new nutrients and would be indispensable for the entry of molecules larger than 520 Da, but such carriers have not been yet described [20].

Throughout the cycle, the size of the vesicles increases, as they accumulate growing numbers of bacteria inside [20, 84]. The surface of the inclusion membrane also increases, while it intercepts biosynthetic transport pathways of the host cell membrane and acquires the ability to fuse with a subset of Golgi derived vesicles [20, 84]. Within 20 hours of cycle, reticular bodies continue their replication and each body can give rise to a thousand of new bacteria [20]. As this process occurs, the inclusion becomes increasingly overloaded with bacteria and as such they are obligated to leave the inclusion [19, 20]. This may be the reason for the reticular bodies to turn into intermediate bodies and new infectious elementary bodies, which occurs about 36 hours after infection [19]. During the final stage, at 50 hours of cycle, the host cell and the inclusion undergo a process of lysis or, very often, the elementary bodies are released by reverse endocytosis [20], which leaves the host cell intact, allowing persistence of a chronic and silent infection [19].

After treatment with cytokines, antibiotics or restriction to particular nutrients [19, 85], this cycle may undergo a modification with the emergence of "persistent" bacteria [85-86]. This kind of bacterium does not complete its continuing transformation from reticular bodies to infectious elementary form. Instead, it remain with low metabolic activity [19]. These RB are morphologically aberrant, appearing with a dilated oval shape within inclusions of small size [20, 85-86]. Excessive accumulation of chromosomes is due to the continuous DNA replication of the bacteria that lack the ability to divide [20]. These persistent forms of *Cp. psittaci* are associated with chronic infections, and it has been shown that aberrant reticular bodies can quickly develop into normal forms and subsequently into infective elementary bodies [85-86]. The way this bacteria model passes through such transformations between aberrant forms and normal forms of reticular bodies is not yet completely understood [75, 87-88].

3. Epidemiology

Parrots were the first animals linked to *Cp. psittaci* in 1929-1930 and 1930-1938 when they were confirmed to be the source of outbreaks of psittacosis [33]. However, thereafter it became clear that this disease was not confined to these birds. In 1939, the agent was isolated from two pigeons in South Africa and later two new cases of psittacosis arose in citizens who contacted with pigeons in the U.S. [89]. Ducks and turkeys are given as possible sources of infection since the early fifties, although in the seventies there was a large decline in the prevalence of bacteria, but without ever ceasing [20]. Confirmation of new U.S. cases of chlamydiosis in turkeys in the following decade [20] and in Europe, already in the nineties [90,91], proved the continuing problematic status of this disease. In the last thirty years it was reported several cases in humans who have contracted the disease through direct contact with ducks [92-95] and more recently the number of these cases increased dramatically [96].

Studies on *Chlamydophila*'s prevalence increased and psittacosis was classified as an endemic disease in Belgium [97-98] and other European countries, such as France and Germany [97].

Psittacines and pigeons are the most disturbing cases, being the range of prevalence within the first, 16% to 81% and mortality frequently above 50% [99-101]. Other studies have shown that parrots are the largest sources of *Cp. psittaci*, especially when they are in captivity [102-103].

The wild pigeons have a broad seropositivity that ranges from 12.5% up to 95.6%. These data were obtained from studies conducted from 1966 to 2005 [20,104-105]. The seropositivity in this species is alarming, once they live in urban and rural areas throughout the world, in close contact with human [60]. Carrier pigeons are reported as having a lower seropositivity than wild pigeons, between 35.9 and 60% [20].

Kaleta and Taday (2003) reported that seabirds are more often infected with *Cp. psittaci* than other birds like chickens, quails and pheasants, but virtually all species of birds can contract the disease, even without apparent symptoms, such as for instance, the cranes and seagull. Psittacosis in arthropods can be detected, however without initiation of infection in these animals [106].

Although the horizontal transmission is the most common way of infection [24], the vertical transmission was also described [18].

Chlamydophila psittaci are most excreted in the faeces [21, 107], nasal [12] and oral discharges of infected animals [108]. Sareyyupoglu and collaborators (2007) indicates that excretion of the bacteria may occur intermittently in sub-clinical infections for a long time, being activated in situations of stress such as transportation and handling [21] or nutritional restrictions and egg laying [108]. Bacteria are found in the powder of feathers [106], in excrements, secretions and respiratory exudates from infected animals, and when dry, become spread in the air [20-21] being the aerosol transmission extremely feasible [109]. The contact of non infected animals with bacteria or its proximity to animals with *Cp. psittaci* gain greater importance, being this an essential criteria for the development of new infections [22].

Animals become infected by ingestion [110] or inhalation of the bacteria [13, 60], and the isolation of this agent is much more substantial from choanal and throat swabs collection rather than from faeces collection [111], especially in the early stages of the disease [20]. Thus, contamination by aerosol exudates must be considered the primary form of infection [89].

Birds who share contaminated water are also susceptible of infection [18], as well as predators eating carcasses contaminated with *Cp. psittaci* [108]. The nest environment is also very susceptible to disease transmission, since this is a place where are deposited loads debris that may contain multiple bacteria [20]. Granivorous animals, such as pigeons or pheasants, that are often found in corrals or stables contaminated with faeces, and also grain storage areas can become infected by inhalation of dust from grain or from aerosols of faeces [18, 20].

Ectoparasites such as fleas, mites and lice may also serve as vectors for the transmission of disease from animal to animal [112].

4. Clinical signs and pathology

After 4 hours of infection via aerosol, bacteria can be found in the respiratory system of the animal [113].

This disease may be acute, sub-acute, chronic or subclinical [113], being the last one found when the animal is showing no signs of disease, and elimination of the bacteria can occur intermittently due to stress [21], inadequate nutrition or other diseases [108]. These animals are persistently infected and named as "source of infection" to other animals [20]. The acute form, in turn, is a generalized form, affecting all the organs of the animal [113].

General clinical signs of disease and highlights of the most common within the species are listed on table 1, being generally flu-like symptoms, CNS disorders, pericarditis, sacculitis and occasionally shock and death, signs of infection [18, 20,113].

Table 1. General clinical signs of disease (adapted from [18,20,113].

	Clinical signs
Overall	Difficulty breathing, fever, lethargy, anorexia, ruffled feathers, diarrhoea, oral and nasal discharges, decreased egg laying, polyuria, pericarditis, sacculitis, pneumonia, lateral nasal adenitis, peritonitis, hepatitis and splenitis, occasionally shock and death.
Species	
Psittacines	Anorexia, diarrhoea, difficulty breathing, sinusitis, conjunctivitis, yellowish droppings and, perhaps, CNS disorders.
Pigeons	Signs appear only when there is another competitor disease. Acute Infection - anorexia, diarrhoea, conjunctivitis, rhinitis, swollen eyelids and a decrease in flight performance. Chronic Infection - lameness, stiff neck, opisthotonos, tremor and convulsions.
Turkeys	D serotype of the bacteria - Anorexia, cachexia, diarrhoea gelatinous yellow-green, low egg production, conjunctivitis, sinusitis, sneezing and mortality between 10 and 30%. B serotype of the bacteria - Anorexia and green manure
Ducks	It affects mostly the young ones. Agitation, unsteady gait, conjunctivitis, serous to purulent nasal discharge and depression.
Chickens	Blindness, anorexia and occasionally death.

Chlamydophila psittaci post-mortem lesions are not specific enough to be able to differentiate this disease from other systemic diseases [113]. The severity of injury depends on several factors including the virulence of serotype, the susceptibility and age of the host, the form and time of exposure and the presence of concurrent diseases [18].

In most cases of psittacosis, lesions are limited to three structures: spleen, liver and air sacs [113]. Table 2 summarizes the post-mortem lesions in these specific organs and points additional possible lesions of *Cp. psittaci* found in animals [18, 108,113].

Table 2. Post-mortem lesions in specific organs (Adapted from [18,108,113]).

Spleen	**Size**: Increased (splenomegaly). **Colour:** blackish, sometimes with greyish white necrotic foci and petechial haemorrhages. **Consistency**: soft. Perivascular sheaths of macrophages in the arterioles transforming the architecture of the organ. Increased macrophages numbers and decreased number of lymphocytes.
Liver	**Size**: Increased (hepatomegaly). **Colour**: Colour ranging from yellow to green. **Consistency**: friable. **Acute infection** – often the presence of a multifocal necrosis is the only sign of disease, and the other organs show no alterations **Subacute or chronic infections** - hyperplasia of the biliary ducts and sinus histiocytosis with mononuclear cell and heterophils infiltrate. Increased activity of Kupffer cells, stimulated by hemosiderin accumulation.
Air Sacs	**Acute and subacute infections** – changes in thickness of the membranes that were covered with fibrinous or fibrinopurulent exudate. Chronic infections - presence of pyogranulomatous infections or diffuse granulomas on serous surfaces.
Intestine	Lymphocytic enteritis.
Kidney	Acute necrosis and nephritis with inflammatory infiltrate of mixed type.
Injuries and/or changes in other organs	Infectious pericarditis, myocarditis, adenitis and peritonitis. Pneumonia although not frequent is possible. Inflammation of adrenals and gonads sporadically found. Brain injuries are rare. Medium increase in granulocytic cells series in spinal cord.

5. Diagnostic techniques

There are several available methods for the diagnosis of *Chlamydophila psittaci*, including the agent direct visualization with a specific staining technique, isolation of the agent followed by agent identification, detection of bacteria specific antigen or genes in samples and, finally, serology tests that identify antibodies against this organism [20,89].

a. Harvesting and storage of samples

Sampling should be carried out aseptically to avoid contaminating bacteria [89]. At necropsy, the main structures to isolate this bacterium are the air sacs, spleen, pericardium, heart, areas of hyperemia of the intestine, liver and kidney. On live animals the choanal, oropharyngeal and cloacal swabs are the principal material for *Chlamydophila psittaci* search [52,89,111]. Other samples can be taken from blood, conjunctiva and peritoneal exudates [20].

The samples for subsequent isolation of *Cp. psittaci* must be handled carefully to prevent the loss of infectivity of bacteria during transport and handling, but also due to its high zoonotic potential [89]. Thus, the safety of the operator must be respected (use of gloves, gown and mask) and the samples and swabs are placed in SPG (sucrose phosphate glutamate) transport medium, which is also suitable for bacteria of the Rickettsia genus [89, 114]. SPG is formed according to Table 3 [115].

Table 3. Composition of SPG [115].

Sucrose	74.6 g / L
K2HPO4	1.237 g / L
Glutamic Acid	0.721 g / L
Fetal calf serum	10%
Streptomycin	100 µg / mL
Vancomycin	100 µg / mL
Nnystatin	50 µg / mL
Gentamicin	50 µg / mL

SPG is also used for samples dilution and freezing, if they will be processed with adelay of four or more days after harvest; otherwise samples should not be frozen [89, 114]. Freezing of material must be performed within the first 24 hours, in a stabilized 7.2 pH phosphate-buffered saline medium and kept at a minimum temperature of -20 ° C [89, 114]. Spencer and Johnson (1983) report that *Cp. psittaci* can survive in SPG to just over 30 days at 4 ° C, but their infectivity decreased by 1.55% [115]. Detection of *Cp. psittaci* in the blood, liver, spleen and kidney is only possible two whole days after, whereas in faeces is only possible beyond the 72nd hour [113].

b. *Chlamydophila psittaci identification*

Giemsa cytological staining

Chlamydophila psittaci can be identified by direct observation of the organism using different staining techniques such as the Giemsa, Stamp and Gimenez stainings [116]. Giemsa staining could be performed from faeces, exudates, or liver and spleen cytologies [20]. Although cytological staining can be useful and quick, it is less sensitive and less specific than immunochemical staining or molecular detection methods [18, 20]. With Giemsa staining the methanol fixed material can be observed under the microscope. Inside the cells a basophilic inclusion composed by EB and IB located near the nucleus is found in infected cells [117]. Hayashi visualized bacteria using this technique, once isolated from organs such as liver, spleen, kidney, heart and intestine [118]. This technique is a powerful tool in the *Chlamydia* diagnosis, but it requires a vast experience from the observer.

Gimenez staining

This staining is often used, although it is not specific to this bacterium and has reduced sensitivity. Other agents beyond *Chlamydophila* (for instance, *Coxiella burnetii, Helicobacter pylori*) are stained red with Gimenez staining in contrast to background in light green [119].

This staining technique is based on carbol-fuchsin (basic fuchsin) reactions contrasting the background with malachite green [120]. The Gimenez staining technique is considered as a rapid diagnostic for the detection of *Cp. psittaci* on dead birds [121]. Some authors compared the use of DGMB (dark-ground methylene blue) staining with MZN (modified Ziehl-Neelsen) and DGG (Giemsa dark-ground) using infected goat foetal membranes, concluding that DGMB is a more specific staining for *Chlamydia* elementary bodies than MZN and DGG [123]. Woodland and colleagues (1982) developed a new staining technique for inclusions of *Chlamydia psittaci* and *Chlamydia trachomatis* and concluded that it was significantly better sensitivity than Giemsa staining. This technique consists on using a methyl green staining with neutral red and washing at pH 5.0 [124].

c. Immunohistochemistry

Immunohistochemistry is a method based on specificity of immune complex formation by the specific antibodies union with their specific antigen, being the IgG much more frequently used in comparison to IgM [20]. Nevertheless, a variability in Immunohistochemistry methods exits, and the choice of appropriated variations depends mainly on the available equipment and characteristics of existing antibody, since virtually all techniques on paraffin sections are suitable for detection of *Cp. psittaci* [20].This technique is more sensitive than routine histochemical staining; however, the user experience is essential to the identification of the bacteria. The body morphology of the agent must be remembered to avoid false positives in situations of cross-reactions with other bacteria and fungi [125]. In some cases, hemosiderin can lead an inexperienced user into errors, directing him into an incorrect positive diagnosis. Antigen positive tissues and sections stained with hematoxylin-eosin must be used as control [20].The antibody used in this method could be polyclonal [126] or monoclonal for the genus of the family *Chlamydophila* [127]. Some antibodies detect the specific epitope of the family Chlamydiaceae, located in the LPS of the bacteria [128]. Other authors reported the degree of sensitivity of this technique with peroxidase-antiperoxidase in the identification of *Chlamydia* and point out the positive samples to Chlamydiae when unapparent to the hematoxylin-eosin technique [129].

d. Serological Tests

Serological tests are still widely used, yet these are not particularly useful for the disease diagnosis on birds, since they show a high prevalence of bacteria [106] and *Chlamydophila psittaci* antibodies are maintained in circulation for months or even years. Due to lack of information and studies on the direct identification of bacteria by serological tests in some birds, these tests are still viewed with some uncertainty concerning the interpretation of the results [20].A positive diagnosis does not mean active infection, but confirms that the animal had contact with the bacteria in the past [12, 114]. Further, in case of acute infections, these tests easily lead to false negative results since the serum sample may be carried out before the seroconversion [18], which is necessary to the method efficiency. Another reason for false negatives is the treatment of animals with antibiotics that reduce or delay the antibody response [12].The serological methods most usually used include the methods of elementary body agglutination (EBA), the complement fixation test (CF), the indirect immunofluorescence (MIF) and commercial ELISA tests [22, 114, 130].

Methods of elementary body agglutination (EBA)

EBA detects IgM [12], therefore diagnosing recent (acute) cases of infection [121]. A negative result does not mean, however, that the animal is not infected, having this technique a very reduced sensitivity [20].

Complement fixation test (CF)

Although CF is the most used serological method [26, 89, 114, 130], it has several disadvantages in the use in psittacines because the immunoglobulins do not fixate the complement [131-132]. In such cases, an indirect test for complement fixation using the spot-*Chlamydophila psittaci* IF (bioMérieux, Basingstoke, Hants) reagent [89] or other serological test such as MIF should be used [114].. This test has also low sensitivity [114] and the technique is very laborious, being discarded whenever multiple samples need to be tested at same time [20].

Micro-indirect immunofluorescence (MIF)

This method detects all isotopes of immunoglobulin produced against the genus *Chlamydophila*. Thus, it is widely used in the detection of antibodies against *C. trachomatis*, *Cp. psittaci* and *Cp. pneumoniae* serotypes in serum or plasma [20]. The indirect immunofluorescence test seems to be more sensitive than the complement fixation test and histochemical techniques, albeit it shows cross-reactivity with other chlamydial species [20].

Direct fluorescent antibody (FA)

The preferably staining method to detect the *Chlamydophila* is the direct FA [89,133]. In this method, an anti-chlamydia fluorescein-conjugated is applied to the smear [134] following the incubation for 30 minutes at 37 ° C [20]. Thereafter, the slides are washed up with PBS and distilled water, dried on air and finally mounted with a resinous compound like Entellan® [20]. The inclusions of the bacteria show a bright green under ultraviolet microscopy [96].

ELISA technique

The primary purpose of a great number of commercial ELISA developed in the last 25 years was for *Chlamydia trachomatis* in humans, but such tests are also suitable for diagnosing *Chlamydophila psittaci*, as they are specific to the LPS antigen of all species of the family Chlamydiales [1,27,135-136]. Commercial ELISA tests were, over the years, widely inquired and several studies about the low specificity and high sensitivity of these methods came up [20], with the first dramatically reducing in situations where the prevalence of the bacterium is low and hence where there is a low number of detected bodies [136]. In fact, it takes hundreds of bacteria so that the results are positive [20]. One of the major disadvantages of this technique is the possible occurrence of false positives, since have cross-reaction with other bacterias (such *Acinetobacter calcoaceticus*, *Escherichia coli*, *Staphylococcus aureus* and *Klebsiella pneumoniae)* have been demonstrated in humans [34,137]. Nevertheless, the development and improvement of these commercial tests increased with the use of monoclonal antibodies and advanced blockers methods [20, 136] that improve the specificity and reduced the false positive cases. There are already available specific commercial ELISA tests for *C. trachomatis*, *Cp. pneumonia*, *Cp. abortus* antibodies [132,138-139], and for *Chlamydophila psittaci's* as well [101]. These methods are as reliable as the indirect immunofluorescence tests, but are faster, easier to perform and less expensive [20], as well as more sensitive than the complement fixation technique, easier to standardize and, above all, more suitable for large epidemiological studies [22,101]. They also do not depend on the viability of the elementary bodies, or of soluble antigens in secretions [136]. An ELISA based on a recombinant ELISA (rMOMP ELISA) was developed and tested, giving a sensitivity and specificity of 100% in cases of psittacosis [18,140].

In our opinion, Immunocomb® (Biogal, Kibbutz Galed, Israel) commercial kit is nowadays the most suitable ELISA test available, as it has a nearly 100% sensibility and specificity [101]. This performance is enjoyable, but the labourer must understand that the choice for the most suitable laboratorial test depends on each case (Figure 2).

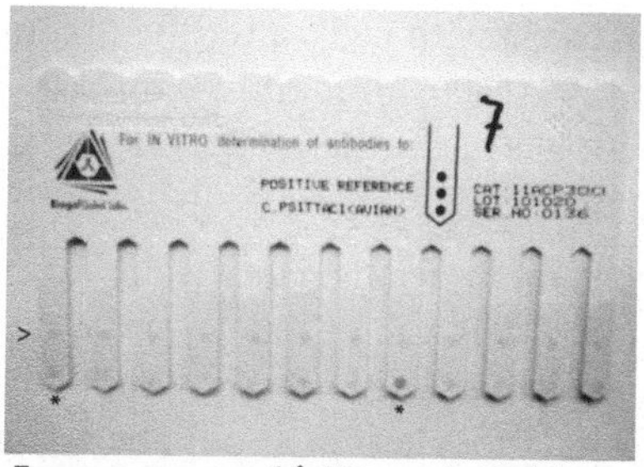

Figure 2. Commercial kit Immunocomb® (Biogal, Kibbutz Galed, Israel) ELISA test, with the reference sample (>) and examples of strong positive animals (*).

e. Isolation of *Cp. psittaci*

Isolation of bacteria may be performed from tissue and faecal specimens or scrapings [145]. A 20% to 40% homogenized suspension sample is prepared using diluents such as phosphate buffer (PBS) at pH 7.2 and the culture media [20,146]. When samples are inoculated within 24 hours after harvested and not frozen, these solvents are used with antibiotics [20]. Whenever samples are chilled or frozen, a transport media such as SPG or Bovarnick's should be used as stabilization agent [15,147].

Before cell cultures or animal inoculation, potentially contaminated samples must be treated by three possible methods: with antibiotics [133], followed or not by low speed centrifugation [148] or filtration [133,149]. The sample is afterwards submitted to a standard procedure, where it is homogenized in diluent containing 1 mg/ml streptomycin, 1mg/ml of vancomycin and 1mg/ml kanamycin [20]. It's possible to select other antibiotics, however penicillin, tetracycline and chloramphenicol should be avoided, since they inhibit the growth of these bacteria [148]. If the sample is slightly contaminated, before the inoculation into the cell culture or on the test animal, samples must be homogenized in an antibiotic solution and remain there for 24 hours [150]. In case of deep contamination of samples, such as faecal samples, they must be homogenized in an antibiotic solution and then subjected to centrifugation at 1000-2000x *g* for 30 min [148]. Thereafter the upper and lower layers must be discarded and the supernatant inoculated into the culture fluid cells or laboratory animals. In case of persistent contamination, the sample should be subjected to filtration pores of 450 to 800 micrometre [148].

f. Cell culture and embryonated SPF eggs

The cell culture is the method of choice used to isolate *Chlamydophila psittaci* [7]. Although other cultures can be used, the most frequently used are the BGM (*Buffalo green monkey*), McCoy, Vero, HeLa or L-929 [24]. In a 1992, a study reports that, within these, BGM has the highest sensitivity [151].

Bacteria can be isolated from cells that have its normal cell cycle of replication, but stable cell lines without reproduction are more satisfactory, since they provide additional nutrients for the *Cp. psittaci* replication and are much easier to observe [148]. For that, suppression of the cells is made by irradiation or by cytotoxic chemicals such as 5-iodo-2-deoxiodine [149], cytocalasine, B, cycloheximide, cycloheximide and emetine hydrochloride (0.5 - 2.0mg/ml) [148]. The type of material used will mainly depend on the available material in the laboratory [20].

To increase the binding of bacteria with cells, after the inoculation of the bacterium into the cell line a centrifugation (500-1500x *g*) for 30-90 minutes is needed [150]. This union will be stronger when incubation is performed at 35°C to 39°C [152]. Cultures are checked for bacteria on days 2, 3, 4 and 5 [148].

Some laboratories use chicken embryos to isolate the organism [96, 153], usually injecting up to 0.3 ml of inoculum in the yolk sac of 6 days embryos [89]. Thereafter, bacterium replicates, which leads to the death of the embryo within a maximum period of 12 days. In case of failure, two additional inoculations should be made before considering the *Cp. psittaci* sample as negative [20].

Usually, the organism causes vascular congestion in the yolk sac membranes, which is homogenized in a 20% suspension membrane [20]. This suspension may be frozen in order to preserve bacteria or inoculated into new eggs or cell culture monolayers [148]. The identification of inclusions is done through cytological or immunohistochemical methods [152], like the indirect fluorescent antibody technique, the immunoperoxidase technique [129], or by histochemical stainings [134] such as Gimenez and Macchiavello based-stains, allowing the visualization of the bacteria [20].

Fixation of monolayer cells was made with acetone for 2 to10 minutes, after transport media has been removed and washed with PBS [154-155]. If the support is made of plastic material, alcohol should be used instead of acetona for fixation [156].

g. Polymerase chain reaction (PCR)

Molecular methods such as PCR allow the direct detection of *Chlamydophila psittaci* from clinical specimens within one day [157]. In literature, the amplification is made from the ribosomal RNA gene region [128,158,159] and the gene encoding the antigen, known as omp1 or ompA [132, 160].

The quality and quantity of extracted DNA is essential for the sensitivity of the test [20]. The efficient extraction of DNA samples and removal of PCR inhibitors ensure the proper functioning of the method [20]. The efficient extraction of DNA is much more difficult in bacteria, when compared to viruses, since bacteria possessing outer membranes are very resistant to destruction [20].

There are several methods of commercial DNA extraction capable of extracting *Chlamydophila* DNA. The test QIAamp® DNA Mini Kit (Qiagen) was reported as being the one with best results for pharyngeal scrapings, whereas the test High Pure PCR Template Preparation Kit® (Roche) was the top performer for faecal and chloacal samples [20].

These commercial tests are suitable when working with PCR inhibitors [20]. They also contain a particular reagent for the bacterial and eukaryotic cells lysis. One of these reagents is GIT (Guanidine IsoThiocyanate) [20].

The cellular RNA is digested with an RNase and then the lysate is centrifuged in a mini-column, where the DNA is joined to a solid phase that can be modified by silica hydroxy-apatite or special filters membranes. Then, the elution takes place by immersing DNA of high purity and free of PCR inhibitors [20]. Cold storage leads to a rapid loss of DNA from organisms, so samples with low levels of target DNA often become negative. To avoid this problem, DNA stabilizers are used in PCR analysis [161]. Some reagents are available commercially as the RNA/DNA Stabilization Reagent for Blood/Bone Marrow® from Roche Applied Science [161,162].

In 2005, a PCR assay proved sensitive enough to detect *Chlamydophila psittaci* in samples from birds [97]. Sachse and colleagues (2005) detected the bacteria based on the amplification, resulting on a specific ompA product for the genus, followed by a second amplification using a specific primer for the genus and a specific primer for the species. At the end, it is created a specific amplicon for *Chlamydophila psittaci* [20, 163].

The PCR results are visualized by electrophoresis and the sensitivity of PCR-EIA was set at 0.1 IFU (infection forming unit) [97].

These tests are in progress and recently new types of PCR emerged. One such case is the SYBR Green-based real-time PCR that targets the rDNA spacer of *Chlamydophila psittaci* [20]. This test detects 10rDNA copies/ml of extracted DNA and all ompA genotypes of the bacteria [20].

h. DNA microarray-based detection

Sachse and colleagues (2005) developed a method to identify *Chlamydia* and *Chlamydophila* spp. species. This test was developed through the platform ArrayTube (CLONDIAG® chip technologies) and it obtained specific hybridization patterns for the species in all organisms of the Chlamydiaceae family. Thus, this study proved this test is a viable alternative for the identification of ambiguous *Chlamydia* cell culture, and a possibility for detection of these microorganisms from tissues [163].

Table 4 below summarizes the advantages and disadvantages of some methods for diagnosis of *Chlamydophila psittaci* [20].

It is our opinion that there's no better diagnostic test for *Clamidophila psittaci* but a more suitable or adequate to each case instead, for different biologic material sampling and laboratorial conditions. If the goal is to define *Chlamydophila*'s prevalence in a large group of animals, PCR should be the first choice, although more reliable tests imply more expensive tests. If the investment had limitations, an ELISA test can be the most adequate choice for the diagnosis. If the group of animals is just of some units, then cultured cells can be a possibility if the proper laboratory conditions are available.

Table 4.Advantages and disadvantages of some methods for diagnosis of *Chlamydophila psittaci* (Adapted from [20]).

Diagnostic methods	Advantages	Inconveniences
Cytological staining	- easy - cheap - quick - no sophisticated equipment needed - dead and live bacteria can be demonstrated	- non-specific - less sensitive - non-automated - interpretation by experienced person
Immunocytochemistry	- more sensitive and specific than cytology - easy - quick - dead and live bacteria can be demonstrated	- cross-reaction with other bacteria (when MAb is against LPS) - interpretation by experienced person - more expensive - fluorescence microscope required - non-automated

Diagnostic methods	Advantages	Inconveniences
Immunohistochemistry	- automation possible - detection in the morphological context	- more labour intensive than immunocytochemistry - histology laboratory required - MAb detecting *Cp.psittaci*-specific antigen in formalin-fixed samples needed - more time consuming than immunocytochemistry - more expensive
Antigen-ELISA	- quick - multiple samples can be tested at once - quantification - easy - dead and live bacteria can be demonstrated	- commercial kits often insensitive - non-specific if the target is LPS or Hsp60 - ELISA reader needed
Culture	- propagation for further investigations - more specific than direct antigen detection - direct evidence of live bacteria - quantification of live bacteria	- transport and storage of samples is critical - BSL3 laboratory - time consuming - expensive - labour intensive - trained personnel required - not all strains can be cultured
Molecular diagnosis (PCR, Micro array)	- highly sensitive - highly specific - quick - automation possible - multiple samples can be tested at once - possibility of direct typing on clinical samples - can be quantitative - can detect live and dead bacteria	- expensive - specialized equipment needed - trained personnel needed
Serology: antibody ELISA	- easy - quick - multiple samples can be tested at once - quantification is possible - automation possible - valuable for epidemiological research	- convalescent sera (retrospective diagnosis) - not a proof that the organism is still present - tests detecting antibodies against LPS, hsp60 or whole organisms are non-specific - less sensitive than molecular diagnosis - ELISA reader needed

6. Treatment

Treatment of psittacosis is performed with medication, being tetracycline the drug of choice [12, 148]. In cases developing in pregnant women or in children under the age of 9 years, the use of tetracycline or doxycycline is contraindicated, being the use of erythromycin the most suitable. Treatment of the patient should be made for at least 14 consecutive days using the drug of choice [164]. In birds, tetracycline or doxycycline should be given over a period of 7 weeks in the feed or on medicated seed [165].

7. Prevention

a. Vaccines

Today there are still no vaccines available against avian chlamydiosis [148]. Attempts on DNA vaccines have reduced signs of disease, injuries and excretion of bacteria. However, a complete protection of individuals remains distant [98]. Currently, treatments and strategies for reducing contamination of these bacteria are the best way to control the disease [12].

b. Disinfection

Chlamydophila psittaci can survive up to 30 days in faeces and cage materials or beds, so regular cleaning of equipment and places where animals are infected is essential [127]. Bacteria of the family *Chlamydiae* are quite sensitive to chemical that affecting the lipid contents or the integrity of the cell walls. Most disinfectants used as detergents inactivate *Cp. psittaci* bacteria, such as a 1 to 1000 ammonium quaternary, 1 to 100 chlorophenol, 70% isopropyl alcohol and 1% lysol [12, 113].

8. Public health concerns

Chlamydophila psittaci is a zoonosis, hence it is an organism capable of producing infection in humans [14, 24, 166]. Man is mainly infected by the dispersed bacteria in the inhaled air, after faeces, urine or secretions of the respiratory system of infected animals dry [21]. The direct contact with infected animals may also lead to infection [4], so that the post mortem examination and manipulation of cultures should be done properly, using appropriate safety equipment and the use of flow laminar chambers [23].

This disease has particular significance in public health, since parrots are common pets in our houses, even in schools or nursing places [148]. The risk of contracting the disease increases with the contact with these animals, but also in day-to-day activities, for example mowing the lawn, shrubs or others without a suitable container for this purpose, exposing individuals to the bacteria [16, 167]. Psittacosis can also be transmitted from person to person, however this process is believed to be uncommon [167-168].

The incubation period is usually between 5-14 days [12]. In humans, signs of psittacosis can vary greatly, ranging from cases where they are completely unapparent to situations where it can be found signs of systemic disease with severe interstitial pneumonia and encephalitis [12, 170]. Infected humans may develop headaches, chills, discomfort and myalgia [12]. Respiratory involvement is common and a number of cases have been documented [171-174]. This disease is, however, rarely fatal if patients are provided with proper treatment, so an awareness of the dangers of psittacosis and rapid evaluation of the case are vital [12, 123].

Chlamydophila psittaci was associated with ocular lymphoma [174], however, this subject is still matter of debate and disagreement and conflicting reports have been published [175,176]. The true greatness of this disease is very far from knowing, since cases where psittacosis is diagnosed and individuals have severe signs of disease are only a tiny fraction of the total occurrences. Cases where the disease is less severe, unnoticed or misdiagnosed infections due to similar symptoms with other respiratory pathogens or asymptomatic infections remain in the shadow of *Cp. psittaci* infection in humans [103, 162].

9. Conclusion

Psittacosis is a disease that is virtually throughout the world and is a zoonosis. This fact must be present in all healthcare professionals, being veterinarians or doctors.

Psittacines are the most commonly affected animals and this fact must be an alert for veterinarians to pay special caution during its manipulation. Owners and handlers of exotic birds should as well learn how to prevent this disease, as they are a potential risk group for infection.

The number of infected animals by *Chlamydophila psittaci* is underestimated [106] and new cases of outbreaks continue to appear worldwide, some of which often die facing this disease [20].

A more feasible, fast and easy diagnostic method and universally accorded is yet to be implemented.

Altogether, control of this disease should be stricter and information about its maleficence worldwide known.

References

1. Everett KD, Bush RM, Andersen AA. Emended description of the order Chlamydiales, proposal of Parachlamydiaceae fam. nov. and Simkaniaceae fam. nov., each containing one monotypic genus, revised taxonomy of the family Chlamydiaceae, including a new genus and five new species, and standards for the identification of organisms. International Journal of Systematic Bacteriology 1999;49(Pt 2) 415-440.
2. Dickx V, Vanrompay D.Chlamydia psittaci in a chicken and turkey hatchery results in zoonotic transmission. Journal of Medical Microbiology 2011;60(Pt 6) 775-779.
3. Ciftçi B, Güler ZM, Aydoğdu M, Konur O, Erdoğan Y. Familial outbreak of psittacosis as the first Chlamydia psittaci infection reported from Turkey. Tüberkulöz Toraks 2008;56(2) 215-220.
4. Beeckman DS, Vanrompay DC. Zoonotic Chlamydophila psittaci infections from a clinical perspective. Clinical Microbiology and Infection 2009;15(1) 11-17.
5. Fraeyman A, Boel A, Van Vaerenbergh K, De Beenhouwer H. Atypical pneumonia due to Chlamydophila psittaci: 3 case reports and review of literature. Acta Clinica Belgica 2010;65(3) 192-196.
6. Pennycott TW, Dagleish MP, Wood AM, Garcia C. Chlamydophila psittaci in wild birds in the UK. Veterinary Record 2009;164 (5) 157-158.
7. Dahlhausen B, Radabaugh CS. Detection of Chlamydia psittaci infection in pet birds using a molecular based diagnostic assay. In: Proceedings of the Annual Conference of the Association Avian Veterinarians Reno, NV. 1997;p. 191–198; 1997.
8. Maluping RP, Oronan RB, Toledo SU. Detection of Chlamydophila psittaci antibodies from captive birds at the Ninoy Aquino Parks and Wildlife Nature Center, Quezon City, Philippines. Annals of Agricultural and Environmental Medicine 2007;14(1) 191-193.

9. Voigt A, Schöfl G, Heidrich A, Sachse K, Saluz HP.Full-Length De Novo Sequence of the Chlamydophila psittaci Type Strain, 6BC. Journal of Bacteriology 2011;193(10) 2662-2663.

10. Reinhold P, Sachse K, Kaltenboeck B. Chlamydiaceae in cattle: Commensals, trigger organisms, or pathogens? Veterinary Journal 2011;189(3) 257-267.

11. Sprague LD, Schubert E, Hotzel H, Scharf S, Sachse K. The detection of Chlamydophila psittaci genotype C infection in dogs. Veterinary Journal 2009;181(3) 274-279.

12. Smith KA, Bradley KK, Stobierski MG, Tengelsen LA. Compendium of measures to control Chlamydophila psittaci (formerly Chlamydia psittaci) infection among humans (psittacosis) and pet birds, 2005. Journal of American Veterinary Medical Association 2005;226(4) 532-539.

13. Berk Y, Klaassen CH, Mouton JW, Meis JF. An outbreak of psittacosis at a bird-fanciers fair in the Netherlands. Nederlands Tijdschrift voor Geneeskdunde 2008; 152(34) 1889-1892.

14. Gaede W, Reckling KF, Dresenkamp B, Kenklies S, Schubert E, Noack U, Irmscher HM, Ludwig C, Hotzel H, Sachse K. Chlamydophila psittaci infections in humans during an outbreak of psittacosis from poultry in Germany. Zoonoses and Public Health 2008; 55(4)184-188.

15. Dickx V, Beeckman DS, Dossche L, Tavernier P, Vanrompay D. Chlamydophila psittaci in homing and feral pigeons and zoonotic transmission. Journal of Medical Microbiology 2010;59(Pt 11) 1348-1353.

16. Fenga C, Cacciola A, Di Nola C, Calimeri S, Lo Giudice D, Pugliese M, Niutta PP, Martino LB. Serologic investigation of the prevalence of Chlamydophila psittaci in occupationally-exposed subjects in eastern Sicily. Annals of Agricultural Environmental Medicine 2007;14(1) 93-96.

17. Geigenfeind I, Haag-Wackernagel D. Detection of Chlamydophila psittaci from feral pigeons in environmental samples: problems with currently available techniques. Integrative Zoology 2010;5(1) 63-69.

18. Vanrompay D, Ducatelle R, Haesebrouck F. Chlamydia psittaci infections: a review with emphasis on avian chlamydiosis. Veterinary Microbiology1995; 45(2-3) 93-119.

19. Hammerschlag MR. The intracellular life of chlamydiae. Seminars in Pediatric Infectious Diseases 2002;13(4) 239-248.

20. Harkinezhad T. Molecular epidemiology of Chlamydophila psittaci in psittacine birds and humans and prevention by DNA vaccination. PhD thesis, Ghent University, Ghent, Belgium; 2008.

21. Sareyyupoglu B, Cantekin Z, Bas B. Chlamydophila psittaci DNA detection in the faeces of cage birds. Zoonoses and Public Health 2007;54(6-7) 237-242.

22. Magnino S, Haag-Wackernagel D, Geigenfeind I, Helmecke S, Dovc A, Prukner-Radovcić E, Residbegović E, Ilieski V, Laroucau K, Donati M, Martinov S, Kaleta EF. Chlamydial infections in feral pigeons in Europe: Review of data and focus on public health implications. Veterinary Microbiology 2009;135(1-2) 54-67.

23. Dvorak G, Spickler AR, Roth JA. Handbook for zoonotic diseases of companion animals. Iowa: Iowa State University; 2008.
24. Andersen AA, Vanrompay D. Avian chlamydiosis. Revue Scientifique et Technique 2000;19(2) 396-404.
25. Raso TF, Carrasco AO, Silva JC, Marvulo MF, Pinto AA. Seroprevalence of antibodies to Chlamydophila psittaci in zoo workers in Brazil. Zoonoses and Public Health 2010;57(6) 411-416.
26. Griffiths PC, Plater JM, Horigan MW, Rose MP, Venables C, Dawson M. Serological diagnosis of ovine enzootic abortion by comparative inclusion immunofluorescence assay, recombinant lipopolysaccharide enzyme-linked immunosorbent assay, and complement fixation test. Journal of Clinical Microbiology 1996;34(6) 1512-1518.
27. Baud D, Regan L, Greub G. Comparison of five commercial serological tests for the detection of anti-Chlamydia trachomatis antibodies. European Journal of Clinical Microbiology and Infectious Diseases 2010;29(6) 669-675.
28. McPhee SJ, Erb B, Harrington W. Psittacosis. Western Journal of Medicine 1987;146: 91-96.
29. Vanrompay D, Van Nerom A, Ducatelle R, Haesebrouck F. Evaluation of five immunoassays for detection of Chlamydia psittaci in cloacal and conjunctival specimens from turkeys. Journal of Clinical Microbiology 1994;32(6) 1470-1474.
30. Moschioni C, Faria HP, Reis MAS, Silva EU. Pneumonia grave por Chlamydia psittaci. Jornal Brasileiro de Pneumologia 2001;27(4) 219-222.
31. Pospischil A. From disease to etiology: historical aspects of Chlamydia-related diseases in animals and humans. Drugs Today (Barc) 2009;45(Suppl B) 141-146.
32. Muschiol S. Small Molecule Inhibitors of Type III Secretion and their Effect on Chlamydia Development. Thesis for doctoral degree (Ph.D.), Department of Microbiology, Tumor and Cell Biology, Karolinska Institutet and Swedish Institute for Infectious Disease Control, Stockholm, Sweden; 2009.
33. Hagan WA, Bruner DW, Timoney JF. Hagan and Bruner's microbiology and infectious diseases of domestic animals. 8ª ed. Cornell University Press: 361; 1988.
34. Taylor-Robinson D, Thomas BJ. The role of Chlamydia trachomatis in genital-tract and associated diseases. Journal of Clinical Pathology 1980;33(3) 205-233.
35. Zhang X, Yuan Z, Guo X, Li J, Li Z, Wang Q. Expression of Chlamydophila psittaci MOMP heat-labile toxin B subunit fusion gene in transgenic rice. Biologicals 2008;36(5) 296-302.
36. Andrews BE, Major R, Palmer SR. Ornithosis in poultry workers. Lancet 1981;1(8221) 632-634.
37. Marsilio F, Di Martino B, Di Francesco CE, Meridiani I. Diagnosis of ovine chlamydial abortions by PCR-RFLP performed on vaginal swabs. Veterinary Research Communications 2005;29(Suppl 1) 99-106.
38. Pospischil A, Thoma R, Hilbe M, Grest P, Zimmermann D, Gebbers JO. Abortion in humans caused by Chlamydophila abortus (Chlamydia psittaci serovar 1). Schweizer Archiv für Tierheilkdunde 2002;144(9) 463-466.

39. Sachse K, Grossmann E. Chlamydial diseases of domestic animals- zoonotic potential of the agents and diagnostic issues. Deutsch Tierärztliche Wochenschrift 2002;109(4) 142-148.

40. Meijer A, Brandenburg A, de Vries J, Beentjes J, Roholl P, Dercksen D. Chlamydophila abortus infection in a pregnant woman associated with indirect contact with infected goats. European Journal of Clinical Microbiology and Infectious Diseases 2004;23(6) 487-490.

41. Bodetti TJ, Jacobson E, Wan C, Hafner L, Pospischil A, Rose K, Timms P. Molecular evidence to support the expansion of the hostrange of Chlamydophila pneumoniae to include reptiles as well as humans, horses, koalas and amphibians. Systematic and Applied Microbiology 2002;25(1) 146-152.

42. Jacobson ER, Heard D, Andersen A. Identification of Chlamydophila pneumoniae in an emerald tree boa, Corallus caninus. Journal of Veterinary Diagnostic Investigation 2004;16(2) 153-154.

43. Soldati G, Lu ZH, Vaughan L, Polkinghorne A, Zimmermann DR, Huder JB, Pospischil A. Detection of mycobacteria and chlamydiae in granulomatous inflammation of reptiles: a retrospective study. Veterinary Pathology 2004;41(4) 388-397.

44. Myers GS, Mathews SA, Eppinger M, Mitchell C, O'Brien KK, White OR, Benahmed F, Brunham RC, Read TD, Ravel J, Bavoil PM, Timms P. Evidence that human Chlamydia pneumoniae was zoonotically acquired. Journal of Bacteriology 2009;191(23) 7225-7233.

45. Lutz-Wohlgroth L, Becker A, Brugnera E, Huat ZL, Zimmermann D, Grimm F, Haessig M, Greub G, Kaps S, Spiess B, Pospischil A, Vaughan L. Chlamydiales in guinea-pigs and their zoonotic potential. Journal of Veterinary Medicine A. Physiology, Pathology, Clinical Medicine 2006;53(4) 185-193.

46. Wang Y, Nagarajan U, Hennings L, Bowlin AK, Rank RG. Local host response to chlamydial urethral infection in male guinea pigs. Infection and Immunity 2010;78(4) 1670-1681.

47. Gaede W, Reckling KF, Schliephake A, Missal D, Hotzel H, Sachse K. Detection of Chlamydophila caviae and Streptococcus equi subsp. zooepidemicus in horses with signs of rhinitis and conjunctivitis. Veterinary Microbiology 2010;142(3-4) 440-444.

48. Pantchev A, Sting R, Bauerfeind R, Tyczka J, Sachse K. Detection of all Chlamydophila and Chlamydia spp. of veterinary interest using species-specific real-time PCR assays. Comparative Immunology Microbiology and Infectious Diseases 2010;33(6) 473-484.

49. Gruffydd-Jones T, Addie D, Belák S, Boucraut-Baralon C, Egberink H, Frymus T, Hartmann K, Hosie MJ, Lloret A, Lutz H, Marsilio F, Pennisi MG, Radford AD, Thiry E, Truyen U, Horzinek MC. Chlamydophila felis infection. ABCD guidelines on prevention and management. Journal of Feline Medicine Surgery 2009;11(7) 605-609.

50. Hartmann AD, Hawley J, Werckenthin C, Lappin MR, Hartmann K.Detection of bacterial and viral organisms from the conjunctiva of cats with conjunctivitis and upper respiratory tract disease. Journal of Feline Medicine and Surgery 2010;12(10) 775-782.

51. Sandmeyer LS, Waldner CL, Bauer BS, Wen X, Bienzle D. Comparison of polymerase chain reaction tests for diagnosis of feline herpesvirus, Chlamydophila felis, and Mycoplasma spp. infection in cats with ocular disease in Canada. Canadian Veterinary Journal 2010;51(6) 629-633.

52. Burns RE, Wagner DC, Leutenegger CM, Pesavento PA. Histologic and molecular correlation in shelter cats with acute upper respiratory infection. Journal of Clinical Microbiology 2011;49(7) 2454-60.

53. Browning GF. Is Chlamydophila felis a significant zoonotic pathogen? Australian Veterinary Journal 2004;82(11) 695-696.

54. Devereaux LN, Polkinghorne A, Meijer A, Timms P. Molecular evidence for novel chlamydial infections in the koala (Phascolarctos cinereus). Systematic and Applied Microbiology 2003;26(2) 245-253.

55. Kauffold J, Henning K, Bachmann R, Hotzel H, Melzer F.The prevalence of chlamydiae of bulls from six bull studs in Germany. Animal Reproduction Science 2007;102(1-2) 111-121.

56. Greco G, Corrente M, Buonavoglia D, Campanile G, Di Palo R, Martella V, Bellacicco AL, D'Abramo M, Buonavoglia C. Epizootic abortion related to infections by Chlamydophila abortus and Chlamydophila pecorum in water buffalo (Bubalus bubalis). Theriogenology 2008;69(9) 1061-1069.

57. Berri M, Rekiki A, Boumedine KS, Rodolakis A. Simultaneous differential detection of Chlamydophila abortus, Chlamydophila pecorum and Coxiella burnetii from aborted ruminant's clinical samples using multiplex PCR. BMC Microbiology 2009;9: 130.

58. Mohamad KY, Rodolakis A. Recent advances in the understanding of Chlamydophila pecorum infections, sixteen years after it was named as the fourth species of the Chlamydiaceae family. Veterinary Research 2010;41(3) 27.

59. Holzwarth N, Pospischil A, Mavrot F, Vilei EM, Hilbe M, Zlinszky K, Regenscheit N, Pewsner M, Thoma R, Borel N. Occurrence of Chlamydiaceae, Mycoplasma conjunctivae, and pestiviruses in Alpine chamois (Rupicapra r. rupicapra) of Grisons, Switzerland. Journal of Veterinary Diagnostic Investigation 2011;23(2) 333-337.

60. de Lima VY, Langoni H, da Silva AV, Pezerico SB, de Castro AP, da Silva RC, Araújo JP Jr. Chlamydophila psittaci and Toxoplasma gondii infection in pigeons (Columba livia) from Sao Paulo State, Brazil. Veterinary Parasitology 2011;175(1-2) 9-14.

61. Huchzermeyer FW, Gerdes GH, Foggin CM, Huchzermeyer KD, Limper LC. Hepatitis in farmed hatchling Nile crocodiles (Crocodylus niloticus) due to chlamydial infection. Journal of the South African Veterinary Association 1994;65(1) 20-22.

62. Read TD, Myers GS, Brunham RC, Nelson WC, Paulsen IT, Heidelberg J, Holtzapple E, Khouri H, Federova NB, Carty HA, Umayam LA, Haft DH, Peterson J, Beanan MJ, White O, Salzberg SL, Hsia RC, McClarty G, Rank RG, Bavoil PM, Fraser CM. Genome sequence of Chlamydophila caviae (Chlamydia psittaci GPIC): examining the role of niche-specific genes in the evolution of the Chlamydiaceae. Nucleic Acids Research 2003;31(8) 2134-2147.

63. Azuma Y, Hirakawa H, Yamashita A, Cai Y, Rahman MA, Suzuki H, Mitaku S, Toh H, Goto S, Murakami T, Sugi K, Hayashi H, Fukushi H, Hattori M, Kuhara S, Shirai M. Genome sequence of the cat pathogen, Chlamydophila felis. DNA Research 2006;13(1) 15-23.

64. Siarkou VI, Stamatakis A, Kappas I, Hadweh P, Laroucau K. Evolutionary Relationships among Chlamydophila abortus Variant Strains Inferred by rRNA Secondary Structure-Based Phylogeny. PLoS One 2011;6(5) e19813.

65. Friis RR. Interaction of L cells and Chlamydia psittaci: entry of the parasite and host responses to its development. Journal of Bacteriology 1972;110(2) 706-721.

66. Peterson EM, de la Maza LM. Chlamydia parasitism: ultrastructural characterization of the interaction between the chlamydial cell envelope and the host cell. Journal of Bacteriology 1988;170(3) 1389-1392.

67. Nixdorff K, Gmeiner J, Martin HH.Interaction of lipopolysaccharide with detergents and its possible role in the detergent resistance of the outer membrane of Gramnegative bacteria. Biochimica et Biophysica Acta 1978;510(1) 87-98.

68. Liu X, Afrane M, Clemmer DE, Zhong G, Nelson DE. Identification of Chlamydia trachomatis outer membrane complex proteins by differential proteomics. Journal of Bacteriology 2010;192(11) 2852-2860.

69. Myeong-Gu Y, Young-Ju K, Yeal P. Partial Characterization of the Pathogenic Factors Related to Chlamydia trachomatis Invasion of the McCoy Cell Membrane. The Journal of Microbiology 2003;41: 137-143.

70. Sandbulte J, TerWee J, Wigington K, Sabara M. Evaluation of Chlamydia psittaci subfraction and subunit preparations for their protective capacities. Veterinary Microbiology 1996;48(3- 4) 269-282.

71. Costerton JW, Poffenroth L, Wilt JC, Kordová N. Ultrastructural studies of the nucleoids of the pleomorphic forms of Chlamydia psittaci 6BC: a comparison with bacteria. Canadian Journal of Microbiology 1976;22(1) 16-28.

72. Barbour AG, Amano K, Hackstadt T, Perry L, Caldwell HD. Chlamydia trachomatis has penicillin-binding proteins but not detectable muramic acid. Journal of Bacteriology 1982;151(1) 420-428.

73. Popov V, Eb F, Lefebvre JF, Orfila J, Viron A. Morphological and cytochemical study of Chlamydia with EDTA regressive technique and Gautier staining in ultrathin frozen sections of infected cell cultures: a comparison with embedded material. Annals de Microbiologie (Paris) 1978;129 B(3) 313-337.

74. Murata M, Azuma Y, Miura K, Rahman MA, Matsutani M, Aoyama M, Suzuki H, Sugi K, Shirai M. Chlamydial SET domain protein functions as a histone methyltransferase. Microbiology 2007;153(Pt 2) 585-592.

75. Hogan RJ, Mathews SA, Kutlin A, Hammerschlag MR, Timms P. Differential expression of genes encoding membrane proteins between acute and continuous Chlamydia pneumoniae infections. Microbial Pathogens 2003;34(1) 11-16.

76. Popov VL, Kirillova FM, Orlova OE. Surface structure of the elementary bodies of Chlamydia. Zhurnal Mikrobiologii, Epidemiologii i Immunobiologii 1984;(5) 30-33.

77. Nichols BA, Setzer PY, Pang F, Dawson CR.New view of the surface projections of Chlamydia trachomatis. Journal of Bacteriology 1985;164(1) 344-349.

78. Chang JJ, Leonard KR, Zhang YX. Structural studies of the surface projections of Chlamydia trachomatis by electron microscopy. Journal of Medical Microbiology 1997;46(12) 1013-1018.

79. Hodinka RL, Wyrick PB. Ultrastructural study of mode of entry of Chlamydia psittaci into L-929 cells. Infection and Immunity 1986;54(3) 855-863.

80. Rockey DD, Fischer ER, Hackstadt T. Temporal analysis of the developing Chlamydia psittaci inclusion by use of fluorescence and electron microscopy. Infection and Immunity 1996;64(10) 4269-4278.

81. Escalante-Ochoa C, Ducatelle R, Charlier G, De Vos K, Haesebrouck F. Significance of host cell kinesin in the development of Chlamydia psittaci. Infection and Immunity 1999;67(10) 5441-5446.

82. Allan I, Pearce JH. Differential amino acid utilization by Chlamydia psittaci (strain guinea pig inclusion conjunctivitis) and its regulatory effect on chlamydial growth. Journal of General Microbiology 1983;129 (7) 1991-2000.

83. Bannantine JP, Rockey DD, Hackstadt T. Tandem genes of Chlamydia psittaci that encode proteins localized to the inclusion membrane. Molecular Microbiology 1998;28(5) 1017-1026.

84. Hackstadt T, Scidmore-Carlson MA, Shaw EI, Fischer ER.The Chlamydia trachomatis IncA protein is required for homotypic vesicle fusion. Cellular Microbiology 1999;1(2) 119-130.

85. Beatty WL, Morrison RP, Byrne GI. Persistent chlamydiae: from cell culture to a paradigm for chlamydial pathogenesis. Microbiological Reviews 1994;58(4) 686-699.

86. Harper A, Pogson CI, Jones ML, Pearce JH. Chlamydial development is adversely affected by minor changes in amino acid supply, blood plasma amino acid levels, and glucose deprivation. Infection and Immunity 2000;68(3) 1457-1464.

87. Belland RJ, Nelson DE, Virok D, Crane DD, Hogan D, Sturdevant D, Beatty WL, Caldwell HD. Transcriptome analysis of chlamydial growth during IFN-gamma-mediated persistence and reactivation. Proceedings of the National Academy of Sciences of United States of America 2003;100(26) 15971-15976.

88. Gieffers J, Rupp J, Gebert A, Solbach W, Klinger M. First-choice antibiotics at subinhibitory concentrations induce persistence of Chlamydia pneumoniae. Antimicrobial Agents and Chemotherapy 2004;48(4) 1402-1405.

89. Saif YM. Diseases of Poultry. 11ª ed. Wiley-Blackwell Publishing; 2003.

90. Ryll M, Hinz KH, Neumann U, Behr KP. Pilot study of the occurrence of Chlamydia psittaci infections in commercial turkey flocks in Niedersachsen. Deutsch Tierärztliche Wochenschrift 1994;101(4) 163-165.

91. Sting R, Lerke E, Hotzel H, Jodas S, Popp C, Hafez HM. Comparative studies on detection of Chlamydophila psittaci and Chlamydophila abortus in meat turkey flocks using cell culture, ELISA, and PCR. Deutsch Tierärztliche Wochenschrift 2006; 113(2) 50-54

92. Newman CP, Palmer SR, Kirby FD, Caul EO.A prolonged outbreak of ornithosis in duck processors. Epidemiology and Infection 1992;108(1) 203-210.

93. Hinton DG, Shipley A, Galvin JW, Harkin JT, Brunton RA. Chlamydiosis in workers at a duck farm and processing plant. Australian Veterinary Journal 1993;70(5) 174-176.

94. Goupil F, Pellé-Duporté D, Kouyoumdjian S, Carbonnelle B, Tuchais E. Severe pneumonia with a pneumococcal aspect during an ornithosis outbreak. Presse Médicale 1998;27(22) 1084-1088.

95. Lederer P, Muller R. Ornithosis-studies in correlation with an outbreak. Gesundheitswesen 1999;61(12) 614-619.

96. Yang J, Ling Y, Yuan J, Pang W, He C. Isolation and characterization of peacock Chlamydophila psittaci infection in China. Avian Diseases 2011;55(1) 76-81.

97. Van Loock M, Verminnen K, Messmer TO, Volckaert G, Goddeeris BM, Vanrompay D. Use of a nested PCR-enzyme immunoassay with an internal control to detect Chlamydophila psittaci in turkeys. BMC Infectious Diseases 2005;5: 76.

98. Verminnen K, Beeckman DS, Sanders NN, De Smedt S, Vanrompay DC. Vaccination of turkeys against Chlamydophila psittaci through optimised DNA formulation and administration. Vaccine 2010;28(18) 3095-3105.

99. Raso Tde F, Júnior AB, Pinto AA. Evidence of Chlamydophila psittaci infection in captive Amazon parrots in Brazil. Journal of Zoo and Wildlife Medicine 2002;33(2) 118-121.

100. Dvorak G, Spickler AR, Roth JA. Handbook for zoonotic diseases of companion animals. Iowa: Iowa State University; 2008.

101. Morais J. Avaliação da seropositivade de Chlamydophila psittaci em psitacídeos de três Instituições Zoológicas do Norte de Portugal. Master thesis, University of Trás-os-Montes-e-Alto-Douro, Vila Real, Portugal; 2012.

102. Chahota R, Ogawa H, Mitsuhashi Y, Ohya K, Yamaguchi T, Fukushi H. Genetic diversity and epizootiology of Chlamydophila psittaci prevalent among the captive and feral avian species based on VD2 region of ompA gene. Microbiology and Immunology 2006;50(9) 663-678.

103. Vanrompay D, Harkinezhad T, van de Walle M, Beeckman D, van Droogenbroeck C, Verminnen K, Leten R, Martel A, Cauwerts K. Chlamydophila psittaci transmission from pet birds to humans. Emerging Infectious Diseases 2007;13(7) 1108-1110.

104. Tanaka C, Miyazawa T, Watarai M, Ishiguro N. Bacteriological survey of feces from feral pigeons in Japan. Journal of Veterinary Medical Science 2005;67(9) 951-953.

105. Prukner-Radovcić E, Horvatek D, Gottstein Z, Grozdanić IC, Mazija H. Epidemiological investigation of Chlamydophila psittaci in pigeons and free-living birds in Croatia. Veterinary Research Communications 2005;29 (Suppl 1) 17-21.

106. Kaleta EF, Taday EM. Avian host range of Chlamydophila spp. based on isolation, antigen detection and serology. Avian Pathology 2003;32(5) 435-461.

107. Olsen B, Persson K, Broholm KA. PCR detection of Chlamydia psittaci in faecal samples from passerine birds in Sweden. Epidemiology and Infection 1998;121(2) 481-484.

108. Center for Food Security and Public Health. Avian chlamydiosis. 2009. www.cfsph.iastate.edu/Factsheets/pdfs/chlamydiosis_avian.pdf (Accessed of 25 August 2011).

109. Van Droogenbroeck C, Beeckman DS, Verminnen K, Marien M, Nauwynck H, Boesinghe Lde T, Vanrompay D. Simultaneous zoonotic transmission of Chlamydophila psittaci genotypes D, F and E/B to a veterinary scientist. Veterinary Microbiology 2009;135(1-2) 78-81.

110. Lemus JA, Fargallo JA, Vergara P, Parejo D, Banda E. Natural cross chlamydial infection between livestock and free-living bird species. PLoS One 2010;5(10) e13512.

111. Andersen AA. Comparison of pharyngeal, fecal, and cloacal samples for the isolation of Chlamydia psittaci from experimentally infected cockatiels and turkeys. Journal of Veterinary Diagnostic Investigation 1996;8(4) 448-450.

112. hewen PE. Chlamydial infection in animals: a review. Canadian Veterinary Journal 1980;21(1) 2-11.

113. Longbottom D, Coulter LJ. Animal chlamydioses and zoonotic implications. Journal of Comparative Pathology 2003;128(4) 217-244.

114. Timms P. Chlamydiosis in birds, wild and domestic animals. In: Australian standard diagnostic techniques for animal diseases, ed LA Corner and TJ Bagust. East Melbourne: Commonwealth of Australia, CSIRO, p.1-8. 1993.

115. Spencer WN, Johnson FW. Simple transport medium for the isolation of Chlamydia psittaci from clinical material. Veterinary Record 1983;113(23) 535-536.

116. Reyes CV. Diff-Quik cytologic recognition of Chlamydophila psittaci in orolabial lesions of Stevens-Johnson Syndrome. Acta Cytologica 2010;54(5) 692-694.

117. Iwamoto K, Masubuchi K, Nosaka H, Kokubu T, Nishida K, Toshida T, Yamanaka M. Isolation of chlamydia psittaci from domestic cats with oculonasal discharge in Japan. Journal of Veterinary Medical Science 2001;63(8) 937-938.

118. Hayashi Y, Kato M, Ito G, Yamamoto K, Kuroki H, Matsuura T, Yamada Y, Goto A, Takeuchi T. A case report of psittacosis and chlamydial isolation from a dead pet bird. Nihon Kyobu Shikkan Gakkai Zasshi 1990;28(3) 535-540.

119. Godfroid J, Nielsen K, Saegerman C. Diagnosis of brucellosis in livestock and wildlife. Croatian Medical Journal 2010;51(4) 296-305.

120. Bancroft J. Gamble M. Theory and Pratice of Histological Techniques, 5th ed. Edinburg: Churchill Livingstone; 2002.

121. Arizmendi F, Grimes JE. Comparison of the Gimenez staining method and antigen detection ELISA with culture for detecting chlamydiae in birds. Journal of Veterinary Diagnostic Investigation 1995;7(3) 400-401.

122. Erbeck DH, Nunn SA. Chlamydiosis in pen-raised bobwhite quail (Colinus virginianus) and chukar partridge (Alectoris chukar) with high mortality. Avian Diseases 1999;43(4) 798- 803.

123. Thomas R, Davison HC, Wilsmore AJ. Use of the IDEIA ELISA to detect Chlamydia psittaci (ovis) in material from aborted fetal membranes and milk from ewes affected by ovine enzootic abortion. British Veterinary Journal 1990;146(4) 364-367.

124. Woodland RM, Malam J, Darougar S. A rapid method for staining inclusions of Chlamydia psittaci and Chlamydia trachomatis. Journal of Clinical Pathology 1982;35(6) 642-644.

125. Thomas NJ, Hunter DB, Atkinson CT. Infectious diseases of wild birds. 1st ed. Blackwell Pub. 303-316; 2007.

126. Dlugosz A, Törnblom H, Mohammadian G, Morgan G, Veress B, Edvinsson B, Sandström G, Lindberg G. Chlamydia trachomatis antigens in enteroendocrine cells and macrophages of the small bowel in patients with severe irritable bowel syndrome. BMC Gastroenterology 2010;10: 19.

127. chautteet K, Vanrompay D. Chlamydiaceae infections in pig. Veterinary Research 2011;42(1) 29.

128. Everett KD, Andersen AA. Identification of nine species of the Chlamydiaceae using PCR-RFLP. International Journal of Systematic Bacteriology 1999;49(Pt 2) 803-813.

129. Moore FM, Petrak ML. Chlamydia immunoreactivity in birds with psittacosis: localization of chlamydiae by the peroxidase-antiperoxidase method. Avian Diseases 1985;29(4) 1036-1042.

130. OIE Terrestrial Manual. Avian Chlamydiosis. Chapter 2.3.1; 2012.

131. Schmeer N, Krauss H, Apel J, Adami M, Müller HP, Schneider W, Perez-Martinez JA, Rieser H. Analysis of caprine IgG1 and IgG2 subclass responses to Chlamydia psittaci infection and vaccination. Veterinary Microbiology 1987;14(2) 125-135.

132. Kaltenboeck B, Heard D, DeGraves FJ, Schmeer N. Use of synthetic antigens improves detection by enzyme-linked immunosorbent assay of antibodies against abortigenic Chlamydia psittaci in ruminants. Journal of Clinical Microbiology 1997;35(9) 2293-2298.

133. Bevan BJ, Bracewell CD. Chlamydiosis in birds in Great Britain. 2. Isolations of Chlamydia psittaci from birds sampled between 1976 and 1984. Journal of Hygiene (London) 1986;96(3) 453-458.

134. Lewis VJ, Thacker WL, Cacciapuoti AF. Detection of Chlamydia psittaci by immunofluorescence. Applied Microbiology 1972;24(1) 8-12.

135. Gutiérrez J, Mendoza J, Fernández F, Linares-Palomino J, Soto MJ, Maroto MC. ELISA test to detect Chlamydophila pneumoniae IgG. Journal of Basic Microbiology 2002;42(1) 13-18.

136. Sachse K, Vretou E, Livingstone M, Borel N, Pospischil A, Longbottom D. Recent developments in the laboratory diagnosis of chlamydial infections. Veterinary Microbiology 2009;135(1- 2) 2-21.

137. Demaio J, Boyd RS, Rensi R, Clark A. False-positive Chlamydiazyme results during urine sediment analysis due to bacterial urinary tract infections. Journal of Clinical Microbiology 1991;29(7) 1436-1438.

138. Hoymans VY, Bosmans JM, Van Renterghem L, Mak R, Ursi D, Wuyts F, Vrints CJ, Ieven M. Importance of methodology in determination of Chlamydia pneumoniae seropositivity in healthy subjects and in patients with coronary atherosclerosis. Journal of Clinical Microbiology 2003;41(9) 4049-4053.

139. Tiran A, Tiesenhausen K, Karpf E, Orfila J, Koch G, Gruber HJ, Tsybrovskyy O, Tiran B. Association of antibodies to chlamydial lipopolysaccharide with the endovascular presence of Chlamydophila pneumoniae in carotid artery disease. Atherosclerosis 2004;173(1) 47-54.

140. Verminnen K, Van Loock M, Hafez HM, Ducatelle R, Haesebrouck F, Vanrompay D. Evaluation of a recombinant enzyme-linked immunosorbent assay for detecting Chlamydophila psittaci antibodies in turkey sera. Veterinary Research 2006;37(4) 623-632.

141. Persson K, Haidl S. Evaluation of a commercial test for antibodies to the chlamydial lipopolysaccharide (Medac) for serodiagnosis of acute infections by Chlamydia pneumoniae (TWAR) and Chlamydia psittaci. APMIS 2000;108(2) 131-138.

142. Harkinezhad T, Geens T, Vanrompay D. Chlamydophila psittaci infections in birds: a review with emphasis on zoonotic consequences. Veterinary Microbiology 2009;135 (1-2) 68-77.

143. Morais J, Coelho AC, Soeiro V, Nunes P, Alvura N, Pires MA. Seropositivdade de Chlamydophila psittaci em aves Ara. II Encontro de Formação da Ordem dos Médicos Veterinários, Lisboa; 2011a.

144. Morais J, Coelho AC, Soeiro V, Nunes P, Alvura N, Pires MA. Seropositivade de Chlamydophila psittaci em psitacídeos. II Simpósio Selvagens Exóticos, University of Trás-os-Montes-e-Alto-Douro, Vila Real, Portugal; 2011b.

145. Sanderson TP, Andersen AA. Evaluation of an enzyme immunoassay for detection of Chlamydia psittaci in vaginal secretions, placentas, and fetal tissues from aborting ewes. Journal of Veterinary Diagnostic Investigation 1989;1(4) 309-315.

146. Ossewaarde JM, Rieffe M, de Vries A, Derksen-Nawrocki RP, Hooft HJ, van Doornum GJ, van Loon AM. Comparison of two panels of monoclonal antibodies for determination of Chlamydia trachomatis serovars. Journal of Clinical Microbiology 1994;32 (12) 2968–2974.

147. Bovarnick MR, Miller JC, Snyder JC. The influence of certain salts, amino acids, sugars, and proteins on the stability of rickettsiae. Journal of Bacteriology 1950;59(4) 509-522.

148. OIE Terrestrial Manual. Chapter 2.3.1: 431-442; 2008.

149. Bevan BJ, Cullen GA, Read WM.Isolation of Chlamydia psittaci from avian sources using growth in cell culture. Avian Pathology 1978;7(2) 203-211.

150. OIE Manual. Chapter B/066: 1-12;1990.

151. Vanrompay D, Ducatelle R, Haesebrouck F. Diagnosis of avian chlamydiosis: specificity of the modified Gimenez staining on smears and comparison of the sensitivity of isolation in eggs and three different cell cultures. Zentralblatt für Veterinärmedizin B 1992;39(2) 105-112.

152. Clark VL, Bavoil PM. Interaction of pathogenic bacteria with host cells. Academic Press, Inc: 378-382; 1994.

153. Trávnicek M, Balascák J, Balatý B, Dravecký T. Isolation of Chlamydia psittaci from bull ejaculate. Veterinární Medicína (Praha) 1980;25(11) 669-673.

154. Hahon N, Zimmerman WD. Intracellular survival of viral and rickettsial agents in acetone at -60 C. Applied Microbiology 1969;17(5) 775-776.

155. Pursell AR, Cole JR Jr.Procedure for fluorescent-antibody staining of virus-infected cell cultures in plastic plates. Journal of Clinical Microbiology 1976;3(5) 537-540.

156. Atala A, Lanza RP. Methods of tissue engineering. San Diego: Academic Pr; 2002.

157. Cunningham R, Jenks P, Northwood J, Wallis M, Ferguson S, Hunt S. Effect on MRSA transmission of rapid PCR testing of patients admitted to critical care. Journal of Hospital Infection 2007;65(1) 24-28.

158. Messmer TO, Skelton SK, Moroney JF, Daugharty H, Fields BS. Application of a nested, multiplex PCR to psittacosis outbreaks. Journal of Clinical Microbiology 1997;35(8) 2043- 2046.

159. Madico G, Quinn TC, Boman J, Gaydos CA. Touchdown enzyme time release-PCR for detection and identification of Chlamydia trachomatis, C. pneumoniae, and C. psittaci using the 16S and 16S-23S spacer rRNA genes. Journal of Clinical Microbiology 2000;38(3) 1085-1093.

160. Yoshida H, Kishi Y, Shiga S, Hagiwara T. Differentiation of Chlamydia species by combined use of polymerase chain reaction and restriction endonuclease analysis. Microbiology and Immunology 1998;42(5) 411-414.

161. DeGraves FJ, Gao D, Kaltenboeck B. High-sensitivity quantitative PCR platform. Biotechniques 2003;34(1) 106-110, 112-105.

162. Harkinezhad T, Verminnen K, Van Droogenbroeck C, Vanrompay D. Chlamydophila psittaci genotype E/B transmission from African grey parrots to humans. Journal of Medical Microbiology 2007;56(Pt 8) 1097-1100.

163. Sachse K, Grossmann E. Chlamydial diseases of domestic animals- zoonotic potential of the agents and diagnostic issues. Deutsch Tierärztliche Wochenschrift 2002;109(4) 142-148.

164. Domino F. The 5-Minute Clinical Consult. 19th edition. Philadelphia: Lippincott Williams & Wilkins; 2011.

165. Boden E. Black's Veterinary Dictionary. MBE, HonAssocRCVS, MRPharmS; 2005.

166. Seth-Smith HM, Harris SR, Rance R, West AP, Severin JA, Ossewaarde JM, Cutcliffe LT, Skilton RJ, Marsh P, Parkhill J, Clarke IN, Thomson NR. Genome sequence of the zoonotic pathogen Chlamydophila psittaci. Journal of Bacteriology 2011;193(5) 1282- 1283.

167. Telfer BL, Moberley SA, Hort KP, Branley JM, Dwyer DE, Muscatello DJ, Correll PK, England J, McAnulty JM. Probable psittacosis outbreak linked to wild birds. Emerging Infectious Diseases 2005;11(3) 391-397.

168. Hughes C, Maharg P, Rosario P, Herrell M, Bratt D, Salgado J, Howard D. Possible nosocomial transmission of psittacosis. Infection Control and Hospital Epidemiology 1997;18(3) 165- 168.

169. Ito I, Ishida T, Mishima M, Osawa M, Arita M, Hashimoto T, Kishimoto T. Familial cases of psittacosis: possible person-to-person transmission. Internal Medicine 2002;41(7) 580- 583.

170. O'Shea H. Combating chlamydiosis. Bioengineered Bugs 2010;1(4) 282-283.

171. Chorazy M, Nasiek-Palka A, Kwaśna K. The case of 57-year-old patient with ornithosis. Wiadomósci Lekarskie 2006;59(9-10) 716-719.

172. Strâmbu I, Ciolan G, Anghel L, Mocanu A, Stoicescu IP. Bilateral lung consolidations related to accidental exposure to parrots. Pneumologia 2006;55(3) 123-127.

173. Haas LE, Tjan DH, Schouten MA, van Zanten AR. Severe pneumonia from psittacosis in a bird-keeper. Nederlands Tijdschrift voor Geneeskdunde 2006;150(3) 117-121.

174. andeli V, Ernest D. A case of fulminant psittacosis. Critical Care and Resuscitation 2006;8(1) 40-42.

175. Chanudet E, Zhou Y, Bacon CM, Wotherspoon AC, Müller-Hermelink HK, Adam P, Dong HY, de Jong D, Li Y, Wei R, Gong X, Wu Q, Ranaldi R, Goteri G, Pileri SA, Ye H, Hamoudi RA, Liu H, Radford J, Du MQ. Chlamydia psittaci is variably associated with ocular adnexal MALT lymphoma in different geographical regions. Journal of Pathology 2006;209(3) 344-351.

176. Zhang GS, Winter JN, Variakojis D, Reich S, Lissner GS, Bryar P, Regner M, Mangold K, Kaul K. Lack of an association between Chlamydia psittaci and ocular adnexal lymphoma. Leukemia and Lymphoma 2007;48(3) 577-583.

Chapter 6

The Endocrine Glands in the Dog: From the Cell to Hormone

1. Introduction

The animal body represents one of the more complex and perfect systems of nature. Despite its complexity and its functionality, which is incredibly effective, the control of its basic functions is performed by only two systems: the nervous system and endocrine system. The nervous system is associated with electrical and chemical signals that are transmitted at high speed, resulting in rapid organic activities. The endocrine system acts through the synthesis and release of chemical messengers and is responsible for several functions of the organism, in a slower, but more durable way.

Endocrinology is the science that studies the internal secretions produced by endocrine glands. Endocrine glands are distributed throughout the body and secrete chemical messengers – hormones, in response to an internal or external stimulus. These hormones are released directly into the bloodstream – endocrine mechanism, in contrast to exocrine glands, which use a ductal system to release their secretions in locations that lead, ultimately, to the exterior of the body – exocrine mechanism.

Hormones are transported through the bloodstream to target organs, where they will exert a physiological control, even in low concentrations, coordinating a multiplicity of organic functions and maintaining homeostasis.

The main endocrine glands in the animal body include pituitary gland, thyroid, parathyroid, pancreas, adrenal (Figure 1), and gonads (ovaries and testes).

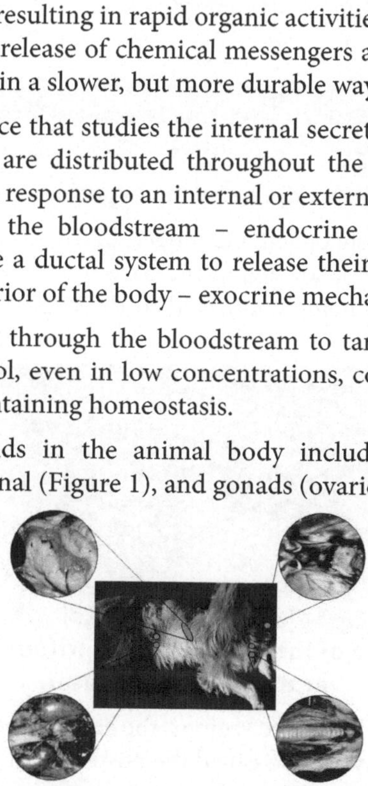

Figure 1.Schematic location of main endocrine glands. Top right figure represents pituitary gland; top left figure represents pancreas; bottom right figure represents thyroid and parathyroid glands; bottom left figure represents adrenal glands.

2. Hypothalamic-pituitary axis

The hypothalamus, located at the base of the ventral diencephalon is limited rostrally by the optic chiasm, caudally by the mammillary processes, laterally by the temporal lobes and dorsally by the thalamus. Ventrally, it continues through the infundibulum which connects it to the pituitary gland. Although not considered a real endocrine gland, the hypothalamus coordinates all pituitary activity by the release of a number of peptides and amines that control the secretion of hormones in the pituitary gland (also named hypophysis). Their terminology ends in RH that means releasing hormone (GnRH - gonadotrophin releasing hormone; CRH - Corticotrophin releasing hormone; TRH - Tirotrophin releasing hormone; PRH - Prolactin releasing hormone; GHRH - Growth hormone releasing hormone). Table 1 summarizes the major hormones produced by this hypothalamic-pituitary axis.

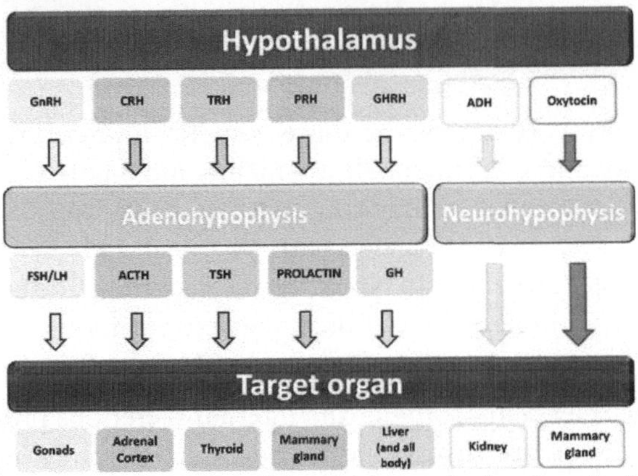

Table 1. Hormones produced by the hypothalamic-pituitary axis.

The pituitary is a small oval shaped gland, lodged in the *sella turcica*, a small depression of the sphenoid bone, which is located at the base of the brain and positioned next to the optic chiasm (Figure 2), being connected to the hypothalamus by a funnel-shaped hypophyseal stalk [1,2].

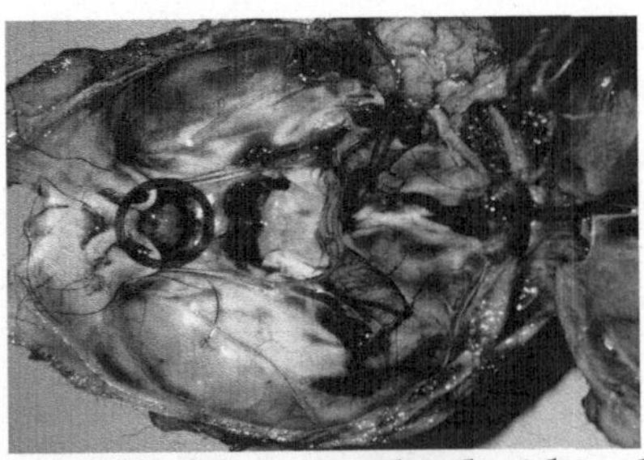

Figure 2.Location of the pituitary gland within the sella turcica, next to the optic chiasm.

The pituitary gland is divided into two regions, the adenohypophysis, or anterior pituitary gland, and the neurohypophysis, also called the posterior pituitary gland or pars nervosa.

The adenohypophysis, in turn, is divided in three sections: pars distalis, pars tuberalis and pars intermedia (Figure 3) [3].

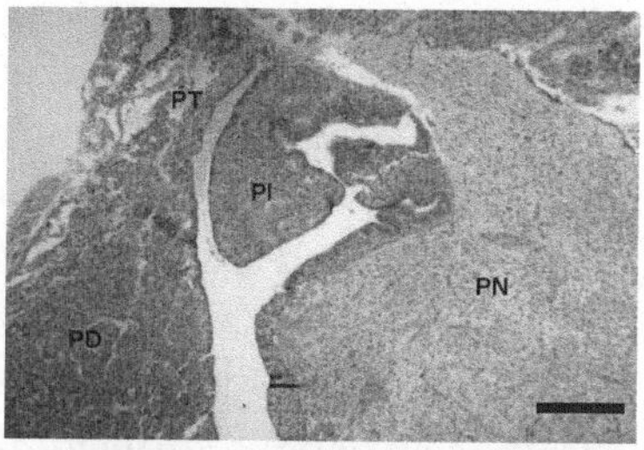

Figure 3.Divisions of the pituitary gland in the dog. PT, pars tuberalis; PI, pars intermedia; PD, pars distalis; PN, pars nervosa. HE. Bar = 100 μm.

❖ The parenchyma of the pars distalis is composed by chromophilic cells, acidophilic or basophilic, arranged in cords, nests or follicles (Figure 4) and by small, round endocrine cells, without evident granules - chromophobe cells which means that they have low tinctorial affinity, also known as principal cells, reserve cells or C cells [4]. Chromophilic cells secrete somatotropic hormone (also known as somatotropin - STH or growth hormone - GH), prolactin (PRL), adrenocorticotropic hormone (ACTH), follicle-stimulating hormone (FSH), luteinizing hormone (LH) (which is also called interstitial cell-stimulating hormone or ICSH in males), thyrotropin or thyroid-stimulating hormone (TSH), melanocyte-stimulating hormone (MSH) and lipotropines [4]. Somatotropin promotes epiphyseal growth [6] and protein production, whereas prolactin leads to mammary gland development and milk secretion. ACTH acts on the adrenal gland cortex, resulting in an increased release of adrenocortical hormones [7]. FSH and LH are gonadotropic hormones, with different effects in males and females [8,9]. TSH acts on the thyroid gland, stimulating its secretion [10]. Lipotropines have the same precursor molecule as ACTH (propiomelanocortin - POMC) [3,5] and, after cleavage, can originate β-MSH and β-endorfine, a pain blocking agent [3] (Table 2).

Also, considering its secretion, chromophilic cells of pars distalis, may be classified in four types:

Lactotrophs or lactotropic cells which secrete PRL (acidophilic) [11].

Corticotropes or corticotropic cells which secrete ACTH (basophilic) [12].

Gonadotropes or gonadotropic cells which secrete gonadotropins LH and FSH (basophilic) [13].

Thyrotrophs or thyrotropic cells which secrete TSH (basophilic) [14].

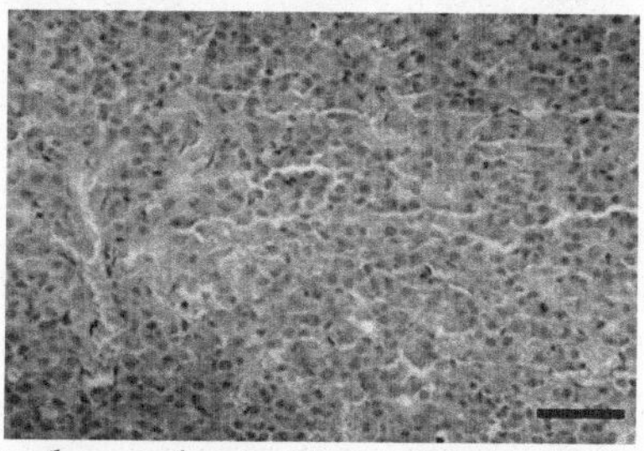

Figure 4.Adenohypophysis. Pars distalis. HE. Bar = 25 μm.

The chromophobe cells are also arranged in clusters or cords and their low tinctorial affinity probably indicates that these cells may correspond to depleted cells of any of the above types described or a state of partial degranulation. However, some of the chromophobe cells may also be undifferentiated, nonsecretory cells [4, 15].

- The pars tuberalis is composed by cuboidal weakly basophilic cells, arranged in cords, nests or follicles and its function is not yet well established [4]. Studies suggest that one of its primary functions, in seasonal mammals (e.g. sheep), is to mediate photoperiod influences in prolactin secretion variations through an unidentified factor called tuberalin i.e. tuberalin performs hormonal control, both in gene expression and in the release of prolactin from lactotrophs in the pars distalis [3].
- The pars intermedia is more developed in domestic animals than in man, consisting of nonspecific basophilic cells, arranged mainly in cords and nests, but also in follicles (Figure 5), which secrete MSH [4] that in turn, promotes distribution of melanin granules, and therefore, darkening of skin [10].

The neurohypophysis is devoid of endocrine cells, being composed of demielinized neurons (Figure 6) whose bodies are in the supraoptic and paraventricular nuclei of the hypothalamus, constituting the storage of the hypothalamic hormones: antidiuretic hormone (ADH), also called vasopressin, oxytocin and neurophysins. These hormones are produced in the hypothalamus, transported through the hypothalamic-pituitary axis and stored in the neurohypophysis, until a stimulus induces their release [4, 16] (Table 2).

ADH has several effects on the body, particularly in terms of water saving and in increasing blood pressure. Oxytocin stimulates contraction of the myoepithelial cells of the mammary gland, causing the ejection of milk. It also binds to the smooth muscle cells of the uterus, promoting uterine contractions during parturition [10] (Table 2).

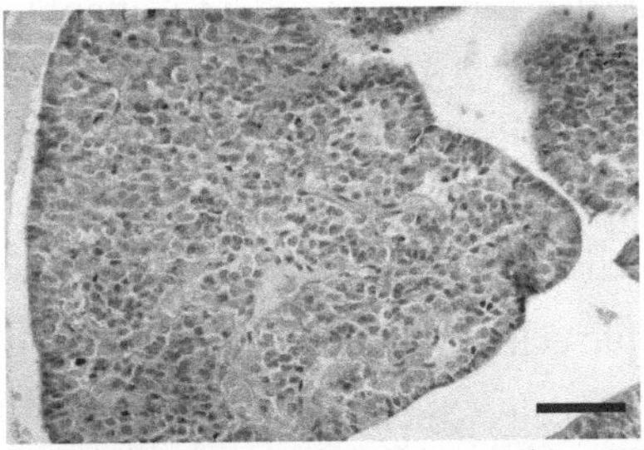

Figure 5.Adenohypophysis. Pars intermedia. HE. Bar = 25 μm.

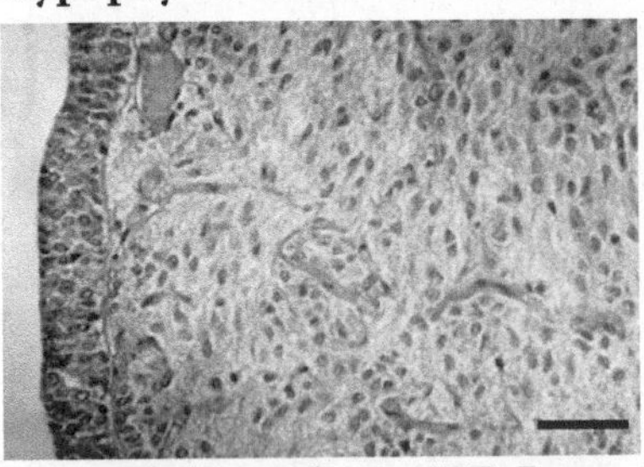

Figure 6. Neurohypophysis. HE. Bar = 25 μm.

Endocrine gland		Hormone	Function	Secretion control is made by
Pituitary	Anterior	GH	Stimulates liver to produce growth factors that stimulate bone and cartilage growth	GHRH (Hypothalamus)
Pituitary	Anterior	Prolactin	Stimulates mammary gland growth and milk production	--------
Pituitary	Anterior	ACTH	Stimulates adrenal cortex to produce hormones (glucocorticoids and mineralocorticoids)	CRH (Hypothalamus)
Pituitary	Anterior	FSH	· Stimulates development of follicles · Stimulates the production of sperm in the seminiferous tubules of the testes	GnRH (Hypothalamus)
Pituitary	Anterior	LH	Stimulates development of ovaries	Oestrogen secreted by Graafian follicles
Pituitary	Anterior	ICSH	Stimulates testosterone production by the interstitial cells of the testes	GnRH (Hypothalamus)
Pituitary	Anterior	TSH	Stimulates thyroid gland to produce hormones (T3, T4, calcitonin)	TRH (Hypothalamus)
Pituitary	Anterior	MSH	Promotes distribution of melanin granules	--------
Pituitary	Posterior	ADH	Stimulates retention of water, increasing its permeability at distal convoluted tubules and collecting ducts of the nephrons	Status of the extracelular fluid and bood plasma
Pituitary	Posterior	Oxytocin	Stimulates uterine contractions during parturition and promotes milk ejection reflex in the mammary glands	Suckling by the neonate initiates a reflex arc

Table 2. Hormones produced by the pituitary gland and their functions.

3. Thyroid

Canine thyroid gland is located at cervical ventral region, lateral and ventral to the 5th-8th tracheal rings (Figure 7), being composed by two separate lobes, occasionally connected by an isthmus [17, 18].

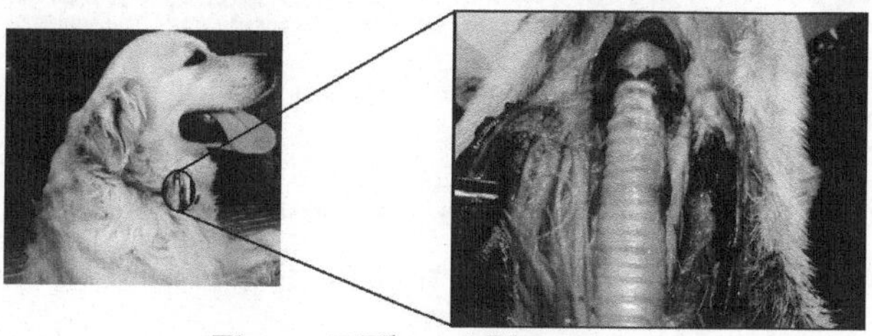

Figure 7.Thyroid location.

In the lobes, the majority of the epithelial cellular population (90%) ranges in height, from low cuboidal to high columnar epithelial cells, which are organized into follicles – follicular cells (Figure 8) [4, 16].

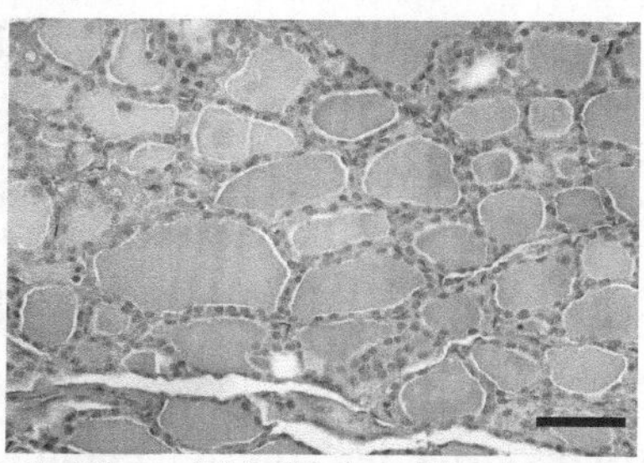

Figure 8. Thyroid follicles. HE. Bar = 25 μm.

The follicle is, therefore, the structural and secretory unit of the thyroid gland, whose center is filled with a colloidal secretion (Figure 9), comprising the hormones triiodothyronine (T3) and thyroxine (T4) [4]. In between the follicles, in a parafollicular position, cells with a pale cytoplasm, and a basal nucleus can be found - parafollicular cells or C cells which produce calcitonin [4, 16, 18].

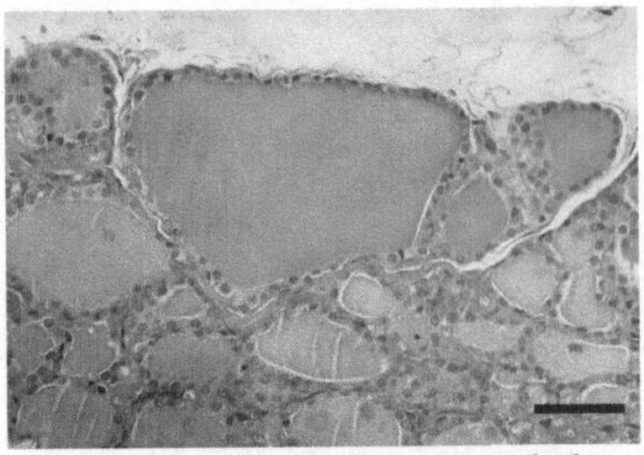

Figure 9. Thyroid follicles. Central colloidal eosinophilic material. HE. Bar = 25 μm.

T4 and T3 have very similar effects in regulating cellular metabolism. Calcitonin assists with the regulation of calcium ion concentration in the blood. It is secreted in response to hypercalcemia, decreasing the resorption of calcium from bones and inhibiting the phosphate reabsortion from renal tubules [10] (table 3).

Due to the action of T3 and T4, thyroid is the main gland, acting in the regulation of metabolism.

Thyroid stimulation is performed by TSH, originated in the adenohypophysis, under stimulation of TRH released by hypothalamus [10].

Endocrine gland	Hormone	Function	Secretion control is made by
Thyroid	T3/T4	Stimulates metabolic rate for growth	TSH (Adenohypophysis)
	Calcitonin	Regulates calcium levels in the blood (decreases the resorption of calcium from bones)	Raised blood calcium levels

Table 3. Hormones produced by thyroid gland and their functions.

4. Parathyroid

Parathyroid glands are salmon-coloured and distinct from the thyroid glands. In the dog there are four parathyroid glands, one external and one internal per each thyroid gland [17, 19, 20].

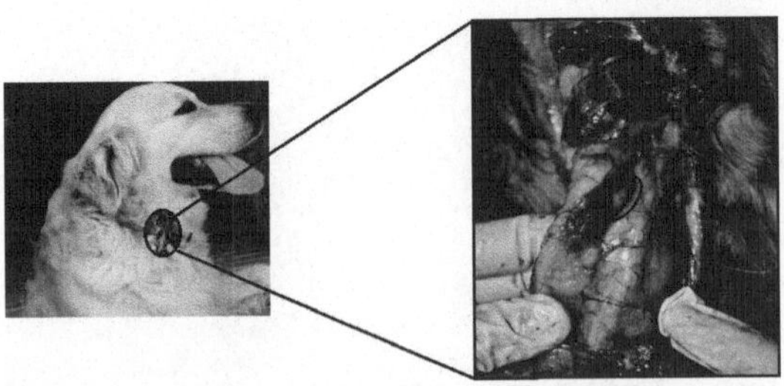

Figure 10. External parathyroid gland location.

External parathyroid glands are capsulated and may be found in varied positions, according to the species, which means that they can be placed between a cranial location to the thyroid gland and the entrance of the chest. In dogs, external parathyroid glands are located very close to the thyroid gland, on its cranial pole and externally to its capsule (Figure 10) [17, 19, 20].

The internal parathyroids are unencapsulated glands. They may be absent in some species or may be found included within the thyroid or close to them. In the dog, internal parathyroid glands are within the thyroid capsule, in the caudal and medial aspects of the thyroid [19, 20].

The parenchyma of parathyroid glands is composed of secretory cells, named chief or principal cells, arranged in cords, clusters, chains or rosettes (Figure 11, Figure 12). In some species, such as cattle and humans, it is also composed by oxyphilic cells, organized in small clusters which have yet no known functions [4]. In dogs, this type of cells were only found in senile animals [21] and were also described in canine parathyroid adenoma [22].

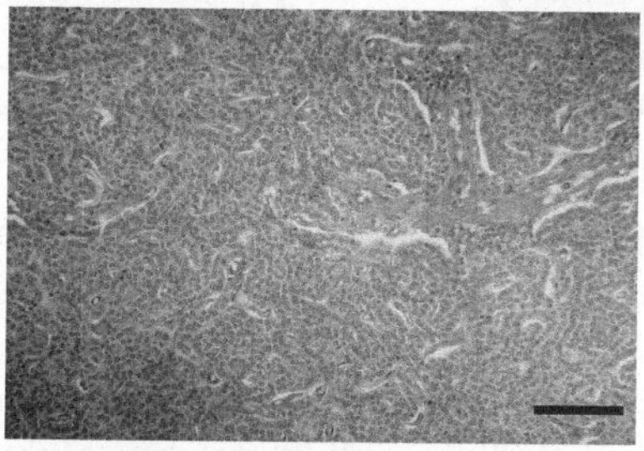

Figure 11. Parathyroid cellular organization in cords, clusters and rosetes. HE. Bar = 50 μm.

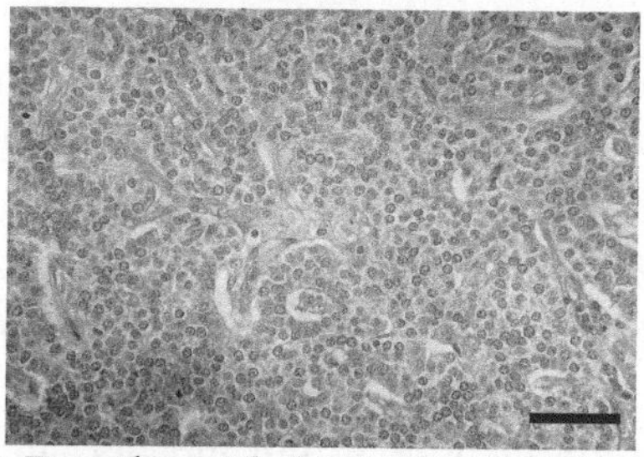

Figure 12. Parathyroid chief cells. HE. Bar = 25 μm.

Chief cells synthesize and secrete PTH. This hormone, together with calcitonin and vitamin D, is involved in the regulation of calcium homeostasis. It is released in response to low blood calcium level [23] due to it's ability to enhance the mobilization of calcium ions from the small intestine and from bone resorption, and also by increasing the simultaneous absorption of calcium and excretion of phosphate from distal convoluted tubules of kidneys [10] (Table 4).

Endocrine gland	Hormone	Function	Secretion control is made by
Parathyroid	Parathormone (PTH)	Stimulates calcium resorption from bones; promotes calcium uptake from the intestine	Low blood calcium levels

Table 4. Hormone production by parathyroid glands.

5. Pancreas

The pancreas is located in the abdominal cavity. In the dog, it is a V-shaped gland with a body and two lobes. It is acutely flexed with the apex nestling close to the cranial flexure of the duodenum. The slender right lobe runs within the mesoduodenum and the thicker but shorter left lobe extends over the caudal surface of the stomach towards the spleen, within the greater omentum (Figure 13) [4, 17].

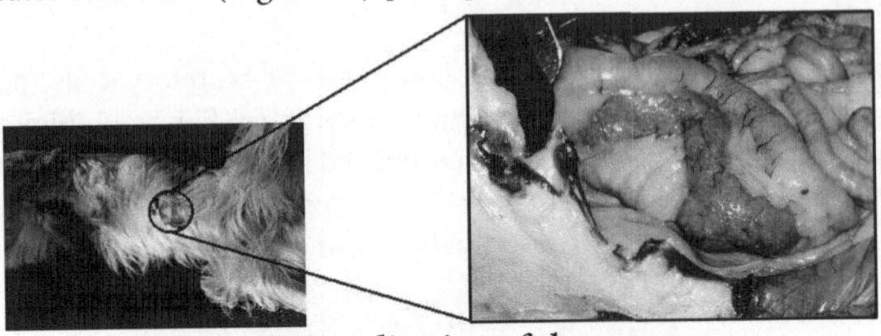

Figure 13. Localization of the pancreas.

The pancreas is one of the mixed glands of the body, since it produces both exocrine (pancreatic juice, important for digestion) and endocrine secretion. The later is produced in the islets of Langerhans, which are randomly scattered in the exocrine parenchyma (Figure 14) [10, 17, 24]. Pancreatic islets are aggregates of endocrine cells required for blood glucose control and diabetes prevention after birth, consisting of polygonal shaped cells, with pale eosinophilic cytoplasm and coarse heterochromatin. Cells are arranged in cords or clusters separated by sinusoids and are subdivided in the following subtypes (Figure 15) [4, 24, 25]:

- ❖ α cells, located peripherally and representing 10-20% of islet cells, secrete glucagon, a hyperglycaemic hormone, as well as cholecystokinin, gastric inhibitory protein and ACTH-endorphin [4, 10, 24, 26].
- ❖ β cells, located in the centre of the islets, are more abundant, representing 60-80% of the islets of Langerhans, and secrete insulin, a hypoglycaemic hormone [4, 10, 24].
- ❖ δ cells, responsible for the production of somatostatin, a hormone responsible for preventing drastic variations in both insulin and glucagon [10, 24, 27]. This hormone is also capable of reducing intestinal motility and secretion of digestive juices. These cells represent about 5-40% of the islets [10, 24].
- ❖ above-mentioned cell types, the endocrine pancreas also contain some minor types of cells, that represent around 5% of the total pancreatic cells. These are divided as follows:
- ❖ F cells, less abundant (2-3%), secrete pancreatic polypeptide (PP), which affects the production of some digestive enzymes and inhibits biliary and pancreatic secretion, as well as, intestinal motility [10, 24].
- ❖ D1 cells, that secrete the vasoactive intestinal peptide (VIP) [4] with important functions in the regulation of intestinal motility and intestinal transport of ions and water [10].
- ❖ EC or enterochromaffin cells, wich secrete secretin, wich stimulates bicarbonate and pancreatic enzyme secretion, and motilin that increases gastric and intestinal motility.

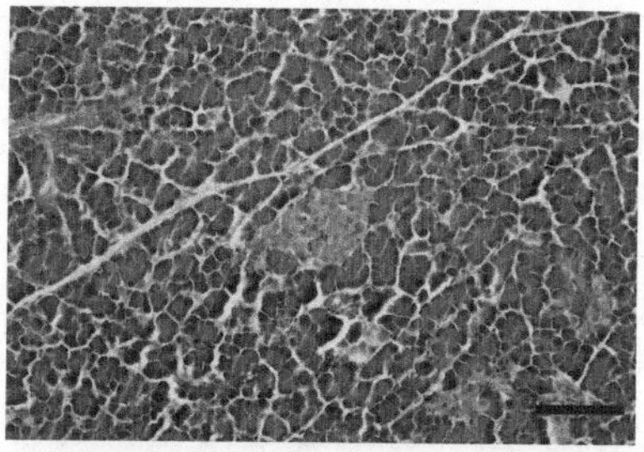

Figure 14. Islets of Langerhans. HE. Bar = 50 μm.

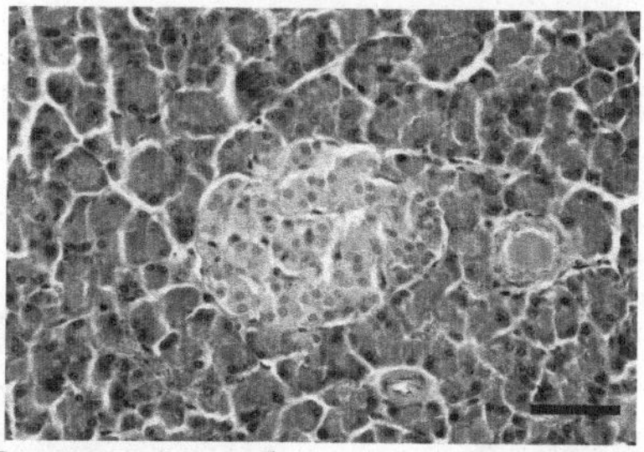

Figure 15. Pancreatic endocrine cells. HE. Bar = 25 μm.

Insulin and glucagon are pancreatic hormones that play pivotal roles in regulating glucose homeostasis and metabolism, which have opposite effects on glycaemia as well as on the metabolism of nutrients [24, 26, 28]. In general, it can be said that:

Insulin – promotes glucose uptake by peripheral tissues, (muscle, liver and adipose tissue) and its accumulation as glycogen and fat, resulting in an anabolic effect [28] and in the removal of glucose from the blood, reducing glycaemia – hypoglycaemic effect [24];

Glucagon – promotes glucose production (catabolic effect) activating liver glycogenolysis and gluconeogenesis, releasing glucose in blood circulation, increasing glucose levels in the blood, promoting glycaemia – hyperglycaemic effect [24, 28].

So, the actions of the two hormones combined contribute to the control of blood glucose.

Glucagon secretion by α-cells is highly regulated by multiple factors, being the most important the glucose and insulin levels. Low glucose levels activate specific channels in the brain and in pancreatic α-cells to generate action potentials of sodium and calcium currents, leading to glucagon secretion. Also, somatostatin inhibits glucagon secretion by inhibiting adenylate cyclase and cAMP production [26].

Endocrine gland	Hormone	Function	Secretion control is made by
Pancreas	Insulin	Increase uptake of glucose into the cell; promotes glycogenesis; lowers blood sugar levels	Raised blood glucose levels
	Glucagon	Promotes glycogenolysis; Increases blood sugar levels	Low blood glucose levels
	Somatostatin	Mild inhibition of insulin and glucagon preventing fluctuations in blood glucose levels. Decreases gut motility and secretion of digestive juices	Blood glucose levels

Table 5.Hormones produced by the pancreas.

Insulin has several physiologic actions that include stimulation of cellular glucose and potassium uptake [29]. Glucose-induced insulin secretion from pancreatic β-cells depends on mitochondrial activation, amongst other factors, like ATP, glutamate and others [30]. Incretin hormones, glucose-dependent insulinotropic polypeptide (GIP) and glucagon like peptide-1 (GLP-1), secreted by cells of the gastrointestinal tract in response to meal ingestion, exert important glucorregulatory effects, including the glucose-dependent potentiation of insulin secretion by pancreatic β-cells [31].

Table 5 summarizes hormones of the pancreas and their functions.

6. Adrenal glands

The adrenal glands are paired organs located against the roof of the abdomen near the thoracolumbar junction, in a position immediately prior to the kidneys and close to their cranial poles (Figure 16). Generally elongated, these glands are often asymmetrical and quite irregular [17].

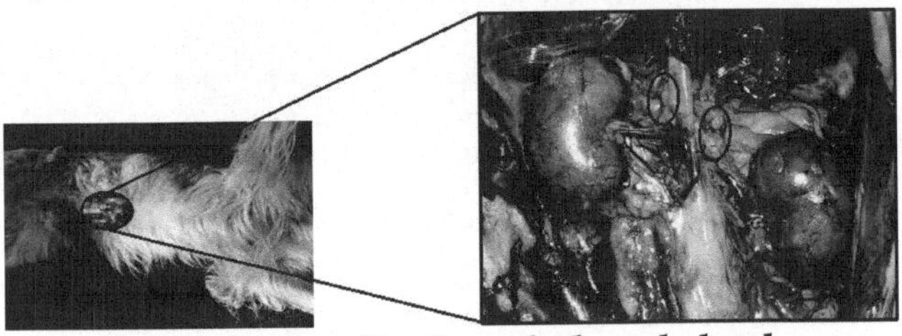

Figure 16. Localization of adrenal glands.

Each of these glands is divided into cortex and medulla. The cortex is yellowish and radially striated, while the medulla is more uniform and darker [17].

Both regions, cortex and medulla, correspond to areas specialized in producing different hormones [4, 32, 34]:

- The cortex consists of polyhedral secretory cells, arranged into two layered thick cords, which originate radially from the medullar zone [4, 33]. It is composed of 3 distinct zones. The outer zone is the *zona glomerulosa*, a thin region that in dogs and cats is composed by cells arranged in an arched or arcuate pattern, therefore also named as *zona arcuata* (Figure 17) [32, 35, 36].

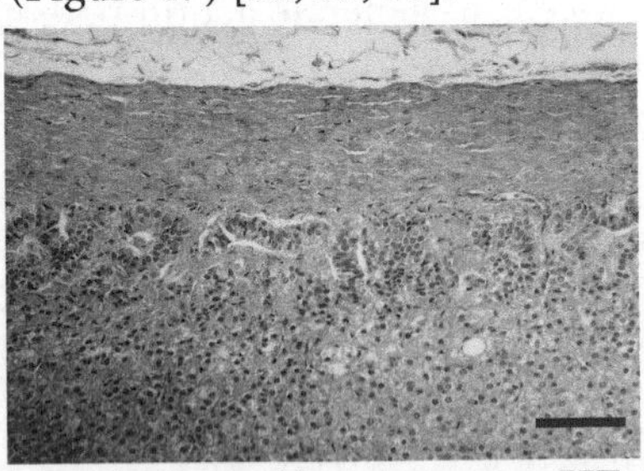

Figure 17. Adrenal cortex. Zona arcuata. HE. Bar = 50 μm.

The *zona glomerulosa* produces mineralocorticoids, particularly the steroid hormone aldosterone [32, 37], which is responsible for increasing sodium retention and water reabsortion in the distal tubules of the kidneys and sodium reabsorption in intestine. Aldosterone also maintains blood concentration and stimulates potassium excretion by the kidneys, thereby, indirectly regulating extracellular fluid volume. A decrease of mineralocorticoids, by loss of this zone or its functional ability, gives rise to water outlet of the blood to the tissues and may result in death, due to retention of high levels of potassium with excess loss of sodium, chloride and water [32].

The *zona fasciculata* is the middle and thickest zone (corresponding to more than 70% of the cortex) and is composed of parallel columns of secretory cells, one to two cells thick, separated by prominent capillaries. The cells are cuboidal or polyhedral, containing vesicular nucleus, frequently binucleated) and foamy cytoplasm (intracellular lipid droplets) (Figure 18). This zone produces glucocorticoids [32, 33, 34, 37].

Glucocorticoids have several functions, including protein catabolism and stimulation of the hepatic gluconeogenesis from amino acids [10, 37]. In dogs, cortisol is the main glucocorticoid produced.

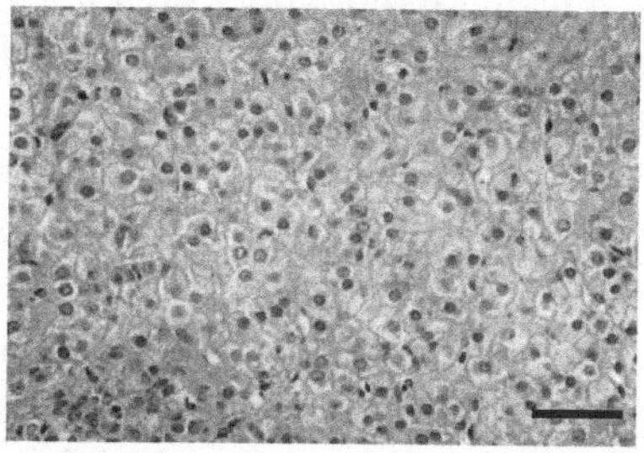

Figure 18. Adrenal cortex. Zona Fasciculata. HE. Bar = 25 μm.

The *zona reticularis* is also composed of polyhedral cells, whose arrangement consists in freely anastomosing cords (Figure 19) [32]. These cells contain less lipid content but have densely granular cytoplasm for which they are called "compact cells" [34]. *The zona reticularis* works as a unit together with the *zona fasciculata*, producing androgens (androstenedione) and also glucocorticoids [34, 37].

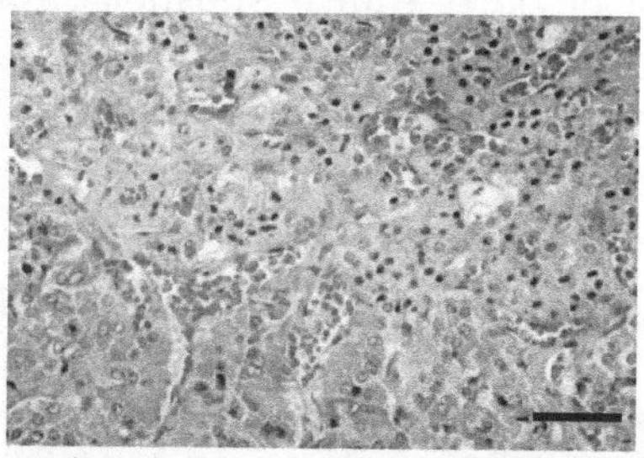

Figure 19. Adrenal cortex. Zona Reticularis. HE. Bar = 25 μm.

The adrenal cortex is stimulated by ACTH, produced in the adenohypophysis. In response, it produces glucocorticoids (e.g. cortisol), mineralocorticoids (e.g. aldosterone) and minor amounts of sex steroids (androgens and estrogens).

- The medulla consists of large columnar or polyhedral secretory cells, randomly distributed, with rich blood supply (Figure 20). The cells have large, vesicular nucleus, basophilic cytoplasm with fine positive chromaffin granules, due to the presence of catecholamines such as epinephrine and norepinephrine, which after exposure to oxidizing agents, such as chromate, yield a brown reaction by the formation of colored polymers [4, 31, 33].

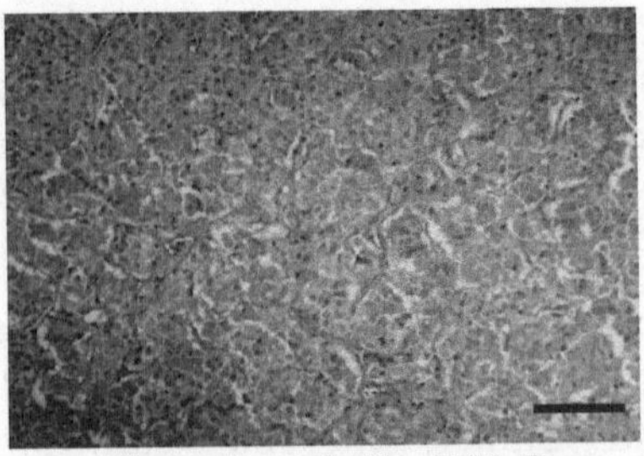

Figure 20. Adrenal medulla. HE. Bar = 50 μm.

The adrenal medulla of dogs has a heterogeneous population of cells [38]. In adults, there are 3 types of adrenal medullary cells (1): epinephrine cells (66–75%), norepinephrine cells (25–33%) and small granule-containing cells (SGC, 1-4%). The adrenal SGC cells of dogs vary from cells with a few granules and a high nucleo-cytoplasmic ratio to cells filled with many granules and a large mass of cytoplasm. Most of the chromaffin granules of these cells are small, ranging from 100 to 200 nm in diameter [39]. The medullary cells produce other peptides in addition to epinephrine and norepinephrine, such as met-enkephalin, substance P, neurotensin, neuropeptide Y, and chromogranin A. The adrenal medulla contains also presynaptic sympathetic ganglion cells, randomly scattered [4, 32].

The first step in the synthesis of epinephrine is the enzymatic conversion of tyrosine to dihydroxyphenylalanine (DOPA) by tyrosine hydroxylase. This is the rate-limiting step of hormone synthesis. DOPA is then converted to dopamine within the cytosol by decarboxylation. Dopamine can also be converted to norepinephrine by hydroxylation. Norepinephrine then leaves the granule to be converted into epinephrine in the cytosol by phenylethanolamine-N-methyltransferase (PNMT), and epinephrine re-enters the granule for storage in the cell. The activity of PNMT is induced by the high local concentration of glucocorticoids in sinusoidal blood from the adrenal cortex [10, 32]. Acute stress, hypoglycemia or other similar situations, result both in catecholamine secretion and in transsynaptic induction of catecholamine biosynthetic enzymes, including tyrosine hydroxylase. Other environmental influences, including growth factors, extracellular matrix, and a variety of hormonal signals that generate cyclic AMP, also may regulate the function of chromaffin cells [32].

In table 6, we can see a summary of some of the hormones produced by adrenal glands and their functions.

Endocrine gland		Hormone	Function	Secretion control is made by
Adrenal	Cortex	Glucocorticoids	Raises glucose levels in the blood, stimulates glucose production by cells, reduce the inflamatory response	Raised blood glucose levels
		Mineralocorticoids	Acts on the distal convoluted tubules of the renal nephrons; regulates uptake of sodium and acid/base balance	Low blood glucose levels
		Sex hormones	(Very small quantities)	———
	Medula	Adrenaline and Noradrenaline	Fear, fight, fright syndrome	Sympathetic nervous system

Table 6. Adrenal glands hormones and functions.

7. Clinical significance

Endocrine diseases, associated to altered functions of endocrine glands, are frequently seen in veterinary practice. The endocrine glands described may be targeted by several conditions summarized in table 7.

Hyperfunction	Primary: most often caused by hyperplasia, cysts or tumours)
	Secondary: most commonly caused by tumours in the pituitary gland which controls the relevant effector gland (e.g. thyroid) or by imbalances in hormonal control (e.g. abnormal accumulation of neurotransmitters that lead to the overproduction of hormones)
Hypofunction	Primary: caused by destruction of secretory glandular cells, developmental abnormalities or genetic defects which determine a decrease in hormones synthesis
	Secondary: caused by a destructive lesion in the pituitary gland which in turn determines hypofunctioning in the respective target gland
Hyperactivity secondary to disorders in other organs, such as secondary hyperparathyroidism due to chronic renal failure or to nutritional imbalances	
Hormone hypersecretion or related substances, with biological or chemical similarity to hormones, commonly secreted by neoplastic cells	
Endocrine dysfunction due to lack of response from target organs or tissues to hormone stimulation, in spite of normal or increased hormone secretion (e.g. diabetes by insulin resistance)	
Endocrine disruption by decreased hepatic hormone degradation (e.g. cirrhosis) or decreased urinary excretion	
Hormone excess due to iatrogenic causes which, directly or indirectly, influences the activity of target organs, leading to the onset of disease (e.g. administration of corticosteroids or prolonged progestogens).	

Table 7. Pathologic conditions affecting endocrine glands.

In dogs, the most common endocrine diseases are summarized in table 8.

Commom Endocrine Diseases In Dogs
Hypothyroidism
Diabetes melitus
Hyperadrenocorticism
Hypoadrenocorticism

Table 8. Most common endocrine diseases in dogs.

- **Hypothyroidism**

Hypothyroidism may result from destruction of the thyroid gland (primary hypothyroidism), decreased hypothalamic secretion of TRH or inadequate pituitary TSH secretion. Over 95% of canine hypothyroidism cases are primary [40, 41]. Two histologic forms of primary hypothyroidism predominate in the dog: lymphocytic thyroiditis and idiopathic atrophy. Regardless of the aetiology, the end result is the same: progressive destruction of the thyroid gland and consequent deficiency of circulating thyroid hormones [40, 41].

Hypothyroidism occurs mainly in middle aged, purebred dogs. Doberman Pinschers and Golden Retrievers are the two breeds most frequently described [42]. Clinical signs associated with hypothyroidism are varied, and behavioural changes are associated with a reduced metabolic rate, dermatological signs, cardiovascular and neuromuscular abnormalities. Obesity, in different grades is always present. Lethargy and cold intolerance are also frequently observed. Seborrhoea, bilateral and symmetrical alopecia, and pyoderma are also common dermatological symptoms. These signs can be accompanied by bradycardia, low voltage ECG complexes and weakness [40, 41, 43, 44].

- **Diabetes mellitus**

Diabetes mellitus is the result of any situation that affects insulin production, insulin transport or the sensitivity of target tissues to insulin [45]. Many factors are known to contribute to the development of diabetes and its complications [46, 47]. These include genetics, diet, sedentary lifestyle, perinatal factors, age, obesity and inflammatory causes [47, 48].

Canine diabetes mellitus is generally classified as insulin dependent or non-insulin dependent based on the need for insulin treatment [40, 48]. Most diabetic dogs are thought to have a disease like human type I diabetes mellitus and are insulin dependent [40, 49, 50]. Unlike human type I diabetes mellitus, which occurs mainly in young human patients, in dogs it is more likely to occur later in life [40, 45, 48]. Dogs do not appear to progress from obesity-induced insulin resistance to type 2 diabetes mellitus, probably because pancreatic beta cells in dogs are either not sensitive to toxicity due mild hyperglycemia or lack other components of the pathophysiology of beta cell failure in type 2 diabetes mellitus [51]. Certain breeds, including Australian Terrier, Keeshounds, Alaskan Malamutes, Finnish Spitzes, Standard and Miniature Schnauzers, Miniature Poodles, and English Springer Spaniels, seem to be at increased risk to develop diabetes. Others, such as Boxers, German Shepherd dogs, Cocker Spaniels and Collies seemed to be at decreased risk [40, 52]. Typical clinical signs are polyuria, polydipsia, polyphagia and weight loss. Exercise intolerance or decreased activity, ketonic breath, recurrent infections (urinary tract, conjunctivitis), cataracts and hepatomegaly can also be present [45].

- **Hyperadrenocorticism**

Hyperadrenocorticism can be spontaneous or iatrogenic. Spontaneous hyperadrenocorticism is associated with inappropriate secretion of ACTH by the pituitary (pituitary-dependent hyperadrenocorticism) or with a primary adrenal disorder (adrenal-dependent hyperadrenocorticism) [40, 53, 54]. Over 80% of dogs with spontaneous hyperdarenocorticism suffer from pituitary dependent hypercorticism, resulting in an over secretion of ACTH [53, 54]. This results in bilateral adrenocortical hyperplasia and excess cortisol production. The negative feedback loop between cortisol and ACTH is lost. Adrenal-dependent hyperadrenocorticism represent the remaining 20% of spontaneous hyperadrenocorticism and is generally associated with unilateral (or occasionally bilateral) adrenal tumours. This is a typical disease of middle age to old animals. Dogs showing pituitary-dependent hyperadrenocorticism exhibit a mean age of 7-9 years old, and those with adrenal-dependent hyperadrenocorticism, a mean age of 11-12 years old. There are some breeds that are most frequently associated with hyperadrenocorticism, but any breed can develop it. Poodles, Daschunds and small Terriers seem to be more predisposed to this disease. Most common clinical signs include polydipsia and polyuria, polyphagia, abdominal distension, liver enlargement, muscle weakness, lethargy, skin changes, alopecia, persistent anoestrus or testicular atrophy, *calcinosis cutis* and neurological signs [54, 55].

- **Hypoadrenocorticism**

Hypoadrenocorticism is a syndrome associated to a deficient production of mineralocorticoid and/or glucocorticoid secretion by the adrenal glands. This can arise from a destruction of more than 90% of both adrenal cortices, causing inability to produce corticosteroids (Primary hypoadrenocorticism or Addison's disease), or from a deficiency in ACTH production by the pituitary (Secondary hypoadrenocorticism) [56, 57]. Besides different pathophysiology, primary and secondary hypoadrenocorticism also exhibit different clinical signs. In dogs, primary hypoadrenocorticism is more representative. It is often associated with idiopathic adrenocortical atrophy, or with some therapeutic or surgical procedures, like mitotane treatment for hyperadrenocorticism or bilateral adrenalectomy. This condition generally affects young and middle age dogs with a median age of 4 years [57]. Great Danes, Portuguese Water Dogs, Rottweilers, Standard Poodles, West Highland White Terrier and Soft-coated Wheaten Terriers are the breeds in greater risk to develop hypoadrenocorticism [56]. Females, especially intact females, are in higher risk. Clinical signs may vary, from mild to severe, regarding the evolution of the disease. Acute hypoadrenocorticism can be life threatening and represents a medical emergency. The animal can be in a hypovolaemic shock, and generally is found in a state of collapse, or collapses when stressed. Weak pulse, bradycardia, abdominal pain, vomiting, diarrhoea, dehydration and hypothermia can also be present. Chronic presentation is more common than the acute disease. Animals with chronic hypoadrecocorticism may present anorexia, vomiting, lethargy, depression and weakness [57].

8. Conclusions

Malfunction of endocrine glands leads to severe multivariate syndromes, requiring a specialized medical approach and appropriate nursing care. For this reason, professionals engaged in clinical veterinary practice need to know animal organic structures and how they function as a whole, including the role of the endocrine system, its glands and their hormones. This systematic approach to endocrine disorders promotes not only a trained professional but a professional with technical and scientific knowledge, enabled with the exact notion of the involved etiopathogenic mechanisms and capable of making a diagnostic and therapeutical difference. This concerted attitude would certainly contribute to improve veterinary medical care to a level of excellence in the care of animal patients.

References

1. Done S., Goody P., Evans S., Stickland N., editors. Color Atlas of Veterinary Anatomy. The dog & Cat. Edinburgh: Mosby; 2004. p2.62, 2.66, 2.67, 2.79.
2. Ningying X., Xiaoling J. Molecular Characterization of Hypothalamo-pituitary-thyroid genes in pig (Sus scrofa). In Perez-Marin C. (ed.) A bird's-eye view of Veterinary Medicine. Rijeka: InTech; 2012. p545-56 http://www.intechopen.com/books/a-bird-s-eye-view-of-veterinary-medicine/molecular-characterization-of-thyroid-peroxidase-gene-in-porcine-sus-scrofa- (accessed the 8 June 2012).

3. Morgan P., Williams L. The pars tuberalis of the pituitary: a gateway for neuroendocrine output. Reviews of Reproduction 1996;(1) 153–61.
4. Banks W.J., editor. Applied Veterinary Histology. St. Louis: Mosby; 1993. p 408-28.
5. Pankov I., Chekhranova M., Karpova S., Iatsyshina S.M., Sazina E. Molecular and genetic study of the role of hormones receptors, and enzymes in regulation of reproduction, lipid metabolism, and other human physiological functions. Vestnik Rossiiskoi Akademii Meditsinskikh Nauk 2005;(9) 6-13.
6. Nilsson A., Ohlsson C., Isaksson O., Lindahl A., Isgaard J. Hormonal regulation of longitudinal bone growth. European Journal of Clinical Nutrition 1994;48(S1) 158-60.
7. Trott J., Schennink A., Petrie W., Manjarin R., Vanklompenberg M., Hovey R. Triennial Lactation Symposium: Prolactin: The multifaceted potentiator of mammary growth and function. Journal of Animal Science 2012;90(5) 1674-86.
8. Perez-Marin C., Moreno M., Calero G. Clinical approach to the repeat breeder cow syndrome. In Perez-Marin C. (ed.) A bird's-eye view of Veterinary Medicine. Rijeka: InTech; 2012. p337-62 http://www.intechopen.com/books/a-bird-s-eye-view-of-veterinary-medicine/clinical-approach-to-the-repeat-breeder-cow-syndrome (accessed the 8 June 2012).
9. Chauvigné F., Verdura S., Mazón M., Duncan N., Zanuy S., Gómez A., Cerda J. Follicle-Stimulating Hormone and Luteinizing Hormone Mediate the Androgenic Pathway in Leydig Cells of an Evolutionary Advanced Teleost. Biology of Reproduction 2012; doi: 10.1095/biolreprod.112.100784.
10. Möstl E. Endocrinología especial. In W. Engelhardt, Breves G (eds.) Fisiología Veterinaria. Zaragoza: Acribia; 2002. p526-38.
11. Macgregor D., Lincoln G. A physiological model of a circannual oscillator. Journal of Biological Rhythms 2008;23(3) 252-64.
12. Tse A., Lee A., Tse F. Ca2+ signaling and exocytosis in pituitary corticotropes. Cell Calcium 2012;51(3-4) 253-9.
13. Choi S.J., Pfeffer R.S. G proteins and autocrine signaling differentially regulate gonadotropin subunit expression in the pituitary gonadotrope. Journal of Biological Chemistry 2012;287(25) 21550-60.
14. Marsili A., Sanchez E., Singru P., Harney J., Zavacki A., Lechan R., Larsen P.R. Thyroxine-induced expression of pyroglutamyl peptidase II and inhibition of TSH release precedes suppression of TRH mRNA and requires type 2 deiodinase. Journal of Endocrinology 2011;211(1) 73-8.
15. Doniach I. Histopathology of the pituitary. Journal of Clinical Endocrinology & Metabolism 1985;14(4) 765-89.
16. Inyushkin A., Orlans H., Dyball R. Secretory cells of the supraoptic nucleus have central as well as neurohypophysial projections. Journal of Anatomy 2009;215(4) 425-34.
17. Dyce K.M., Sack W.O., Wensing C.J.G., editors. Veterinary Anatomy. USA:WB Saunders Company; 1996. p209-15.
18. Ehrhart N., Chapter 118: Thyroid. In: Slatter D.H. (ed) Textbook of small animal surgery. Philadelphia:Saunders; 2003. p1700-10.

19. Flanders J.A., Chapter 119: parathyroid In: Slatter D.H. (ed) Textbook of small animal surgery. Philadelphia:Saunders; 2003. p1711-22.
20. http://www.vsso.org/Parathyroid_Tumors.html (accessed the 30 August 2012).
21. Setoguti T. Electron microscopic studies of the parathyroid gland of senile dogs. American Journal of Anatomy 1977;148(1) 65-83.
22. Baba A.I., Câtoi C. Comparative Oncology. Bucharest: The Publishing House of the Romanian Academy; 2007. Chapter 16, Endocrine Tumors. Available from: http://www.ncbi.nlm.nih.gov/books/NBK9554/ Romanian Academy (accessed the 18 July 2012).
23. Pace V., Scarsella S., Perentes E. Parathyroid gland carcinoma in a Wistar rat. Veterinary Pathology 2003;40(2) 203-6.
24. Carrera J.A.P. Secreciones endocrinas del páncreas. In: Sacristán A.G., Montijano F.C., Palomino L.F.C., Gallego J.G., Silanes M.D.M.L., Ruiz G.S. (eds) Fisiología Veterinaria. Madrid:Mcgraw-Hill; 1995. p1074.
25. Kragl M., Lammert E. Calcineurin/NFATc Signaling: Role in Postnatal β Cell Development and Diabetes Mellitus. Developmental Cell 2012;23(1) 7-8.
26. Ali S., Drucker J. Benefits and limitations of reducing glucagon action for the treatment of type 2 diabetes. American Journal of Physiology - Endocrinology and Metabolism 2009;296 E415–21.
27. Aspinall V., O'Reilly M., Anatomy and Physiology. In: Lane D.R., Cooper B. (eds) Veterinary Nursing. London:Butterworth Heinemann; 2004. p41-4.
28. Quesada I., Tudurí E., Ripoll C., Nadal A. Physiology of the pancreatic α-cell and glucagon secretion: role in glucose homeostasis and diabetes. Journal of Endocrinology 2008;199 5-19.
29. Nguyen T.Q., Maalouf N.M., Sakhaee K., Moe O.W. Comparison of insulin action on glucose versus potassium uptake in humans. Clinical Journal of the American Society of Nephrology 2011;6(7) 1533-9.
30. Akhmedov D., De Marchi U., Wollheim C.B., Wiederkehr A. Pyruvate dehydrogenase E1α phosphorylation is induced by glucose but does not control metabolism-secretion coupling in INS-1E clonal β-cells. Biochimica et Biophysica Acta. 2012;15(10) 1815-24.
31. Nauck M.A. Incretin-based therapies for type 2 diabetes mellitus: properties, functions, and clinical implications. The American Journal of Medicine. 2011;124(1 Suppl) S3-18.
32. Rosol T.J., Yarrington J.T., Latendresse J., Capen C.C. Adrenal gland: structure, function, and mechanisms of toxicity. Toxicologic Pathology 2001;29(1) 41-8.
33. http://www.anatomyatlases.org/MicroscopicAnatomy/Section15/Plate15294.shtml (accessed the 8 June 2012).
34. Galac S., Reusch C., Kooistra H., Rijnberk A. Adrenals. In Rijnberk A., Kooistra H. (eds) Clinical Endocrinology of Dogs and Cats: An Illustrated Text. Dordrecht:Manson Publishing;2010. p93.

35. Engelkin L.R. Review of Veterinary Physiology. Jackson:Teton NewMedia; 2002. p519-23.
36. http://ocw.tufts.edu/Content/4/CourseHome/221047/221064 (accessed the 8 June 2012).
37. Carcagno A.R., 1995. Corteza Adrenal. In: Sacristán A.G., Montijano F.C., Palomino L.F.C., Gallego J.G., Silanes M.D.M.L., Ruiz G.S. (eds) Fisiología Veterinaria. Madrid:Mcgraw-Hill; 1995. p767-80.
38. Verhofstad A.A.J. Kinetics of adrenal medullary cells. Journal of Anatomy 1993;183 315-26.
39. Kajihara H., Akimoto T., Iijima S. On the chromaffin cells in dog adrenal medulla; with special reference to the small granule chromaffin cells (SGC Cells). Cell and Tissue Research 1978;191 1-14.
40. Feldman E.C., Nelson R.W., editors. Canine and Feline Endocrinology and Reproduction. St. Louis: Saunders; 2004. p86-151; 486-538; 252-357.
41. Panciera D.L. Chapter Fourteen: Canine hypothyroidism. In: Torrence A.G., Mooney C.T (eds.) BSAVA Manual of small animal endocrinology. Gloucester: British Small Animal Veterinary Association; 1998. p103-13.
42. Panciera D.L. Hypothyroidism in dogs: 66 cases (1987-1992). J Am Vet Med Assoc. 1994;204(5) 761-7.
43. Dixon R.M., Reid S.W.J., Mooney C.T. Epidemiological, clinical, haematological and biochemical characteristics of canine hypothyroidism. The Veterinary Record, 1999(145) 481-7.
44. Jaillardon L., Martin L., Nguyen P., Siliart B. Serum insulin-like growth factor type 1 concentrations in healthy dogs and dogs with spontaneous primary hypothyroidism. The Veterinary Journal 2011:190 e95-9.
45. Graham P.A. Chapter Twelve: Canine diabetes mellitus. In: Torrence A.G. and Mooney C.T (eds) BSAVA Manual of small animal endocrinology. 2nd edition, 1998. p83-96.
46. Mega C., Teixeira de Lemos E., Vala H., Fernandes R., Oliveira J., Mascarenhas-Melo F., Teixeira F., Reis F. Diabetic nephropathy amelioration by a low-dose sitagliptin in an animal model of type 2 diabetes (Zucker Diabetic Fatty rat). Experimental Diabetes Research 2011; doi:10.1155/2011/162092.
47. King G.L. The role of inflammatory cytokines in diabetes and its complications. J Periodontol 2008;79(8)Suppl 1527-34.
48. Guptill L., Glickman L., Glickman N. Time Trends and Risk Factors for Diabetes Mellitus in Dogs: Analysis of Veterinary Medical Data Base Records (1970–1999). The Veterinary Journal 2003;165 240-7.
49. Bennet N. Monitoring techniques for diabetes mellitus in the dog and the cat. Clinical Techniques in Small Animal Practice, 2002;17(2) 65-9.
50. Declue A.E., Nickell J., Chang C.H., Honaker A. J. Upregulation of proinflammatory cytokine production in response to bacterial pathogen-associated molecular patterns in dogs with diabetes mellitus undergoing insulin therapy. Journal of Diabetes Science and Technology. 2012;6(3) 496-502.

51. Verkest K.R., Rand J.S., Fleeman L.M., Morton J.M. Spontaneously obese dogs exhibit greater postprandial glucose, triglyceride, and insulin concentrations than lean dogs. Domest Anim Endocrinol. 2012;42(2) 103-12.
52. Hoenig M. Comparative aspects of diabetes mellitus in dogs and cats. Molecular and Cellular Endocrinology 2002;197 221-9.
53. Peterson M.E. Diagnosis of Hyperadrenocorticism in Dogs. Clin Tech Small Anim Pract 2007;22 2-11.
54. Herrtage M.E.Chapter Ten. Canine Hyperadrenocorticism. In: Torrence A.G., Mooney C.T (eds) BSAVA Manual of small animal endocrinology. Gloucester: British Small Animal Veterinary Association; 1998. p55-73.
55. Grecco D. Hyperadrenocorticism Associated with Sex Steroid Excess. Clin Tech Small Anim Pract 2007;22(1) 12-7.
56. Herrtage M.E. Chapter Eleven: Hypoadrenocorticism. In: Torrence A.G. and Mooney C.T (eds) BSAVA Manual of small animal endocrinology. Gloucester: British Small Animal Veterinary Association; 1998. p75-82.
57. Grecco D. Hypoadrenocorticism in Small Animals. Clin Tech Small Anim Pract 2007;22(1) 32-5.

Chapter 7

Sex Steroid Hormones and Tumors in Domestic Animals

1. Introduction

Sex steroid hormones play a role in the development and control of animal tumours, particularly in those arising in their target organs. Due to their incidence and prevalence, mammary tumours of female dogs and cats are among the most frequently studied with focus on the role of ovarian oestrogen and progesterone. In these tumours, sex steroid hormones have been shown to act during the three steps of the carcinogenesis cascade: initiation, promotion and progression. Experimental data have shown the mutagenic effect of oestrogens [1] while epidemiologic and clinical studies highlighted the role of ovarian hormones as promoters on mammary tumours in both the dog and the cat [2-9]. Finally, oestrogens and progesterone further act during tumour progression. Their role in the last two steps of carcinogenesis makes it possible to control the evolution of the disease.

Studies on the role of ovarian hormones during tumour progression depend on the capability of demonstrating the presence of oestrogen receptors (ER) and progesterone receptors (PR) in tumours. Earlier studies on the field were published in the seventies of the 20th century, all related to mammary gland tumours. Some of these studies revealed the presence of unoccupied hormone receptors in tissue homogenates from mammary tumours of dogs and cats [10-13]. However, actual knowledge comes from the late nineties, when different groups of researchers standardized immunohistochemical (IHC) methods of analysis for ER and PR in feline and canine tissues [14-19]. Once the IHC analysis revealed the presence of sex steroid hormones receptors in mammary tumours, several studied analyzed their value as favourable prognostic indicators [18, 20-25] adding new data to the well-known similarities between and human and animal mammary tumours [26]. However, the important role of ER and PR as predictive factors of response to endocrine treatment of breast cancer has been rarely analyzed in animal tumours although recent studies based on the blockade of PR in canine mammary carcinomas and reproductive tract tumours of female and male dogs and cats support their value in the control of these diseases [27-30].

Mammary gland tumours are the most frequent tumours in female dogs and the third in the cat. However, they are not the only tumours known to be sex steroid-dependent. Tumours of the reproductive tract of female and male dogs and cats and some skin appendages can be defined as hormone-dependent on the basis of the IHC expression of ERα and PR [31, 32]. In addition, epidemiological and clinical studies support the role of steroid hormones as tumour promoters [28]. The most common tumours in the genital tract of the bitch are benign smooth muscle tumours of the vagina, vulva and perineal skin. Their hormone-dependence is similar to that of mammary gland tumours as the majority of canine genital tract leiomyomas express PR and also respond to neoadjuvant treatments with the PR antagonist aglepristone with a reduction in size [28].

In the dog, and to a lesser extent in the cat, benign and malignant sebaceous gland neoplasias are among the most common skin tumours. Studies concerning the role of sex steroid hormones during tumour promotion and progression are scarce but do show there is ER and PR expression in sebaceous gland tumours of dogs. Therefore, not only androgens but also progesterone and estrogens may regulate hormone-related physiology. In fact, preclinical studies indicate partial clinical remission after chemical castration in old dogs with hepatoid gland tumours and heart failure [30].

2. Methods for studying steroid hormone receptors

Immunohistochemical (IHC) methods based on antigen-antibody reactions are widely used today to detect steroid hormone receptors in tumours. New specific antibodies have been developed against a range of steroid hormone receptors, enabling reliable detection by ordinary light microscopy. Traditionally, however, steroid hormone receptors were detected by biochemical assay based on the binding of radiolabelled ligands to unoccupied receptors. Among the most commonly used biochemical techniques was the dextran-coated charcoal (DCC) method [33], which – until the late nineties – provided all the data available on steroid hormone receptor expression in mammary carcinomas in female domestic animals. Biochemical techniques, however, were not without drawbacks: they had to be applied to frozen tissue samples, were very expensive, needed specialised equipment and were not widely accessible. For this reason, published research on the use of these techniques was scanty. The development of monoclonal antibodies highly specific to oestrogen receptor (ERα) and progesterone receptor (PR) proteins enabled the development of immunohistochemical techniques based on the binding of receptors to specific antibodies [34-37]. These techniques offered several major advantages over biochemical methods [38-40]:

- They could be applied to tissue samples routinely processed for histopathology and could be performed in the pathology laboratory, rendering them both more accessible and less costly.
- They provided information regarding the specific location of ER and PR, enabling analysis of the relationship between receptor expression and tissue structures in normal and/or tumoural mammary glands, thus avoiding the false-positive findings common in biochemical examinations.
- They furnished information on all the receptors present in tissue samples, irrespective of the occupation status.

The process of standardizing IHC methods of ER and PR detection in animal tissues involved the use of commercially available antibodies raised against human antigens first as antibodies raised against canine and feline antigens were not produced. Then, these

IHC methods for detecting ER and PR in formalin-fixed, paraffin wax-embedded tissue samples needed to be validated before they could be routinely implemented, as stipulated by the "National Institutes of Health Consensus Conference on Estrogen Receptors in Breast Cancer" (NIHCC), held in 1979. The first step in the validation procedure was the comparison of ER and PR detection using both biochemical and IHC techniques and the correlation of IHC results with those of the gold-standard radioligand-binding assays in order to evaluate their specificity and sensitivity. In 1999, Graham et al. [15] analysed ERα expression in formalin-fixed, paraffin-embedded tissue samples from canine mammary tumours using biochemical and IHC methods, reporting good correlation between the two. In 2000 and 2002, Martín de las Mulas et al. [17, 19] validated the IHC method for the detection of ERα and PR detection, respectively, in formalin-fixed, paraffin-embedded tissue samples from feline mammary tumours using the avidin-biotin-peroxidase complex (ABC) method, and compared their findings with those obtained using the DCC biochemical method; reported agreement between the two methods was 72.7% for ERα and 95.6% for PR. The IHC technique used demonstrated good specificity (true-negatives) and sensibility (true-positives) (Table 1).

Table 1. Specificity and sensibility of an IHC method for detecting ER and PR, versus a biochemical method (DCC) in feline mammary carcinomas [17, 19].

DCC versus IHC	ERα	PR
SPECIFICITY	95.6%	89.4%
SENSIBILITY	47.6%	87.5%

Second, the NIHCC (1979) also recommended the clinical validation of technically validated IHC methods since the presence of ER and/or PR in human breast cancer was known to be a favourable prognostic indicator as well as a predictive marker of the response to adjuvant hormone therapy [41, 42]. The prognostic value of the IHC expression of ERα and PR expression in canine mammary carcinoma has been demonstrated in the dog and the cat [18, 20-25]. Finally, preclinical and clinical studies of our group have shown that the PR antagonist Aglepristone produces partial clinical remission of canine mammary carcinoma [29].

At present, IHC methods are routinely used in a number of veterinary laboratories for the detection of ER and PR. However, no consensus has yet been reached regarding tissue preparation, the antibodies and techniques to be used, and the evaluation of results. New image-analysis systems may help to objectively evaluate receptor expression and to standardise the results obtained by different pathologists [43]. The guidelines issued by the American Society of Clinical Oncology/College of American Pathologists to improve the accuracy of immunohistochemical ERα and PR testing in breast cancer and their utility as predictive markers of the response to hormone therapy may serve as a model for veterinary pathologists [44].

3. Mammary gland tumours in dogs and cats

Mammary gland tumours are the most common neoplasms in female dogs and the third most common in female cats, but are rare in other domestic animals. Between 41% and 53% of mammary tumours in dogs and between 85% and 93% in cats are malignant. Most authors agree that these tumours account for around 50% and 17% of all neoplasms in dogs and cats, respectively, with an incidence of 205 and 25.4 per 100.000 dogs and cats at risk. Median age at tumour presentation is 10-12 years in both species [45]. Tumours develop almost exclusively in females, appearing only rarely in males [46-48]. Breed is also a risk factor: mammary tumours are more common in pure-bred than in mixed-breed animals, and some breeds – including Poodles, Boxers, Beagles, a number of Spaniel breeds, and Siamese cats – display a higher incidence than others [45, 49-51]. Other risk factors are more controversial, or have been the subject of less research: diet, exposure to radiation, family background and individual history of benign and malignant mammary lesions. The action of ovarian hormones – oestrogens and progesterone – on mammary gland tissue during different stages of development is also a risk factor associated with the development of mammary tumours, while breeding-related factors such as parity, age at first gestation, number of pregnancies, pseudopregnancy and changes in the oestrous cycle, do not appear to influence the risk of developing mammary tumours, although not all authors agree on this [45].

The development of mammary tumours in female dogs and cats is clearly hormone-dependent, and they offer a good spontaneous model of human breast cancer. The preventive effects of castration on the development of mammary tumours in both species have been reported [52-54]. Early ovariectomy in dogs and cats has a protective effect against both benign and malignant mammary tumours, the intensity of that effect depending on the number of cycles before spaying. In dogs spayed before the first oestrus, the risk of developing a mammary tumour is 0.05 %, compared to 8% after the first oestrus and 26% after the second oestrus; the protective effect of spaying disappears after the age of 2.5 years. In cats, spaying before 6 months of age reduces the risk of mammary carcinoma by 91% with respect to unspayed cats, while spaying before 1 year of age cuts the risk by 86%.

While prolonged administration of oestrogens has not been shown to increase the incidence of mammary tumours [55,56], administration of medroxyprogesterone acetate and progestins over a prolonged period to young female dogs increases the risk of mainly benign mammary tumours; the intensity of that risk depends on the dosage received and on the regularity or irregularity of treatment [6]. A number of authors, however, also report an increased incidence of malignant tumours [7]. The risk of developing a malignant tumour rises following long-term experimental administration of oestrogens combined with high-dose progestins as shown by experimental studies to analyze the effects of the pill [55, 57], and following the administration of drugs with combined progestagenic-oestrogenic activity to control the signs of oestrus [6-9]. Thus, prolonged administration of high-dose (125 x human dose) of a progestational compound (lynestrenol) prompted the development of breast cancer in 40% of intact treated dogs [6]. By contrast, a combined regime of low-dose progestagen+oestrogen appears to afford some protection [6]. Cats treated with synthetic progestins or oestrogen-progestin combinations displayed a threefold higher risk of developing benign and malignant mammary tumours than untreated cats [58].

The role played by ovarian steroid hormones during tumour progression (i.e., once the tumours are detected clinically) has been studied through their expression of ERα and PR. Early studies using biochemical methods of ERα and PR analysis showed that between 65% and 92% of mammary tumours contain hormone receptors [17, 19]. With IHC methods, differential expression between benign and malignant tumours has been observed in dogs and cats as the expression was higher in the former. However, data concerning ERα expression in mammary carcinomas are very different among different laboratories. Thus, in the dog, 7% [59], 10% [16], 11% [14], 22% [20], 24% [15], 59% [60, 61], 87.5% [18] and 92.6% [62] of canine mammary carcinomas have been shown to express ERα (Figure 1). Concerning PR expression, reported data are the following: 14% [63], 33% [14], 42%-52% [62, 64], 60% [16] and 66% [20](Figure 2). In the cat, 7% and 17% of in situ carcinomas expressed ERα and PR, respectively [59] while invasive carcinomas expression figures range from 10% [65] to 25% [17] for ERα and from 38.5% and 43% for PR [19, 65]. Many of these studies point to progesterone, and not oestrogens, as the sex steroid hormone driving proliferation in mammary gland tumours as all benign tumours of the canine mammary gland and 2/3 of malignant tumours express PR [14, 16, 20, 22].

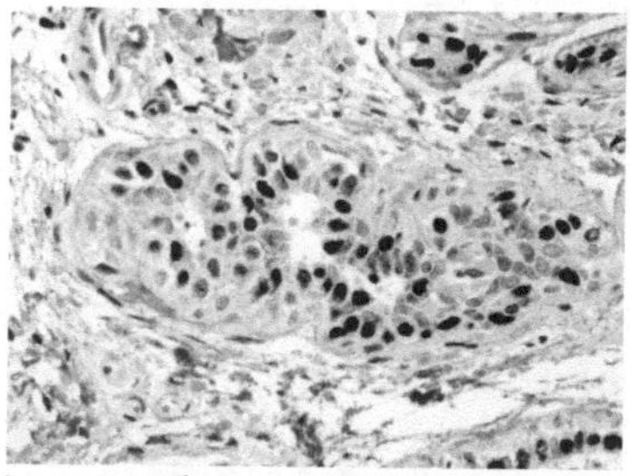

Figure 1. Details of a canine simple carcinoma showing expression of ERα in the nucleus of luminal epithelial cells (brown colour). ABC. 40X.

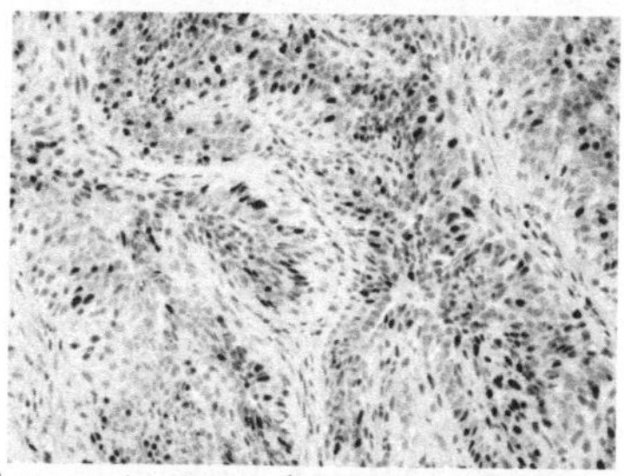

Figure 2. Canine simple carcinoma showing PR expression in the nucleus of neoplastic epithelial cells. (brown colour). ABC. 20X.

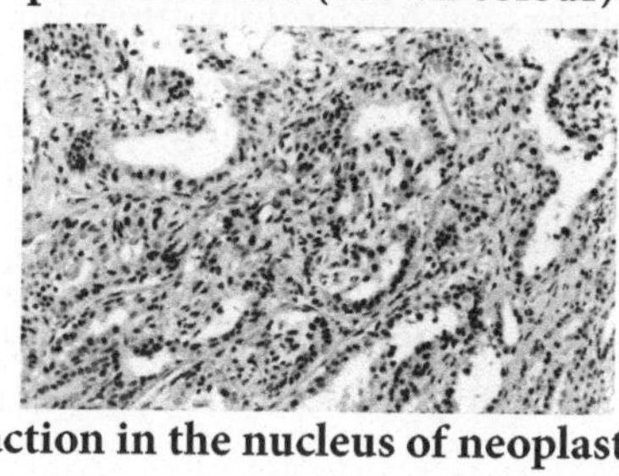

Figure 3. ERβ immunoreaction in the nucleus of neoplastic epithelial cells of canine mammary carcinoma. ABC. 20X.

After the cloning of a second ER in rats and humans, designated ERβ [66, 67], it became known that currently reported data correlated with the isoform α of ER (ERα). Our group was the first to publish data on the expression of the second isoform of the ER (ERβ) in mammary tissues of dogs [68], and one more study has been performed up to date [69].

ERβ expression was observed in the ductal and acinar epithelium of normal mammary glands and in one third of mammary tumours. Expression was greater in benign than in malignant tumours [68]. Among malignant tumours, ERβ expression was greater in complex and mixed tumours than in simple carcinomas, indicating that ERβ may also be a prognostic factor of these tumours (Figure 3).

The prognostic value of steroid hormone receptor activity in malignant tumours (lower risk of relapse and metastasis, together with greater survival time) is now widely accepted after several univariate and multivariate prognostic studies using IHC methods for detection of ER and PR [18, 20-25]. In a study using IHC techniques to detect ER and PR expression in 228 tumours (155 malignant and 73 benign) from 100 bitches, Martín de las Mulas et al. [20] found that a total of 76% of tumours (96% benign and 66% malignant) expressed ERα and/or PR. In seven cases with lymph node metastasis, both the primary tumours and their metastases were ERα and PR negative, indicating a loss of hormone influence and thus greater aggressiveness. Expression of PR alone in 66% of malignant tumours suggested that PR played a more important role than ERα in tumour proliferation.

Surgery is the treatment of choice for feline and canine mammary tumours. Treatment with drugs such as tamoxifen has been tested in dogs with mammary carcinoma, but is not recommended due to their considerable side effects; these drugs are therefore not currently in use [70]. Ovariohysterectomy (OHE) performed at the time of surgery does not appear to produce any clear benefit in dogs with mammary carcinoma [71, 72]. The only adjuvant treatment administered at present is chemotherapy, and results are not wholly satisfactory [45].

In 1998, Cappelletti et al. [73] reported different ERα and PR counts in tumours analysed before and after treatment with a range of drugs including tamoxifen, concluding that malignant mammary neoplasms were sensitive to steroid hormone treatment. A feline dysplasia of the mammary gland, the feline fibroadenomatous change, is highly sensitive to Alizin®, a PR antagonist [74, 75]. The fact that all benign tumours and two thirds of malignant tumours in dogs express mainly PR [16, 17, 22] points to the potential use of progesterone receptor antagonists as a neoadjuvant and/or adjuvant treatment for these tumours. A recent study performed by our group [29] has shown that administration of the PR receptor antagonist Aglepristone (Alizin®, Virbac, France) as neoadjuvant treatment in female dogs inhibits the proliferation of PR-expressing mammary carcinomas. Twenty-seven non-spayed bitches with mammary tumours were treated with Alizin® before surgical tumour removal. Tumour tissue samples were analysed before and after treatment, and PR expression was reduced following treatment (36.4% versus 59.1% prior to treatment). The proliferative index (PI) was also analysed before and after treatment, using the avidin-biotin-peroxidase complex technique and a proliferative marker (Ki67). A significant decrease in the PI was recorded in tumours expressing PR, while no change was observed in those not expressing PR, suggesting that the PR antagonist Aglepristone inhibited tumour proliferation in PR-positive tumours by blocking the PR.

4. Female and male reproductive-tract tumours in dogs and cats

4.1. Female reproductive tract

The actual incidence of female reproductive-tract tumours is difficult to ascertain, presumably because a significant percentage of dogs and cats are neutered [76]. These tumours may arise in the vagina, vulva, uterus or ovaries; vulvar and vaginal tumours are the most common (after mammary gland tumours), accounting for 2.4% to 3% of all canine neoplasms [77, 78]. No incidence rates are available for vulvar and vaginal tumours in cats. Uterine tumours are rare in both dogs and cats, accounting for 0.3%-0.4% and 0.2%-1.5% of all canine and feline tumours, respectively [77, 79-84]. Ovarian tumours are also uncommon in dogs and cats; although the true incidence is unknown, the reported incidence in intact bitches is 6.25%, thus representing 0.5% to 1.2% of all canine tumours [85, 86], while reported incidence in cats ranges from 0.7% to 3.6% [87]. The most common neoplasms in the canine female reproductive tract are benign tumours of mesenchymal origin, classified as leiomyomas, fibroleiomyomas, fibromas and polyps depending on the amount of connective tissue present [88,89]. The use of markers for smooth-muscle differentiation (e.g. desmin, calponin, smooth muscle actin) is valuable for the accurate identification of smooth muscle involvement in tumour growth [31, 90, 91] (Figure 4).

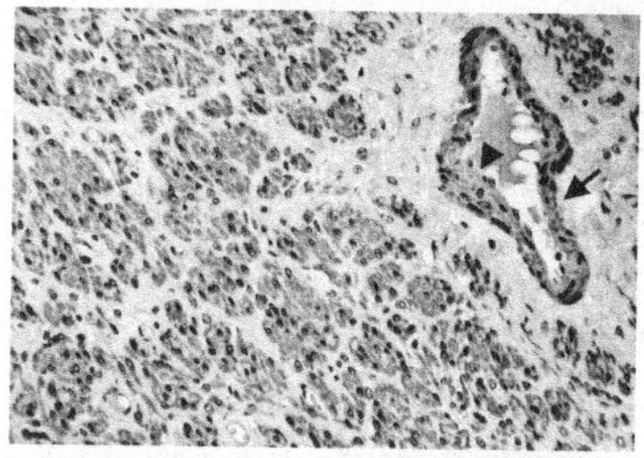

Figure 4. Immunohistochemical detection of the smooth muscle protein calponin in a leiomymoma. Most of the tumour cells show immunoreactive products to calponin antibody in their cytoplasms (brown colour). The vascular smooth muscle cells are also reactive (arrow) while endothelial cells are unreactive (arrowhead). ABC. 20X.

Leiomyoma is among the most common tumours of the female reproductive tract in many domestic species. It is located primarily in the vulva and vagina, followed by the uterus and its incidence is greater in older non-neutered bitches [77, 78]. In two different studies, all dogs diagnosed with leiomyoma were non-neutered bitches [78, 93] and the recurrence rate was 15% in bitches left unneutered after local excision. On the contrary, there was no recurrence in any animal when ovariohysterectomy was performed at the same time as excision. In another study [77], no leiomyomas were diagnosed in ovariectomised bitches under two years old. These epidemiological and clinical findings support the hormone-dependent nature of leiomyomas [88]. In addition, the role of ovarian steroid hormone receptors in the progression of female reproductive tract leiomyomas in the dog has also been demonstrated. Thus, Millán et al. [31] performed the first study on canine leiomyomas from the reproductive tract (uterus, vagina and vulva) demonstrating the IHC expression of ERα and PR in tumour tissue samples. Half of the leiomyomas (50%) expressed ERα and more than three quarters (82.1%) expressed PR (Figure 5).

Finally, a pioneer study of our group reported that the expression of PR in a canine vaginal fibroma was a predictive factor of favourable response to hormone therapy. Aglepritone at a dose of 10 mg/kg injected at days 1, 2, 8, 15, 28 and 35 prompted a progressive reduction in the size of the mass, which measured 9.1 x 5.4 cm on day 1 and 6.4 x 4.7 cm on day 45 [28](Figure 6). The authors evaluated the proliferation index in the same study using a proliferation marker (Ki67), recording similar low values at days 15 and 25 of treatment, suggesting that Aglepristone did not reduce tumour size by reducing the tumour cell proliferation rate but rather through increasing apoptosis. It was therefore concluded that the size of PR-expressing benign tumours of the canine vagina could be reduced by palliative or neoadjuvant therapy with the PR antagonist Aglepristone. These findings regarding steroid hormone receptor expression in canine tumours of the female reproductive tract highlight the potential of hormone therapy in selected cases. In cats, leiomyomas located in the mammary gland and in the perineal region are reported to express ERα and PR [27]; however, no research has yet focussed on the expression of steroid hormone receptors in feline leiomyomas located in the vagina, vulva or uterus.

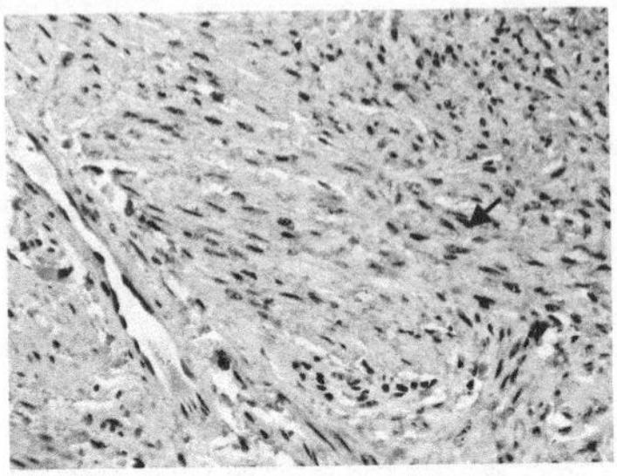

Figure 5. Immunohistochemical detection of ERα in a leiomyoma. Most of the tumour cells show immunoreactive products to ER antibody in their nucleus (brown colour)(arrow). ABC. 40X.

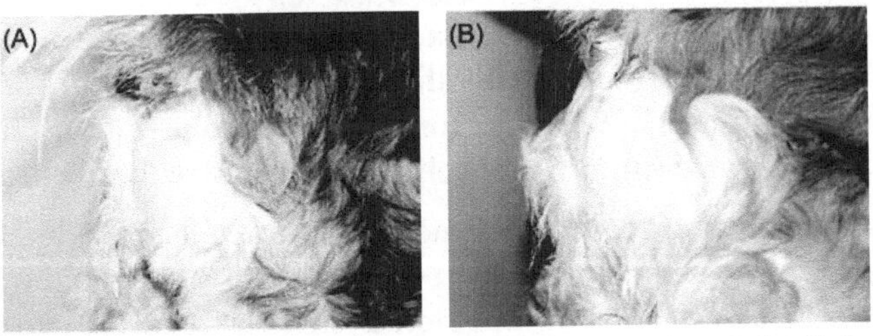

Figure 6. A) Female dog with a perineal mass measuring 9.1 x 5.4 cm. (B) The appearance of the tumour mass 28 days after treatment with aglepristone. The size is reduced to 6.4 x 4.7 cm [28].

4.2. Male reproductive tract

Male reproductive-tract tumours in dogs and cats may arise in the testes, prostate, penis or foreskin. Testicular tumours are the second most common cancer in intact dogs, accounting for roughly 90% of all reproductive-tract tumours [96]. In cats, however, testicular tumours are rare [97]. Prostate tumours are uncommon in dogs, with a reported incidence of between 0.2% to 0.6% [98, 99], and equally rare in cats [97, 100-102]. Many penis and foreskin tumours affect the epithelial surface of these structures, the most common being the transmissible venereal tumour of the penis in dogs [103].

Currently, the only male reproductive-tract tumour in domestic species for which published data is available regarding the possible influence of steroid hormones on tumour development is canine prostate carcinoma. The dog is the only non-primate species that develops spontaneous prostate cancer [104]. Most tumours in this location are of epithelial origin [98, 105] and mainly affect older dogs (average age 10 years), prostate carcinoma being common [98]. The prostate is an androgen-dependent organ [106], and androgens achieve their effect through activation of androgen receptors (AR).

However, there is a good deal of controversy concerning the influence of androgens on the development and biological behaviour of malignant prostate tumours. While some studies have found no evidence that castration has a protective effect against prostate carcinoma [99], others argue that castration before sexual maturity reduces the risk of this malignancy [105]; still others suggest that castration may actually increase the incidence and aggressive behaviour of canine prostate carcinomas [98]. The expression of steroid hormone receptors in tumour tissue samples of canine prostate carcinoma has been rarely studied. The more complete study up to date showed that expression of AR, ERα and ERβ was lower in malignant tumour epithelial cells than in normal prostate tissue and benign lesions, suggesting that oestrogen actions in the prostate are complex and may play a dual role in the aetiology of prostate cancer [32, 107]. This study also demonstrated for the first time that PR expression in canine prostate tumours is greater than in normal prostate tissue [32], although the effect of progesterone at this location still remains to be demonstrated, as does the potential for hormone therapy.

5. Cutaneous tumours in dogs and cats

Tumours of the skin and subcutaneous tissue are the most common neoplasms affecting dogs and the second most common in cats [108]. Incidence rates have been estimated at around 450 per 100,000 dogs and 120 per 100,000 cats [108]. In dogs, most skin tumours are benign, the most frequent being histiocytomas and sebaceous gland adenomas. In cats, however, approximately 50% to 65% of skin tumours are histologically malignant, the most frequently-reported being squamous cell carcinomas [109].

Epidemiological research has identified breed and age as major risk factors for these tumours. A number of authors note a linear increase in risk by a factor of 1.1 per year of increasing age; additionally, pure-bred dogs appear to be twice as likely to develop a malignancy as cross-breeds. When all types of tumours are considered together, no significant sex predilection is apparent [110]. A number of etiological factors – physical, viral, genetic and molecular – have been reported for some skin tumours [111]. Over the last few years, it has become increasingly evident that steroid sex hormones may play an important role in the pathogenesis of these tumours, as they do in mammary tumours. It is well known that oestrogens, progesterone and androgens not only help regulate skin development and function, such as the development and/or physiology of sebaceous glands and hair follicles, but are also involved in the development and biological behaviour of certain skin neoplasms [112].

To date, a number of studies have demonstrated a possible relationship between sex steroid hormones and sebaceous, perianal and hepatoid gland tumours and mast-cell tumours in domestic animals. To better understand this relationship, recent research has focussed on pinpointing the site of action of these hormones and on locating their receptors in both normal and tumour tissues. As a result, biochemical and immunohistochemical studies carried out over the last few years have detected androgen receptors (AR), oestrogen receptor α (ERα) and progesterone receptors (PR) in epidermis, hair follicles and fundamentally in the sebaceous glands of canine skin [113-117]. These results suggest that not only androgens and oestrogens, but also progesterone, may play a major role in the regulation of normal skin appendage function and in the pathogenesis and development of neoplasms.

Sebaceous gland tumours are among the most common skin tumours in the dog. They can be divided into four groups based on histological appearance: sebaceous hyperplasia, sebaceous epitheliomas, sebaceous adenomas and sebaceous adenocarcinomas. They account for between 6.8% to 7.9% of all skin tumours in dogs, and between 2.3% to 4.4% in cats [118]. Canine benign and malignant sebaceous gland neoplasias may provide a suitable experimental model for the study of hormone influences on the development of glandular tumours [114]. As in human skin, specific staining for ERα and PR is seen mainly in the basal cells of normal sebaceous glands [115-117]. However, unlike in human medicine, no data are available regarding the possible involvement of these steroid sex hormones in the pathology of canine and feline skin and the development of cutaneous neoplasms. A single study by the present authors analysed ERα and PR expression in canine sebaceous gland hyperplasias, adenomas/epitheliomas and carcinomas [117], revealing that canine sebaceous glands express both ERα and PR (Figure 7 y 8). Moreover, differences were recorded between types of lesion in the number of cells expressing ERα and PR. Compared with normal sebaceous glands, ERα expression was significantly lower in sebaceous gland epitheliomas and adenocarcinomas, suggesting that ERα plays a key physiological role in the maintenance of normal sebaceous glands, and that a decrease in levels influences the development of both benign and malignant neoplasms. A number of studies indicate that this drop in ERα could be secondary to changes in androgen or oestrogen production, but further research is required to confirm this hypothesis in canine sebaceous glands. The cited study also found that PR expression in adenocarcinomas was significantly lower than in normal and hyperplastic sebaceous glands, suggesting that tumour growth may become less hormone-dependent during the progression phase of carcinogenesis, as reported in certain human mammary tumours. Unlike ERα, the proportion of PR-positive cells did not differ significantly from that found in normal sebaceous glands, a finding also reported in humans [112]. This may indicate that progesterone does not necessarily influence the growth of this type of tumours. Conversely, sebaceous gland carcinomas display a significant loss in PR staining intensity; PR loss may be one factor involved in the pathogenesis of canine sebaceous gland neoplasms.

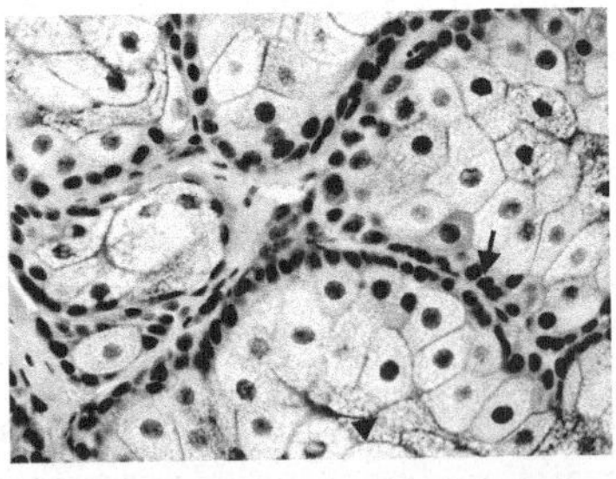

Figure 7. Immunohistochemical localization of PR in sebaceous gland hyperplasia. Nuclear staining is observed in basal cells (arrow) and differentiated sebocytes (arrowhead) [117]. ABC. 40X.

The influence of female sex steroids on their receptors in skin has been highlighted by several studies. When an ovariectomised bitch received a local estradiol (E2) implant, ER levels in the affected skin were found to be six times higher than in control skin [119]. However, despite the considerable amount of work done to date in this field, further research is still required to demonstrate the presence of AR and examine of the effects of these hormones and their pharmacological antagonists on tumour development.

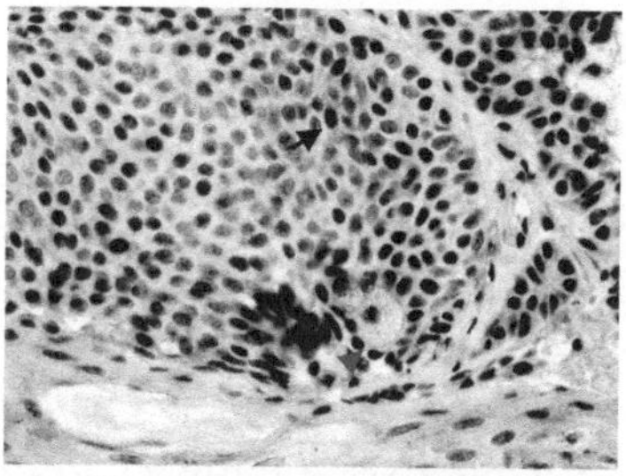

Figure 8. Immunohistochemical localization of PR in a sebaceous gland epithelioma. Nuclear staining is observed in basal cells (arrow) and differentiated sebocytes (arrowhead) [117]. ABC. 40X.

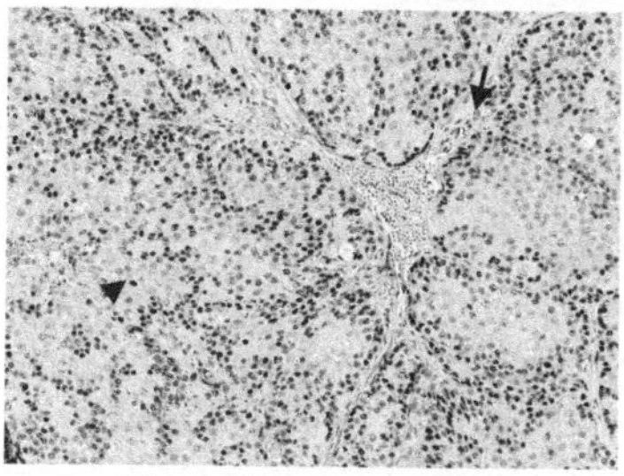

Figure 9. Immunohistochemical localization of ERα in a hepatoid gland adenoma. Nuclear staining is observed in basal cells (arrow) and differentiated hepatoid cells (arrowhead). ABC. 20X.

Other tumours considered clearly hormone-dependent include those arising in the perianal or hepatoid glands, modified sebaceous glands located in the perianal dermis. The most frequently observed tumours of this region in dogs are perianal adenoma, perianal adenocarcinoma and apocrine gland adenocarcinoma of the anal sac. Perianal adenomas account for between 58% and 96% of all canine perianal tumours [120]. Unlike adenomas, perianal gland carcinomas are rare, accounting for between 3% and 17% of all perianal neoplasms [121]. Although found in both male and female dogs, the highest incidence is reported in intact males of mean age 10 or more [122]. This evidence has for years been interpreted as proof of a clear stimulation of tumour development by sex steroid hormones, particularly androgens [123]. Adenomas have been found to be hormone-responsive; a full or partial regression has been observed following castration or oestrogen treatment [113, 120, 124]. In females, perianal adenomas occur almost exclusively in ovariohysterectomised animals whose low oestrogen levels fail to suppress tumour growth. Similarly, testicular interstitial cell tumours – which clinical observation suggests are associated with an increase in systemic androgen levels – occur more frequently in association with perianal tumours [125]. While hormone dependence has been clearly demonstrated in the case of perianal adenomas, there appears to be no link between perianal adenocarcinomas and steroid sex hormones. Perianal gland carcinomas do not regress following castration and are not responsive to hormone therapy with oestrogens [121, 124]. However, receptors for these hormones have been found in normal, hyperplastic and neoplastic perianal glands in dogs (Figure 9). An early report identified androgen-binding sites in perianal adenomas [124]. Research by Pisani *et al.* [126] detected AR expression in all normal and abnormal glands, although in hyperplastic tissues the proportion of positive nuclei was significantly greater than in normal tissue. A similar increase in the percentage of positive-staining nuclei was also observed in perianal epitheliomas, while in adenomas the increase with respect to normal tissue was only slight. In adenocarcinomas, the proportion of AR-positive cells was similar to that observed in benign tumours.

All these observations support the view that therapy based on antagonists of these hormones could prove beneficial in the treatment of these tumours. The present authors have carried out a preliminary clinical trial in order to evaluate the effect of Deslorelin (Suprelorin™ Virbac), a GnRH antagonist, on the clinical response of perianal gland adenomas [127]. This antagonist suppresses pituitary production of the hormones LH and FSH and of steroid sex hormones; its effect has been compared to that of surgical castration. The trial found that subcutaneous deslorelin implants induced complete remission in at least 50% of dogs and a partial response to treatment in a further 29%. This antagonist could thus be considered as a new option for the treatment of perianal gland adenomas.

Finally, the association between mast-cell tumours (MCTs) and steroid sex hormones remains controversial. The role of these hormones in tumour pathogenesis is poorly understood, although some evidence is now available: one study has detected cytosolic receptors for oestrogen and progesterone in canine MCTs [127], while another found that 6 out of 9 MCTs contained no ERα and 3 were questionable [128].

6. Conclusion

Sex steroid hormones are involved in the development of animal tumours with high epidemiological and clinical impact. Research in the field has shown the potential benefits of endocrine manipulations to control tumour progression in a neoadjuvant or adjuvant setting. From a comparative point of view, steroid hormone dependent animal tumors represent an accessible and natural model of human disease.

References

1. Ahern TE, Bird RC, Church Bird AE, Wolfe LG: Expression of the oncogene c-erbB-2 in canine mammary cancers and tumor-derived cell lines. American Journal of Veterinary Research 1996;57 693-696.

2. Dorn CR, Don T, Scheneider R, Hibbard HH. Survey of animal neoplasms in Alameda and Contra Costa Counties, Calif.:II. Cancer morbidity in dogs and cats from Alameda County. Journal of the National Cancer Institute 1968;40 307-318.

3. Schneider R, Dorn CR, Taylor D. Factors influencing canine mammary tumor development and postsurgical survival. Journal of the National Cancer Institute 1969;43 1249-1261.

4. Kwapien RP, Giles RC, Geil RG, Casey HW: Malignant mammary tumors in beagle dogs dosed with investigational oral contraceptive steroids. Journal of the National Cancer Institute 1980; 65 137-144.

5. Giles RC, Kwapien RP, Geil RG, Casey HW. Mammary nodules in beagle dogs administered investigational oral contraceptive steroids. Journal of the National Cancer Institute 1978;60:1351-1364.

6. Misdorp W. Progestagens and mammary tumours in dogs and cats. Acta Endocrinologica (Copenh) 1991;125 27-31.
7. Stovring M, Moe L, Glattre E. A population-based case-control study of canine mammary tumors and clinical use of medroxiprogesterone acetate. Acta Pathologica, microbiologica, et immunologica Scandinavica (APMIS) 1997;105 590-596.
8. Allen HL. Feline mammary hypertrophy. Veterinary Pathology 1973;10 501-508.
9. Loretti AP, Ilha MR, Ordás J, Martín de las Mulas J. Clinical, pathological and immunohistochemical study of feline mammary fibroepithelial hyperplasia following a single injection of depot medroxyprogesterone acetate. Journal of Feline Medicine and Surgery 2005;7(1) 43-52.
10. Mialot JP, Andre F, Martin PH, Cotard MP, Raynaud JP. Etude des recepteurs des hormones steroids dans les tummeurs mammaires de la chienne. I: mise en evidence, caracterisation et relation avec le type histologique. Recueil de Medicine Veterinaire 1982;158; 215-221.
11. Parodi AL, Misdorp W, Mialot JP, Mialot M, Hart AA, Hurtrel M, Salomon JC. Intratumoral BCG and Corynebacterium parvum therapy of canine mammary tumours before radical mastectomy. Cancer Immunology Immunotherapy 1983;15(3) 172-7.
12. Martin PM, Cotard M, Mialot JP, André F, Raynaud JP. Animal models for hormone-dependent human breast cancer. Relationship between steroid receptor profiles in canine and feline mammary tumors and survival rate. Cancer Chemotherapy and Pharmacolgy 1984;12(1) 13-17.
13. Sartin EA, Barnes S, Kwapien RP, Wolfe LG. Estrogen and progesterone receptor status of mammary carcinomas and correlation with clinical outcome in dogs. American journal of Veterinary Researche 1992;53 2196-2200.
14. Manzel O, Wurm S, Ueberschär S, Hoppen H-O: Estrogen and Progesterone receptors in histologic sections of canine mammary tumours in correlation to histologic type: conference proceedings, September 28, 1995, Edinburgh, Unite Kindong, ECVP; 1995.
15. Graham JC, O'Keefe DA, Gelberg HB. Immnunohistochemical assay for detecting estrogen receptors in canine mammary tumors. Am J Vet Res 1999;60(5) 627-630.
16. Geraldes M, Gärtner F, Schmitt F. Immunohistochemical study of hormonal receptors and cell proliferation in normal canine mammary glands and spontaneous mammary tumours. Veterinary Record 2000;146 403–406.
17. Martin de las Mulas J, van Niel M, Millán Y, Blakenstein MA, van Mil F, Misdorp W. Immunohistochemical analysis of estrogen receptors in feline mammary gland benign and malignant lesions: comparison with biochemical assay. Domestic Animal Endocrinology 2000;18 111-125.
18. Nieto A, Peña L, Pérez-Alenza MD, Sánchez MA, Flores JM, Castaño M: Immunohistologic detection of estrogen receptor alpha in canine mammary tumors: clinical and pathologic associations and prognostic significance. Veterinary Pathology 2000;37 239–247.

19. Martin de las Mulas J, Niel MV, Millan Y, Ordas J, Blankenstein MA, Mil FV, Misdorp W: Progesterone receptors in normal, dysplastic and tumourous feline mammary glands. Comparison with oestrogen receptors status. Research in Veterinary Science 2002;72 153-161.

20. de las Mulas J, Millán Y, Dios R. A prospective analysis of immunohistochemically determined estrogen receptor alpha and progesterone receptor expression and host and tumor factors as predictors of disease-free period in mammary tumors of the dog. Veterinary Pathology 2005;42 200–212.

21. Millanta F, Calandrella M, Vannozzi I, Poli A. Steroid hormone receptors i normal, dysplastic and neoplastic feline mammary tissues and their prognostic significance. Veterinary Record, 2006;158(24) 821-4.

22. Chang CC, Tsai MH, Liao JW, Chan JP, Wong ML, Chang SC. Evaluation of hormone receptor expression for use in predicting survival of female dogs with malignant mammary gland tumors. Journal of American Veterinary Medical Association. 2009;235(4) 391-396.

23. Ferreira E, Bertagnolli AC, Cavalcanti MF, Schmitt FC, Cassali GD. The relationship between tumour size and expression of prognostic markers in bening and malignant canine mammary tumours. Veterinary and Comparative Oncology. 2009; 7(4) 230-5.

24. Sassi F, Benazzi C, Castellani G, Sarli G. Molecular-based tumour subtypes of canine mammary carcinomas assessed by immunohistochemistry. BMC Veterinary Research. 2010; 6 5.

25. Dolka I, Motyl T, Malicka R, Sapierzynsky E, Fabisiak M. Relationship between receptors for insulin-like growth factor-I, steroid hormones and apoptosis-associated proteins in canine mammary tumors. Polish Journal of Veterinary Sciences, 2011; 14(2) 245-251.

26. Rosen PP, Oberman HA. Tumors of the mammary gland. Washington, D.C: Armed Forces Institute of Pathology; 1993.

27. Martín de las Mulas J, Rollón E, Millán Y, Ordás J, Carrasco L, Reymundo C Perineal leiomyoma expressing steroidal hormone receptors in a queen. Veterinary Record 2002;150(18) 578-9.

28. Rollón E, Millán Y, Martín de las Mulas J. Effects of aglepristone, a progesterone receptor antagonist, in a dog with a vaginal fibroma. Journal of Small Animal Practice 1997;49 41-43.

29. Guil-Luna S, Sánchez-Céspedez R, Millán Y, De Andrés FJ, Rollón E, Domingo V, Guscetti F, Martín de las Mulas J. Aglepristone decreases proliferation in progesterona receptor-positive canine mammary carcinomas. Journal of Veterinary Internal Medicine 2011;25(3) 518-523.

30. Domingo V, De Andrés FJ, Rollón E, Millán Y, Guil-Luna S, Sánchez-Céspedes R, Linares N, Martín de las Mulas J. Clinical response of canine perianal adenomas to subcutaneous implants of Deslorelin: conference proceedings, March 24-26, 2011, Glasgow Annual Congress of European Society of Veterinary Oncology, Glasgow, England. 2011.

31. Millán Y, Gordon A, de los Monteros AE, Reymundo C, de las Mulas JM. Steroid receptors in canine and human female genital tract tumours with smooth muscle differentiation. Journal of Comparative Pathology 2007;136 197-201.

32. Gallardo F, Mogas T, Baró T, Rabanal R, Morote J, Abal M, Reventós J, Lloreta J. Expression of Androgen, Oestrogen α and β, and Progesterone Receptors in the Canine Prostate: Differences between Normal, Inflamed, Hyperplastic and Neoplastic Glands. Journal of Comparative Pathology 2007;136 1-8.

33. Baulieu E-E., Mester J. Steroid hormone receptors. In: De Groot L.J., (ed.). Endocrinology. Philadelphia: W.B. Saunders Co.; 1989. p16-39.

34. Greene GL, Nolan C, Engler JP, Jensen EU. Monoclonal antibodies to human estrogen receptors: Proceeding of the National Academic of Sciences of the USA. 77:5115-5119, 1980.

35. Greene GL, Harris K, Bravo R, Kinders R, Moore B, Nolan C. Purification of T47D human progesterone receptor and immunochemical characterization with monoclonal antibodies. Molecular Endocrinology 1988;2 714-726.

36. al Saati T, Clamens S, Cohen-Knafo E, Faye JC, Prats H, Coindre JM, Wafflart J, Caveriviere P, Bayard F, Delsol G. Production of monoclonal antibodies to human estrogen-receptor protein (ER) using recombinant ER (RER). International Journal of Cancer 1993;55 651-654.

37. Goussard J. Paraffin section immunocytochemistry and cytosol-based ligand-binding assay for ER and PR detection of breast cancer: the time has come for more objectivity. Cancer Letters 1998;132:61-66.

38. De Mascarel I, Soubeyran I, MacGrogan G, Wafflart J, Bonichon F, Durand M, Avril A, Mauriac L, Trojani M, de Coindre JM. Immunohistochemical analysis of estrogen receptors in 938 breast carcinomas. Concordance with biochemical assay and prognostic significance. Applied Immunohistochemistry 1995;3 222-231.

39. MacGrogan G, Soubeyran I, de Mascarel I, Wafflart J, Bonichon F, Durand M, Avril A, Maurac L, Trojani M, Coindre JM. Immunohistochemical Detection of Progesterone Receptors in Breast Invasive Ductal Carcinomas. Applied Immunohistochemistry 1996;4 219-227.

40. Allred DC, Harvey JM, Berardo M, Clark GM. Prognostic and predictive factors in breast cancer by immunohistochemical analysis. Modern Pathology 1998;11 155-168.

41. Balaton AJ, Berthelot N, Cuadrado C, Fillon L, Galland I, Gilles C, Lemoine C, Lucas C, Taluau V. Antigenic retrieval using a pressure cooker. Annales de Pathologie 1996;16(4) 307-309.

42. Goussard J. Value of detection of hormone receptors by biochemical and immunochemical methods in therapeutic decision for breast cancer. Bulletin du Cancer 1996;83(12) 1031-1036.

43. Krecsak L, Micsik T, Kiszler G, Krenacs T, Szabo D, Jonas V, Csaszar G, Czuni L, Gurzo P, Ficsor L, Molnar B. Technical note on the validation of a semi-automated image analysis software application for estrogen and progesterone receptor detection in breast cancer. Diagnostic Pathology 2011; 6: 6. www.diagnosticpathology.org/content/6/1/6

44. Hammond ME, Hayes DF, Dowsett M, Allred DC, Hagerty KL, Badve S, Fitzgibbons PL, Francis G, Goldstein NS, Hayes M, Hicks DG, Lester S, Love R, Mangu PB, McShane L, Miller K, Osborne CK, Paik S, Perlmutter J, Rhodes A, Sasano H, Schwartz JN, Sweep FC, Taube S, Torlakovic EE, Valenstein P, Viale G, Visscher D, Wheeler T, Williams RB, Wittliff JL, Wolff AC. American Society of Clinical Oncology/College of American Pathologists guideline recommendations for immunohistochemical testing of Estrogen and Progesterone Receptors in Breast Cancer. Archives of Pathology and Laboratory Medicine 2010 134(6):907-22.

45. Lana S.E., Rutteman G.R., Withrow S.J. Tumors of the mammary gland. In: Withrow, S.J & MacEwen, B.R. (ed) Small Animal Clinical Oncology. Philadelphia, P.A.: Saunders; 2007. p455-477.

46. Brodey RS, Goldschmidt HH, Roszel JR. Canine mammary gland neoplasms. Journal of the American Animal Hospital Association 1983;19 61-90.

47. Madewell BR, Theilen GH: Tumors of the mammary gland. In: Theilen G.H., Madewell B.R., (ed). Veterinary Cancer Medicine. Philadelphia: Lea & Febiger; 1987. p327-344.

48. Skorupski KA, Overly B, Shofer FS, Goldschmidt MH, Miller CA, Sørenmo KU. Clinical characteristics of mammary carcinoma in male cats. Journal of Veterinary Internal Medicine 2005;19 52-55.

49. Hayes HM, Jr., Milne KL, Mandell CP. Epidemiological features of feline mammary carcinomas. Veterinary Record 1981;108 476-479.

50. Arnesen K, Gamlem H, Glattre J, Grondalen J, Moe L, Nordstoga K. The Norwegian canine cancer register 1990-1998. Report from the project "Cancer in the dog". The European Journal of Companion Animal Practice 2001;11 159-169.

51. Craig LE. Cause of death in dogs according to breed: a necropsy survey of five breeds. Journal of the American Animal Hospital Association 2001;37 438-443.

52. Dorn CR, Don T, Scheneider R, Hibbard HH. Survey of animal neoplasms in Alameda and Contra Costa Counties, Calif.:II. Cancer morbidity in dogs and cats from Alameda County. Journal of the National Cancer Institute 1968;40 307-318.

53. Schneider R, Dorn CR, Taylor D. Factors influencing canine mammary tumor development and postsurgical survival. Journal of the National Cancer Institute 1969;43 1249-1261.

54. Overley B, Shofer FS, Goldschmidt MH, Sherer D, Sorenmo KU. Association between ovarihysterectomy and feline mammary carcinoma. Journal of Veterinary Internal Medicine 2005;19(4) 560-3.

55. Giles RC, Kwapien RP, Geil RG, Casey HW. Mammary nodules in beagle dogs administered investigational oral contraceptive steroids. Journal of the National Cancer Institute 1978;60:1351-1364.

56. Rutteman GR. Contraceptive steroids and the mammary gland: Is there a hazard? Breast Cancer Researche and Treatment 1992;23 29-41.

57. Kwapien RP, Giles RC, Geil RG, Casey HW. Malignant mammary tumors in beagle dogs dosed with investigational oral contraceptive steroids. Journal of the National Cancer Institute 1980;65 137-144.

58. Misdorp W, Romijn A, Hart AA. Feline mammary tumors: a case-control study of hormonal factors. Anticancer Research 1991; 11(5) 1793-1797.
59. Burrai GP, Mohammed SI, Miller MA, Marras V, Pirino S, Addis MF, Uzzau S, Antuofermo E. Spontaneous feline mammary intraepithelial lesions as a model for human estrogen receptor- and progesterone receptor-negative breast lesions. BMC Cancer. 2010;10 156.
60. Sobczak-Filipiak M, Malicka E: Estrogen receptors in canine mammary gland tumours. Polish Journal of Veterinary Sciences 2002;5 1–5.
61. Mouser P, Miller MA, Antuofermo E, Badve SS, Mohammed SI. Prevalence and classification of spontaneous mammary intraepithelial lesions in dogs without clinical mammary disease. Veterinary Patholgy. 2010;47(2) 275-84.
62. Millanta F, Caneschi V, Ressel L, Citi S, Poli A. Expression of vascular endothelial growth factor in canine inflammatory and non-inflammatory mammary carcinoma. Journal of Comparative Pathology. 2010;142(1) 36-42.
63. Toniti W, Buranasinsup S, Kongcharoen A, Charoonrut P, Puchadapirom P, Kasorndorkbua C. Immunohistochemical determination of estrogen and progesterone receptors in canine mammary tumors. Asian Pacific Journal of Cancer Prevention. 2009;10(5) 907-11.
64. Millanta F, Calandrella M, Bari G, Niccolini M, Vannozzi I, Poli A. Comparison of steroid receptor expression in normal, dysplastic, and neoplastic canine and feline mammary tissues. Researche Veterinary Science 2005;79(3) 225-32.
65. Brunetti B, Asproni P, Beha G, Muscatello LV, Millanta F, Poli A, Benazzi C, Sarli G. Molecular Phenotype in Mammary tumours of queens: correlation between primary tumour and lymph node metastasis. Journal of Comparative Pathology.2012 Jul 19.
66. Kuiper GG, Enmark E, Pelto-Huikko M, Nilsson S, Gustaffson JA: Cloning of a novel receptor expressed in rat prostate and ovary. Proc Natl Acad Sci USA 1996;93 5925–5930.
67. Mosselman S, Polman J, Dijkema R: ER-beta: identification and characterisation of a novel human estrogen receptor. FEBS Lett 1996;392 49–53.
68. Martín de las Mulas J, Ordás J, Millán MY, Chacón F, De Lara M, Espinosa de los Monteros A, Reymundo C, Jover A. Immunohistochemical expression of estrogen receptor beta in normal and tumoral canine mammary glands. Veterinary Pathology 2004;41(3) 269-72.
69. Illeraa JC, Perez-Alenza M, Nieto A, Jimenez MA, Silvana G, Dunner S, Peña L. Steroids and receptors in canine mammary cancer. Steroids 2006; 7(1) 541–548.
70. Morris JS, Dobson JM, Bostock DE. Use of tamoxifen in the control canine mammary neoplasia. Veterinary Record 1993;133 539-542.
71. Yamagami T, Kobayashi T, Takahashi K, Sugiyama M: Influence of ovariectomy at the time of mastectomy on the prognosis for canine malignant mammary tumours. Journal of Small Animal Practice 1996;37 462-464.
72. Morris JS, Dobson JM, Bostock DE, O'Farrel E. Effect of ovariohysterectomy in bitches with mamary neoplasia. Veterinary Record 1998;142 656-658.

73. Cappeletti V, Granata G, Miodini P, Coradini D, DiFronzo G, Cairoli F, Colombo G, Nava A, Scanziani E. Modulation of receptor levels in canine breast tumors by administration of tamoxifen and Etretinate either alone or in combination. Anticancer Research 1988;8 1297-1302.

74. Wehrend A, Hospes R, Gruber AD. Treatment of feline mammary fibroadenomatous hyperplasia with a progesterone antagonist. Veterinary Record 2001;148 346-347.

75. Martín de las Mulas J, Millán Y, Bautista MJ, Pérez J, Carrasco L. Oestrogen and progesterone receptors in feline fibroadenomatous change: an immunohistochemical study. Research in Veterinary Science 2000;67 15-21.

76. McEntee MC. Reproductive oncology. Clinical Techniques in Small Animal Practice 2002;17(3) 133-149.

77. Brodey RS, Roszel JF. Neoplasms of the canine uterus, vagina, and vulva: a clinicopathologic survey of 90 cases. Journal of the American Veterinary Medical Association 1967;151 1294-1307.

78. Tacher C, Bradley RI. Vulvar and vaginal tumors in the dog: a retrospective study. Journal of the American Veterinary Medical Association 1983;183 690-692.

79. Cotchin E. Neoplasia in the cat. Veterinary Record 1957;69 425-434.

80. Engle CG, Brodey RS. A retrospective study of 395 felilne neoplasms. Journal of the American Animal Hospital Association 1969;5 21-25.

81. Herron MA. Tumors of the canine genital system. Journal of the American Hospital Association. 1983;19 981-994.

82. Schmidt RE, Langham RF. A survey of feline neoplasms. Journal of the American Veterinary Medical Association 1967;151 1325-1328.

83. Theilen GH., Madewell BR. Tumors of the urogenital tract. In: Theilen GH & Madewell BR (ed) Veterinary Cancer Medicine. Philadelphia: Lea & Febiger; 1979. p567-600.

84. Withrow SJ., Susaneck, SJ. Tumors of the canine female reproductive tract. In: Morrow DA (ed) Current therapy in theriogenology. Philadelphia: WB Saunders; 1986. p521-528.

85. Dow C. Ovarian abnormalities in the bitch. Journal of Comparative Pathology 1960;70 59-69.

86. Cotchin E. Spontaneous uterine cancer in animals. British Journal of Cancer 1964; 18:209-27.

87. Cotchin, E. Some tumors of dogs and cats of comparative veterinary and human interest. Veterinary Record 1959;71 1040-1054.

88. Klein MK. Tumors of the female reproductive system. In: Withrow SJ. & MacEwen EG. (ed) Small Animal Clinical Oncology. Philadelphia: Saunders Elsevier; 2001. p445-454.

89. MacLachlan NJ, Kennedy PC. Tumors of the genital system. In: DJ Meuten (ed) Tumors in domestic animals. Iowa: Iowa State Press; 2002. p547-574.

90. Frost D, Lasota J, Miettinen M. Gastrointestinal stromal tumors and leiomyomas in the dog: a histopathologic, immunohistochemical, and molecular genetic study of 50 cases. Veterinary Pathology 2003;40 42-54.

91. Zhu X –Q, Shi Y –F, Cheng X –D, Zhao C –L, Wu Y –Z. Immunohistochemical markers in differential diagnosis of endometrial stromal sarcoma and cellular leiomyoma. Ginecologic Oncology. 2004;92 71-79.

92. McGinley KM, Bryant S, Kattine AA, Fitzgibbon JF, Googe PB. Cutaneous leiomyomas lack estrogen and progesterone receptor immunoreactivity. Journal of Cutaneous Pathology 1997;24 241-245.

93. Kydd DM, Burnie AG. Vaginal neoplasia in the bitch: a review of 40 clinical cases. Journal of Small Animal Practice 1986;27 255-263.

94. Espinosa de los Monteros A, Millán Y, Ordás J, Carrasco L, Reymundo C, Martín de las Mulas J. Immunolocalization of the smooth muscle-specific protein calponin in complex and mixed tumors of the mammary gland of the dog: assessment of the morphogenetic role of the myoepithelium. Veterinary Pathology 2002;39 247-256.

95. Galac D, Kooistra HS, Dielemn SJ, Cestnik V, Okkens AC. Effecs of aglepristone, a progesterone receptor antagonist, administered during the early luteal phase in non-pregnant bitches. Theriogenology 2004;62 494-500.

96. Hayes HM, Pendergrass TW. Canine testicular tumors: epidemiologic features of 410 dogs. Internal Journal of Cancer 1976;18 482-487.

97. Carpenter JL., Andrews LK., Holsworth J. Tumors and tumor-like lesions. In: Holzworth J. (ed) Diseases of the cat. Philadelphia:WB Saunders; 1987. p406-459.

98. Bell FW, Klausner JS, Hayden DW, Feeney DA, Johnston SD. Clinical and pathologic features of prostatic adenocarcinoma in sexually intact and castrated dogs: 31 cases (1970-1987). Journal of the American Veterinary Medical Association 1991;199 1623-1630.

99. Obradovich J, Walshaw R, Goullaud E. The influence of castration on the development of prostatic carcinoma in the dog: 43 cases (1978-1985). Journal of Veterinary Internal Medicine 1987;1 183-187.

100. Caney SM, Holt PE, Day MJ, Rudorf H, Gruffydd-Jones TJ. Prostatic carcinoma in two cats. Journal of Small Animal Practice 1998;39 140-143.

101. Hubbard BS, Vulgamott JC, Liska WD. Prostatic adenocarcinoma in a cat. Journal of the American Veterinary Medical Association 1990;197 1493-1494.

102. LeRoy BE, Lech ME. Prostatic carcinoma causing urethral obstruction and obstipation in a cat. Journal of Feline Medicine and Surgery 2004;6 397-400.

103. Ndiritu CG. Lesions of the canine penis and prepuce. Modern Veterinary Practice 1979;60 712-715.

104. Lai CL, L´Eplattenier H, van den Ham R, Verseijden F, Jagtenberg A, Mol JA, Teske E. Androgen Receptor CAG repeat Polymorphisms in Canine Prostate Cancer. Journal of Veterinary Internal Medicine 2008;22 1380-1384.

105. Cornell KK, Bostwick DG, Cooley DM, Hall G, Harvey HJ, Hendrick MJ, Pauli BU, Render, JA, Stoica G, Sweet DC, Waters DJ. Clinical and pathologic aspects of spontaneous canine prostate carcinoma: a retrosprective analysis of 76 cases. Prostate 2000;45 173-183.

106. Bell FW, Klausner JS, Hayden DV, Lund EM, Liebenstein BB, Feeney DA, Johnston SD, Shivers JL, Ewing CM, Isaacs WB. Evaluation of serum and seminal plasma markers in the diagnosis of canine prostatic disorders. Journal of Veterinary Internal Medicine 1995;9 149-153.

107. Bonkhoff H, Fixemer T, Hunsicker I, Remberger K. Estrogen receptor expression in prostate cancer and premalignant prostatic lesions. American Journal of Pathology 1999;155 641-647.

108. Vail DM.,Withrow SJ. Tumors of the mammary gland, In: Vail DM.,Withrow SJ (eds.) Small Animal Clinical Oncology. Philadelphia, WB Saunders; 2001. p455-477.

109. Blackwood L. Tumours of the skin and subcutaneous tissues, In: Dobson JM., Lascelles BDX. (eds.) BSAVA Manual of canine and feline oncology. England, BSAVA ; 2011. p130-158.

110. Kaldrymidou H, Leontides L, Koutinas AF. Prevalence, distribution and factors associated with the presence and potential for malignancy of cutaneous neoplasm in 174 dogs admitted to a clinic in northen Greece. Transboundary and emerging diseases 2002; 49(2) 87-91.

111. Goldschmidt MH., Hendrick MJ. Tumors of the skin and soft tissues, In: Meuten DJ. (ed.) Tumors in domestic animals. EEUU, Iowa State Press; 2002. p45-119.

112. Kariya Y, Moriya T, Suzuki T, Chiba M, Ishida K, Takeyama J, Endoh M, Watanabe M, Sasano H. Sex steroid hormones receptors in human skin appendage and its neoplasms. Endocrine Journal 2005; 52(3) 317-325.

113. Chaisiri N, Pierrpoint CG. Steroid-receptor interaction in a canine anal adenoma. Journal of Small Animal Practise 1979; 20(7) 405-416.

114. Brakta-Robia CB, Egerbacher M, Helmreich M, Mitteregger G, Benesch M, Bamberg E. Immunohistochemical localization of androgens and oestrogen receptors in canine hair follicles. Veterinary Dermatology 2002; 13 (2) 113-118.

115. Ginel PJ, Millán Y, Gómez-Laguna J. Localization of oestrogen and progesterone receptors in canine skin. Veterinary Dermatology 2006; 17 353-354 (Abstract).

116. Frank LA, Donnell RL, Kania SA. Oestrogen receptor evaluation in Pomeranian dogs with hair follicle arrest (alopecia X) on melatonin supplementation. Veterinary Dermatology 2006; 17(4) 252-258.

117. Ginel PJ, Lucena R, Millán Y, González-Medina S, Guil-Luna S, García-Monterde J, Espinosa de los Monteros A, Martín de las Mulas J. Expression of oestrogen and progesterone receptors in canine sebaceous gland tumors. Veterinary Dermatology 2009; 21 (3) 297-302.

118. Bostock D. Neoplasm of the skin and subcutaneous tissues in dogs and cats. Brithis Veterinary Journal 1986; 142(1) 1-19.

119. Eigenmann JE, Poortman J, Koeman JP. Estrogen induced flank alopecia in the female dog, evidence for local rather than systemic hyperoestrogenism. Journal of the American Animal Hospital Association 1984; 20 (1) 621-624.

120. Nielsen SW, Aftosmis J. Canine Perianal Gland Tumors. Journal of American Veterinary Medical Association 1964; 144(15) 127-135.

121. Vail DM, Withrow SJ, Schwarz PD, Powers BE. Perianal adenocarcinomas in the canine male: a restrospective study of 41 cases. Journal of American Animal Hopital Association 1990; 26(3) 329-334.

122. Turek, MM., & Withrow, SJ. (2001). Perineal tumors, In: Vail DM.,Withrow SJ (eds.) Small Animal Clinical Oncology. Philadelphia, WB Saunders; 2001. P503-510.

123. Isitor GN, Weinman DE. Origin and early development of canine circumanal glands. American Journal of Veterinary Research 1979; 40 (4) 487-492.

124. Wilson GP, Hayes HM. Castration for treatment of perianal gland neoplasms in the dog. Journal of American Veterinary Medicine Association 1979; 174 (12) 1301-1303.

125. Hayes HM, Wilson GP. Hormone-dependent neoplasms of the canine perianal gland. Cancer Research 1977; 37 (1) 2068-2071.

126. Pisani G, Millanta F, Lorenzi D, Vannozzi I, Poli A. Androgen receptor expression in normal, hyperplastic and neoplastic hepatoid glands in the dog. Research in Veterinary Science 2006; 81 231-236.

127. Elling H, Ungemach FR. Sexual hormone receptors in canine mast cell tumour cytosol. Journal of Comparative Pathology 1982; 92 629-630.

128. Larsen AE, Grier RL. Evaluation of canine mast cell tumors for presence of estrogen receptors. American Journal of Veterinary Research 1989; 50 1779-1780.

Chapter 8

Feline Mammary Fibroepithelial Hyperplasia: A Clinical Approach

1. Introduction

Feline mammary masses are frequently suspected of being mammary tumours. Immediate attention is required as over 80% of mammary tumours in cats are malignant [1,2], albeit mammary masses in cats are less common than in dogs. However, prevalence of mammary tumours is highly variable with the geographic region, as it tends to be lower in areas where most cats are neutered at a young age. Due to the negative prognosis generally attributed to feline mammary tumours, little attention has been paid to benign mammary growths and mastectomy is still often performed to deal with feline mammary fibroepithelial hyperplasia.

Feline mammary fibroepithelial hyperplasia represents a benign, progesterone-associated fibroglandular proliferation of one or more mammary glands that may occur in both the female and male cat [3,4]. It is also named feline hypertrophy, fibroadenomatous changes, mammary hyperplasia or fibroadenoma complex [3-5].

Feline mammary fibroepithelial hyperplasia (FEH) is characterized by the sudden onset of mammary swollen within a short period of 2 to 5 weeks, frequently concerning several mammary glands. When exuberant it is often at the origin of the consultation [6-9]. Ulceration and abscessation of the mammary gland may occur due to gland enlargement and trauma, in chronic situations [9,10].

Feline mammary fibroepithelial hyperplasia is considered to be a benign condition, yet its behaviour and gross appearance is similar to mammary neoplasic lesions, in particular when solitary ulcerated or violaceous lesions are present. Although it rapid growth may cause concern, fibroepithelial mammary lesions are reversible, and the volume of the mammary masses tend to decrease after luteolysis or at the end of exogenous progestagen activity [4,5,11].

Tentative diagnosis of mammary fibroepithelial hyperplasia should be based on the gross appearance of the lesions and on the history despite that most frequently, historic information is limited or incomplete, as a previous occurring estrus is seldom detected. Thus, diagnosis of feline mammary fibroepithelial hyperplasia is a clinical issue, and is not difficult to be established when all the mammary glands show a rapid enlargement, independently of the size of the swollen mammary gland [4,9]. This diagnosis may be further supported by the raised blood progesterone levels or by reported recent progestin treatment. However, when fibroepithelial lesions develop in only one mammary gland, distinguish between hyperplasia and mammary tumour may become more challenging. Biopsies or excision of the mammary lesions are frequently performed. Nevertheless, differential diagnosis with mammary carcinomas has to be carefully established, as around 85% of all mammary neoplasias are malignant [9].

As FEH is a non-neoplastic progesterone-associated disorder, it is possible for most situations to apply medical treatment. Administration of antiprogestins remains the elective medical treatment, and its schedule and duration is usually related to the severity of the problem at presentation. Complete excision of the mammary chain, under the supposition of a mammary tumour, may become a really aggressive surgery. Nowadays, with the available medical options mastectomy should be avoided in case of FEH.

Recurrence of the situation, although possible, remains controversial [6,11-13]. Nevertheless it is an important issue when discussing the therapeutic approach with owners. Ovariohysterectomy remains an option in animals not intent to reproduction and in animals submitted to progesterone-based contraception, even if postponed until mammary glands regress into the normal size.

The objective of this work was to present and discuss the clinical approaches available to establish the diagnosis and the therapeutic options for feline mammary fibroepithelial hyperplasia. The final purpose in the diagnosis and treatment of such disease is not only to confirm that the clinical situation was correctly identified, but also to select the most suitable therapeutic approach to each patient, and also avoiding precipitate mastectomy and other complications of the surgical act, with the minimum repercussions on patients' welfare.

2. Epidemiology of the feline mammary fibroepithelial hyperplasia

Feline mammary fibroepithelial hyperplasia occurs in intact queens of any age, in pregnant females and in female or male cats under progestin treatment [6-8,14]. It predominantly affects younger intact female cats, a segment of the population that also presents an increased ratio of spontaneous ovulation [15,16]. The reported age range for FEH is 6 months to 13 years [17-20]. Not so frequently, the condition may also be seen in aged females, associated or not with a contraceptive treatment, and sporadically in hormonally treated male tomcats. In a local study, the age range for FEH was 10 months to 10 years (the median for the age was 3 years), and the condition was exclusively diagnosed in queens [21]. This contrast with the usual age at presentation in case of mammary neoplasia, which is middle-aged queens, since the risk for mammary tumour increase with the cat age, particularly at 10-12 years [1,22].

Moreover, few reports exist on the occurrence of FEH in males under treatment with antiandrogenic drugs, such as delmadinon acetate (Meisl et al., cited in [8]) and cyproterone acetate [12], frequently used by cat fanciers for eliminating the urine spraying in intact adult tomcats. Infrequently, descriptions of FEH in spayed queens or male cats supposedly not submitted to steroid treatment have been published [11,23], but the doubt remained on the absence of an involuntary hormonal treatment.

It is generally accepted that the incidence of this disturbance may reach up to 20% of the mammary masses detected in cats, its prevalence varying with the country or the region, which reflect cultural differences in the reproductive management of domestic and free-roaming felids. In a study developed in the north of Portugal, based on the excisional material sent for histopathology analysis, the mammary fibroepithelial hyperplasia reach 13% of the feline mammary masses [21]. Nevertheless, according to our experience, incidence of FEH seems to be in regression among the group of animals submitted to progesterone-based contraception, may be due to the fact that most contraceptive treatments are now based in oral, veterinary drugs (such as Megescat®) instead of human design depot products (like Depo-Provera®). Nevertheless, the medroxyprogesterone acetate and the megestrol acetate are the most frequently reported progestin associated to FEH, in particular when the drug is injected [13,14,18,24].

Mammary enlargement is usually observed within 1-2 weeks after estrus or within 2-6 weeks after hormone treatment.

Apparently, no breed predisposition has been suggested for FEH. Even so, the majority of the cases were described in domestic shorthaired cats, which could simply be due to the fact that it may constitute the majority of the population worldwide.

3. Pathogenesis of the feline mammary fibroepithelial hyperplasia

The exact pathogenesis of FEH remains unclear, although sex steroid involvement has been acknowledged for long. Progesterone or its synthetic analogues have being recognized as being at the origin of most of the FEH situations described.

The interaction between the activity of the mammary gland and the sex steroids is recognised for long. In brief, development and growth of the mammary gland is under the control of progesterone, which effects are mainly mediated through the progesterone receptor (PR) on stromal and epithelial cells [25]. Local activation of PR triggers a cascade of specific and sequential series of molecules, specific for each glandular element, which stimulates mammary gland proliferation. In physiological conditions, the cyclic changes between estrogens and progesterone stimulate or repress the cyclic activation of such PR-mediated pathways [25]. A decrease in PR levels is associated to a reduction of progesterone activity. Progesterone has been reported as having a major role in mammary ductal branching [26,27], while estrogens acting via the ER have been associated to ductal elongation and bifurcation [27].

An aberrant regulation or those pathways may be at the origin of the disturbed response to the progesterone stimulation and contribute to the development of mammary gland hyperplastic or neoplastic growth. It is possible that such response may be associated to two factors: the extreme sensitivity of the feline mammary gland to sex steroids action, as referred in older studies (Bässler, cited in [17]); and the fact that the mammary gland is usually very thin when non-pregnant or non-lactating [28].

In a recent study, the two progesterone receptors (PR) isoforms (A and B) have been evidenced in tissue samples from fibroepithelial hyperplasia lesions, with predominant expression in the ductal epithelium. It was also reported a higher expression of PR in the stroma of FEH lesions in comparison to those found in stroma from mammary carcinomas [29]. The presence of estrogen receptors (ER) in FEH lesions remains a subject of controversy, as the number of cases where ER has been detected varies along the reports [20,30,31]. Nevertheless, a slight reduction in ER expression seems to accompany the process. Expression of PR in a progesterone-target tissue is dependant of the previous stimulation by estrogens via ER, while progesterone effects also include the down-regulation of estrogen receptors. So it is also possible that the length of progesterone dominance or the circulating levels of progesterone may influence the amount of ER found in mammary tissue in the available studies.

The potential role of estrogens in the development of fibroepithelial hyperplasia needs clarification, as it may influence the relationship between the progesterone and estrogen receptors in mammary gland tissue. Further, in one recent study the concentrations of estradiol in animals suffering from FEH were higher than values typical for the luteal phase, both in case of the first appearance of fibroepithelial hyperplasia and in recurrences [13].

Progestagens (progesterone and synthetic progestins) influences on feline mammary glands result in the stimulation of the cellular proliferation through PR stimulation. It was proposed that binding of progestagens to PR would enhancement the local GH expression [29,32]. The GH presents a mitogenic action, which is mediated by insulin-like growth factor-1 (IGF-1) [32,33], a molecule shown to possess a strong mitogenic and anti-apoptotic effect on the mammary epithelial cells. The increased expression of GH, GH receptor and IGF-I was demonstrated in FEH lesions [29].

For fibroadenomatous hyperplasia associated to the cyproterone acetate administration it was found that this drug may present a "gestagenic" effect, which it was suggested to contribute to the development of fibroepithelial hyperplasia of mammary glands [12].

Comparative studies of the proliferative index (measured by Ki67/MIB1 expression) in feline fibroepithelial hyperplasia and other mammary tumours showed that, in spite of being a benign disturbance, it shows a very high proliferative index similar to the one observed in invasive mammary carcinomas [34,35]. Fibroepithelial hyperplasia, which exhibits unique morphological and biological features, is characterised by rapid proliferation of epithelium and stroma [35]. Regardless its classification as a hyperplastic lesion, with a favourable biological behaviour, all cases of fibroepithelial hyperplasia exhibited high rates of cell proliferation, with mean values similar to those of carcinomas in accordance with the results of a previous investigation [35].

Despite that increase expression of PR has been found in the FEH lesions in comparison to normal diestrous mammary tissue samples, the blood levels for progesterone are usually within the normal levels for the species [6], although cats may present considerable variation in their progesterone blood levels [36]. This is suggestive that the disease would correspond to a disturbed, exaggerated response of the tissue to the circulating hormones.

4. Morphological and pathological features of mammary fibroepithelial hyperplasia lesions

Macroscopically, FEH lesions appear as firm, well-circumscribed but unencapsulated masses, that may present two types of macroscopic patterns: the solid type, of smooth-surfaced tissue with scant fluid; and the parenchymal, intraductal pattern, with fluid-filled spaces [18]. The two patterns can be combined in the same lesion, or one of them can predominate over the other. The cut surface is solid, diffusely white or grey-white and homogeneous [9,37,38]. Areas containing gelatinous material may be found, disposed as cleft-like spaces created by the enlarged ducts [21,37] (Figure 1). Although necrosis or ulceration are rare [17], they can be found in long lasting situations or whenever the reduction of the mammary gland swelling was attempted by progestin administration.

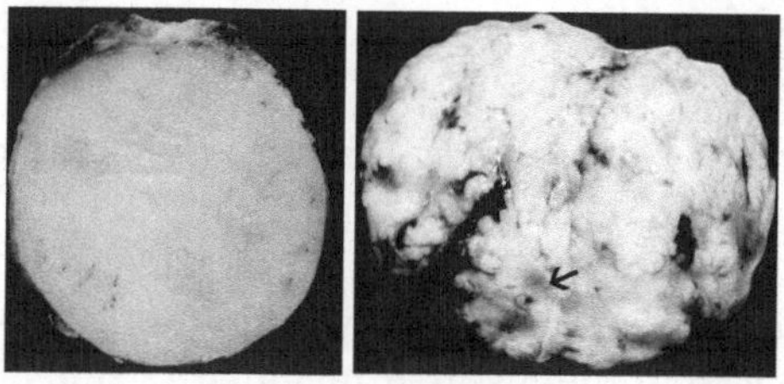

Figure 1. Gross appearance of feline mammary fibroepithelial hyperplasia lesions. On the left, the cut surface of a formalin-fixed lesion showing a solid pattern. On the right, the cut surface of a fresh lesion showing several cleft-like areas (arrow), typical of the intraductal pattern.

Microscopically, the two patterns are similar [18]: the diseased mammary gland is characterized by the proliferation of glandular fibroepithelial elements. The lesions correspond to well-demarcated, non-encapsulated growths within the mammary gland [17,31], with the ducts forming pseudo-acinar or cystic structures, encircled by a loose, myxoid stroma [21]. Although the proportions of epithelial and connective tissue are variable with the lesion and distinct from the one found in the normal gland, the branched ducts and stroma retains its organization in lobular-like units. The branching ductal structures are lined by several layers of epithelial cells and surrounded by markedly proliferating and oedematous connective tissue. Loose periductal connective tissue, that gives higher prominence to the mammary stroma, is loose-textured and merged in the periphery to the more dense collagenous tissue that separates the mammary lobules [9,17,31,37,38]. Mitotic figures are commonly found both in the epithelium and the stroma [17,31], and apocrine differentiation is frequently found within the epithelial component. Further, it is often observed that the cells in the intralobular stroma lack polarity and show indistinct borders [17], and also some degree of cytological atypia, which is reactive [21]. Thereby, a falsely malignant appearance is created, which could be patent in the results for a fine needle aspiration biopsy. An inflammatory infiltrate is seldom found, and when present it is mostly of the lymphoplasmocitary type [21].

5. Clinical presentation

Usually, the main complaint for FEH is the existence of excessive mammary enlargement that evolved rapidly. This in fact characterises the disease.

Feline mammary glands thickness is minimal in cycling females, and also it does not change much until close to parturition [28]. Consequently, for most cases an increase of the volume of the mammary glands, either isolated or multiple, in otherwise clinically healthy animals, draws the attention of the cat owner. Time since the beginning of the mammary enlargement till the animal presentation seems to vary with the form of the FEH. It tends to be shorter in cases of more notorious swelling of multiple glands and may be longer in cases of solitary and smaller lesions.

The major clinical sign is the swollen, firm mammary gland tissue, that can be detected in as multiple, bilateral enlargement of the mammary chains, or develop as a solitary, unique lesion that may develop from any of the mammary glands (Figure 2). The size of the enlarged glands is quite variable, ranging from 1.5 to 18 cm [21]. In our experience, when multiple lesions develop, asymmetrical lesions are more frequently found in non-pregnant females, while females being pregnant tend to develop more homogeneous swellings of the mammary glands (Figure 2).

At the visual inspection, the skin covering the diseased mammary glands may be tense and erythematous, in particular in larger lesions. The nipples can be difficult to find due to the size of the gland. At palpation, the lesions are presented as diffuse, firm and consistent masses, or in some cases they present a soft and more gelatinous, floating consistency. If notorious swelling develops, the diseased mammary glands may become pendulous. In uncomplicated situations and unless the masses are too swollen, the lesions are not painful, although some distress may be elicit during mammary manipulation during the clinical examination. Further, when severe swelling of the mammary glands developed, locomotory problems may arise that may induce some distress with movement or reluctance to walk and a reduction of appetite. Less severe lesions usually evolve in the absence of an inflammatory reaction.

Whatever the dimensions of the mammary glands, when FEH develops in pregnant females, no milk is produced in the diseased glands [23]. Consequently, after parturition, kittens are unable to nurse satisfactorily and usually the owners refer to litter vocalisation, restless and fading, with offspring death over a short-time period in postpartum.

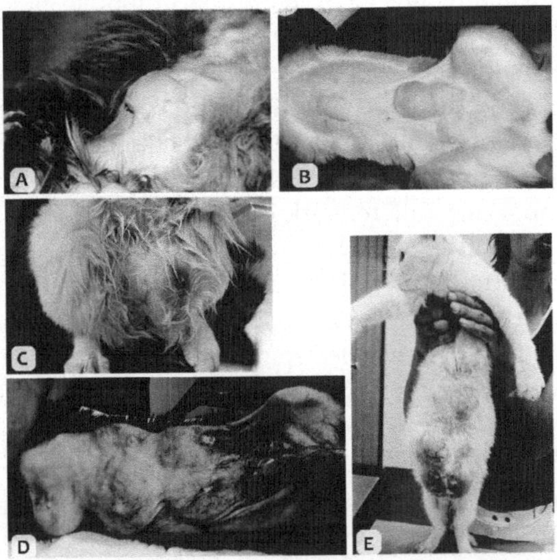

Figure 2. Diverse aspects of feline mammary fibroepithelial hyperplasia. A – A solitary lesion in a female cat submitted to megestrol acetate treatment. B - Multiple lesions showing asymmetric distribution of the diseased mammary glands, which also presented different dimensions, in a young spontaneous-ovulatory queen. C – In larger lesions, the skin around the nipple may be stretched, moist and violet, due to excessive grooming. D – FEH complicated with mastitis and ulceration in a female at post-partum day 6. E – FEH in a peri-partum young female that also showed skin erosion around the nipples of the caudal mammae.

In some severe or prolonged situations, the primary FEH may co-exist with mastitis or ulceration (Figure 2). In our clinic, mastitis is more frequently found in lactating females suffering from FEH. However, ulceration may develop secondary to perfusion problems derived from skin overstretching, with local ischemia, leading to abscessation, or also due to excessive grooming. Ulceration predisposes the diseased gland to mastitis or abscessation and subsequently to systemic illness [10-12]. In such situations, depending on the severity of the process, the skin may be wet, exudative, haemorrhagic and abnormal glandular discharge, with necrotic debris or purulent. Involvement of the regional lymph nodes is possible [10]. Then, the animal may be presented to consultation with fever, lethargy, anorexia, pale mucous membranes and dehydration.

Little information is available on the haematological and blood biochemistry changes in animals suffering from FEH. Nevertheless, in animals suffering from non-complicated mammary fibroepithelial hyperplasia, most parameters analysed (blood haematology and biochemistry) were within the normal range values for the species [11,14]. In animals with FEH co-existing with mastitis and ulceration, it can be found anaemia [10,39], normal to increase packed-cell volume [12,13,39] and the leukocyte count near the maximum normal limit or increased [10,12,39]. All these changes have been associated to inflammation and/or sequestration of fluid within the distended mammary tissue or to patient dehydration.

On what concerns the blood biochemistry, for most cases the values for blood urea and creatinine, or for the hepatic enzymes (such as the alkaline phosphatase, the alanine aminotransferase and the aspartate aminotransferase) were within the normal limits for cats [11-13], or slightly decreased [10].

6. Diagnostic evaluation

6.1. Reaching a tentative diagnosis

Diagnosis of feline mammary fibroepithelial hyperplasia is always a clinical issue, and should be based on the symptoms, the patient signalment and on history [39,40]. Differential diagnoses should include the mammary tumours (adenocarcinoma or carcinoma, mammary adenoma, or mammary sarcoma) and the mammary fibroepithelial hyperplasia.

Usually it is not difficult to establish a diagnosis when multiple glands are enlarged. An important criterion is the rapid onset of the mammary swelling, independently of the size of the swollen mammary gland. Also the age of the female may be suggestive of FEH, as it is more frequently found in young females. The sex of the animal should not be an exclusion criterion, as FEH also develop in males submitted to hormonal treatment for urine spraying or skin conditions. Neither it should be the reproductive status of the cat, as FEH can develop in neutered cats with pyoderma or miliary dermatitis following hormonal treatment with progestins. Moreover, a rapid enlargement of the mammary chains in a early or mid-pregnant females should lead to the suspicion of FEH, as the mammary glands shows little development until near parturition in cats. Unless an excessive swelling of the mammary exits, FEH is painless.

Yet, when fibroepithelial lesions develop in a single mammary gland, distinguishing between hyperplasia and mammary tumour may become more challenging, particularly in mature or older animals. As in other FEH conditions, the lesion develops at a very rapid rate, is frequently painless and although firm it is also turgid with a regular oedematous texture at palpation. Although it should not be considered as a rule, frequently FEH solitary lesions reach larger volumes than those referred to feline mammary tumours [22], and are softener.

Discoloration of the skin underlying FEH lesions was once reported [41], but I was not able to confirm that association in my practice.

Occurrence of FEH indicates that the animal ovulated and endogenous progesterone is raised or that it was treated with progestins. Hence, the mammary fibroepithelial hyperplasia diagnosis may be further supported by determination of blood progesterone levels. However, one should be aware that progesterone levels may be low when the underlying cause are exogenous progestins, because nowadays progesterone analysis are quite specific and may not cross-label with the used progestin molecule. Thus, it is also of utmost importance to determine the existence of a recent progestin treatment.

6.2. Diagnostic endorsements

Biopsies are often referred as being the most acceptable form to confirm the diagnosis of mammary fibroepithelial hyperplasia. However, cytological differentiation between benign and malignant mammary lesions is difficult. The accuracy of cytological differentiation is low, and its specificity has not yet been attributable. Further, the cytological analysis should be interpreted together with the symptoms and the sudden onset of the clinical signs [11].

It should be remembered that mammary fibroepithelial hyperplasia lesions are highly proliferative [34,35] and that some degree of cytological atypia [21] are often described, which along with the described loss of cell polarity [17] and the occurrence of mitosis [17,31], can create a falsely malignant appearance that could biased the diagnosis. Consequently, if a histopathological diagnosis is wanted, an excisional biopsy is preferable to a fine needle aspiration, despite being more expensive.

Diagnosis of FEH in cytological specimens should meet the following criteria: Two different cells (one of uniform epithelial cells and one of spindle-shaped mesenchymal cells) should co-exist, and may display a moderate anisocytosis and anisokaryosis, with only minimal nuclear criteria of malignancy. A large amount of eosinophilic extracellular matrix is expectably found in close proximity to the cells (Mesher, cited in [11]).

Mammary ultrasonography may also be helpful on the diagnosis of feline mammary fibroepithelial hyperplasia. Furthermore it is a rapid and easily performed method for assessment of the mammary gland structure. Generally, the ultrasonographic mammary echogenicity is higher in FEH lesions when compared to normal and lactational feline mammary glands (Figure 3). On ultrasound images, FEH lesions present mainly as a well-circumscribed solid mass of granular, slightly hyperechoic texture, with regularly delimited margins. It is also common to found small cleft-like structures, appearing as irregular anechoic areas, without acoustic enhancement, and small hyperechoic foci scattered within the glands image, which are independent of the form of FEH (multiple or solitary form). The presence of clefts in mammary fibroepithelial lesions provided a more heterogeneous appearance to the ultrasound images. In our practice clefts are more frequently found in animals under progestin treatment. The ultrasound pattern is more homogeneous in solid lesions, whilst when the intraductal pattern dominates, anechoic areas corresponding to clefts of different shapes are found within the mammary gland parenchyma (Figure 4).

Radiology is of little interest in cases of FEH, as for most situations lateral abdominal surveys only shows the enlargement of the mammary glands, an intact body wall and sporadically homogeneous fluid opacity in the diseased mammary glands [10]. In comparison, ultrasonography can bring you more information through the assessment of the lesion echogenicity and pattern. However, when attempting to establish a differential diagnosis with mammary carcinoma, thoracic and abdominal radiographs are advised to screen for possible metastases and calcification.

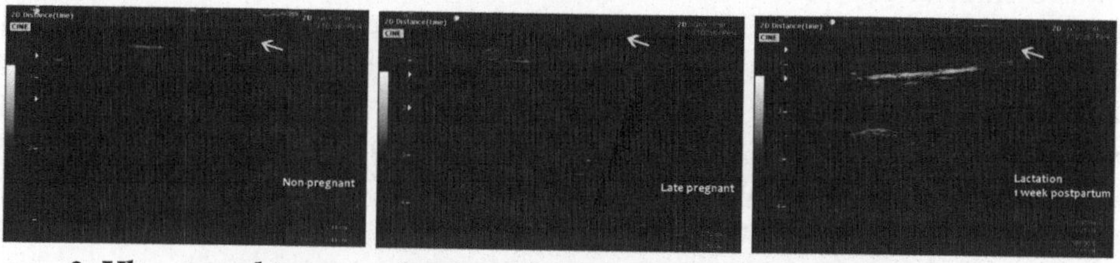

Figure 3. Ultrasound images of normal feline mammary gland in non-pregnant, late pregnant and lactating females (from left to right).

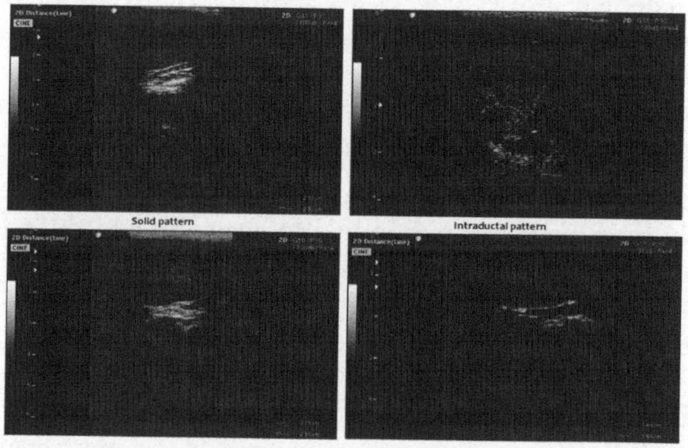

Figure 4. Ultrasound images of feline mammary fibroepithelial hyperplasia lesions. On the left, images from a solid pattern lesion. On the right, images from lesions presenting cleft-like anechoic areas, characteristics of the intraductal pattern.

Finally, confirmation of the tentative diagnosis can also be achieved through the response to Aglepristone treatment. Aglepristone as an antiprogesterone drug can elicit a positive response with a reduction of the mammary swelling and improvement of the clinical condition, which can be obtained around day 3 post-administration (for the doses and schedule, please see next section).

7. Therapeutic approaches

In most animals diagnosed with FEH, the extent of the swelling of the mammary glands and the possibility of necrosis and infection warrant treatment, though this is generally considered as a benign disturbance [23]. Even so, seldom sporadic recovery is observed [6], and when described it usually take several weeks to months.

The feline mammary fibroepithelial hyperplasia being a progesterone-associated disturbance, the therapeutic approach should focus on the removal of the progesterone influences in order to revert the symptoms. Thus, discontinuing of any ongoing hormone therapy is mandatory.

Available approaches should be discussed with the cat owner, including a prevision of the costs for the treatment, the time to full recovery and the possibility for the occurrence of a relapse. For most FEH situations 21-24 days may be needed to fully reversion of the mammary gland enlargement, but it may vary with the selected therapeutic approach.

In addition to the treatment directed to feline mammary fibroepithelial hyperplasia, situations complicated with mastitis and skin ulceration or abscessation or systemic illness, additional. treatment targeting the recovery of the inflammatory condition and the stabilization of the patient may be needed. Adequate broad-spectrum antimicrobial treatment (with Amoxicillin-Clavulanic acid or Cephradine for example), or fluid replacement may be needed. Also, when pain or discomfort exists, short-time treatment with nonsteroidal anti-inflammatory drugs (such as Meloxicam, Ketoprofen or Carprofen) may be used to alleviate the symptoms.

7.1. Surgical approaches

Until the late 90´s decade, ovariectomy or ovariohysterectomy were considered the most suitable treatments [19]. The lateral surgical approach was preferable to the ventral to avoid the trauma of the mammary tissue. Excision of the ovaries usually leads to regression of the mammary tissue within three to four weeks, but in some situations regression was not achieved [11,23].

Mastectomy is discouraged as a first approach to the feline mammary fibroepithelial hyperplasia. Only in animals not responding to spaying or to the medical treatment, partial or total mastectomy may be considered, but the surgery is difficult to perform because of the extensiveness of the mammary glands. A radical mastectomy often leads to complications and is only to be recommended when other options have failed.

7.2. Medical approaches

Nowadays, medical therapeutic approaches are available in most countries. Economic constraints may influence the drug of choice, and this may influence the recovery time. Also, when predicting the recovery time, one should be aware that FEH secondary to exogenous progestin would take longer to regress if antiprogesterone drugs are not selected.

Several studies demonstrated that the progesterone receptor blocker Aglepristone (Alizine®, Virbac, France) can successfully revert FEH [8,11,13,19,23]. Aglepristone is a molecule that competitively binds to the progesterone receptor without activating the hormone response cascade in target tissues. This drug binds to with a 9-fold affinity to progesterone receptor, and according to the manufacturer its residence time in the organism is of 6 days, if administered once in the dose of 20mg/kg or twice at 10mg/kg [23]. Although not licenced to be used in cats, this drug is commonly used to induce abortion or to treat pyometra in this species. By consequence, its application in cats is under the veterinarian responsibility.

Before starting the treatment with Aglepristone it is important to exclude pregnancy, as this drug may elicit abortion of a premature birth. When FEH develops in pregnant females it is mandatory that the therapeutic approaches are discussed with the cat owner in detail, and is important to mention that despite the mammary enlargement, the diseased glands will not produce milk and also that the kittens attempts to nurse may predispose to complications such as mastitis and ulceration, which will worsen the evolution of the primary condition.

Several therapeutic schedules have been described in the literature for Aglepristone in FEH (Table 1). Personally, I prefer to inject 10mg/kg of Aglepristone (Alizine®) on days 1 and 3, subcutaneously (SC), and to re-evaluate the situation a week later. If necessary, a second administration is performed following the same schedule. Rarely (only one situation in 25 cases treated with Alisine®) I needed to perform a third administration (again two doses 48h apart), in a female that was submitted to oral progestin treatment that started during estrus. Reduction of the mammary volume, in particular the mammary thickness, is the major parameter for assessment of the response to treatment. Mammary thickness can be assessed by ultrasonography. By using this schedule, it can be observed a slight reduction in the thickness of the disease mammary glands between days 1 and 3, which is predictive of the expected length of the treatment. For most cases, FEH recovery was obtained in 3 to 4 weeks, with only one situation (the one above mentioned) taking 6 weeks to obtain full regression of the mammary condition.

Varying with the reports, the a mean of 4 to 5 treatments (Table 1) are needed to recover from FEH [23,42], and full recovery was obtained in varying periods that last for 3 to 11 weeks [23].

Occasionally, short-term skin irritation at the site of injection has been reported [23], but it seldom originates a problem.

Table 1. Administration regimens proposed for Aglepristone (Alizine®, Virbac, France) treatments in feline mammary fibroepithelial hyperplasia.

Alizine® doses	Treatment schedule	References
0,33ml/kg/d corresponding to 10mg/kg/d	2 doses, 24h apart; Repeat at week intervals to full recovery	[13]
	4 to 5 consecutive days	[19]
	4 to 5 consecutive days and again on day 7	[8]
	On days 1, 2, 7, 14 and 21	[42]
	2 doses, 24h apart, for 4 consecutive weeks	[23]
0,66ml/kg/d corresponding to 20mg/kg/d	Once a week, for 4 consecutive weeks	
0,33ml/kg/d corresponding to 10mg/kg/d	On days 1, 2 and 7	[40]
0,5ml/kg/d corresponding to 15mg/kg/day		

In some case descriptions, dopamine agonists such as Cabergoline and Bromocriptine were also used for FEH treatment [40]. Though these products were not licenced for cats in some countries, they are commonly used in the feline practice. Vomiting or anorexia are described as side effects in a small proportion of cases, as well as a slight depression of the blood pressure, although these symptoms tend to disappear with continued treatment. Nonetheless, its usefulness in the treatment of feline mammary fibroepithelial hyperplasia remain uncertain, as prolactin has not been described as one of the players in FEH pathogenesis and FEH lesions are negative to prolactin [43]. Nevertheless, such drugs may be helpful when it is need to discontinue the queen lactation, in cases where FEH develops in lactating females.

Cabergoline (Galastop®, Ceva Santé Animale, France) is a dopaminergic agonist that produces a selective and long-lasting inhibitory effect on prolactin secretion, which in turn may be helpful to supress lactation. In dogs and cats it also induces luteolysis, and consequently it may induces abortion. Cabergoline is used for interrupt lactation at a dose of 5μg/kg body weight, *per os* (PO), once daily for 5-7 consecutive days depending on the severity of the situation. It is also used for mastitis treatment. Its use was described in association with castration in a tomcat [11], or in association with aglepristone in an assumed pregnant young queen [44].

Bromocriptine (Parlodel® is the most frequently used pharmacological presentation) is used in the veterinary practice less often than Cabergoline, as it was found to induce abnormal behavioural effects, such as limb flicks, head/body shakes, and hallucinatory-like behaviour as well as excessive grooming [45]. This drug can be used at the dose of 0.25mg/cat/day, PO, for 5 to 7 days. Its use on FEH situations enrols the same concerns as for Cabergoline.

8. Prognosis

Generally, the prognosis for uncomplicated feline mammary fibroepithelial hyperplasia is good. The co-existence of mastitis or ulceration may induce some concern, particularly when the situation was left untreated for a long period. In rare situations, abscess formation and systemic illness worsen the prognosis.

Spontaneous regression of the enlarged mammary glands after removal of the progesterone influences may occur, but it may take up to 11 months. Nevertheless, ovariohysterectomy or withdrawal of the progestin treatment does not always result in regression of the masses. With the available progesterone antagonist, medical treatment of the condition has improved, and regression of the mammary swelling is usually obtained within a 4-8 weeks interval. It is possible that the co-existing mammary abscesses may require the surgical drainage of the abscess content, in a way to hasten the FEH regression [10].

Recurrence of the disease is controversial. Some studies refer that it is rarely observed [11]. However, in the absence of neutering, several reports of FEH in females describe the recurrence of the condition at a variable timing after the initial treatment [6,23,31]. Consequently, recurrence of the mammary lesions is important concern particularly in females that can maintain their full reproductive activity.

Thus, when debating the prognosis with the cat owner, it is important to discuss also the measures need for avoiding the recurrence of FEH. If a progestin administration for contraception was the causative agent it should be advised the cat spaying. This should also be advised whenever the female is not intended for breeding. In cases where the surgery for neutering is decided it can be performed later, when mammary enlargement regressed, making the procedure easier for the surgeon and less traumatic for the cat, avoiding undesirable trauma of the enlarged mammary glands during surgery. If progestin was used as treatment for skin disorders, alternative therapeutics should be found.

9. Concluding remarks

FEH is a progesterone-associated disease that is characterized by a very rapid swelling of mammary gland, which onset is usually within 2 to 4 weeks from the occurrence of an estrus or the administration of a progestin treatment. Occasionally, this primary lesion can be complicated with mastitis, ulceration or abscessation of the diseased mammary glands. Diagnosis of feline mammary fibroepithelial hyperplasia is exclusively a clinical issue, though some complementary methods of diagnosis may be helpful aids to confirm the diagnosis.

Treatment of feline mammary fibroepithelial hyperplasia has undergone major changes in the past three decades, and considerable improvement of cat welfare was achieved with the introduction of successful medical treatment. Nowadays, antiprogesterone drugs are available that ease the therapeutics and hastens a favourable outcome. With these drugs, the treatment targets the major causal mechanism, interrupting the progesterone-mediated pathways of mammary development and growth. Antiprogesterone molecules are now in the first line treatments for FEH, allowing to avoid massive mastectomy, a very aggressive approach to the cat. However, relapses are possible, and most frequently ovariectomy or ovariohysterectomy are advised to avoid recurrence of the problem.

Nevertheless, new studies on molecular pathways involved in the disease might strengthen additional interplaying factors of interest to design additional therapeutic approaches, as well as to highlight the factors underlying the relapses described in the literature in order to improve the medical treatment and the animal welfare.

References

1. Murphy S. 2009. Mammary tumours in cats – causes and practical management. Conference proceedings of the European Society of Feline Medicine - ESFM Feline Symposium, 1st April 2009, Birmingham, UK: 11-15.
2. Giménez F, Hecht S, Craig LE, Legendre AM. 2010. Early detection, aggressive therapy: optimizing the management of feline mammary masses. J Feline Med Surg. 12(3): 214-24.
3. Johnson C. 1994. Diseases of the mammary glands. In: Sherding R. (Ed). The Cat: Diseases and Clinical Management. 2nd Ed. Churchill Livingstone, New York: 1874-5.
4. Johnston S, Root Kustritz M, Olson P. 2001. Disorders of the mammary gland of the Queen. In: Canine and Feline Theriogenology. W.B. Saunders Comp, Philadelphia: 474-85.
5. Hayden D, Johnston S, Kiang D, Johnson K, Barnes D. 1981. Feline mammary hypertrophy/fibroadenoma complex: clinical and hormonal aspects. Am J Vet Res. 42(10): 1699-703.
6. Loretti A, Ilha M, Breitsameter I, Faraco C. 2004. Clinical and pathological study of feline mammary fibroadenomatous changes associated with depot medroxyprogesterone acetate therapy. Arq Bras Med Vet Zootec. 56(2): 270-4.
7. Loretti A, Ilha M, Ordás J, de las Mulas JM. 2005. Clinical, pathological and immunohistochemical study of feline mammary fibroepithelial hyperplasia following a single injection of depot medroxyprogesterone acetate. J Feline Med Surg. 7(1): 43-52.

8. Sontas B, Turna O, Ucmak M, Ekici H. 2008. What is your diagnosis? Feline mammary fibroepithelial hyperplasia. J Small Anim Pract. 49(10): 545-7.

9. Rutteman G, Withrow S, EG M. 2001. Tumours of the mammary gland. In: Withrow S. and MacEwen E. (Ed). Small Animal Clinical Oncology. W.B. Saunders Comp, Philadelphia: 455-77.

10. Burstyn U. 2010. Management of mastitis and abscessation of mammary glands secondary to fibroadenomatous hyperplasia in a primiparturient cat. J Am Vet Med Assoc. 236(3): 326-9.

11. Leidinger E, Hooijberg E, Sick K, Reinelt B, Kirtz G. 2011. Fibroepithelial hyperplasia in an entire male cat: cytologic and histopathological features. Tierarztl Prax Ausg K Kleintiere Heimtiere 39(3): 198-202.

12. Jelinek F, Barton R, Posekana J, Hasonova L. 2007. Gynaecomastia in a tom-cat caused by cyproterone acetate: a case report. Veterinarni Medicina. 52: 521–525.

13. Jurka P., Max A. 2009. Treatment of fibroadenomatosis in 14 cats with aglepristone – changes in blood parameters and follow-up. Vet Rec165: 657-660

14. MacDougall L. 2003. Mammary fibroadenomatous hyperplasia in a young cat attributed to treatment with megestrol acetate. Can Vet J. 44(3): 227-9.

15. Gudermuth DF, Newton L, Daels P, Concannon P. 1997. Incidence of spontaneous ovulation in young, group-housed cats based on serum and fecal concentrations of progesterone. J Reprod Fertil Suppl 51:177–184.

16. Griffin B. 2001. Prolific cats: the estrous cycle. Compend. contin. educ. pract. vet. 23 (12): 1049-1057.

17. Allen HL. 1973. Feline Mammary Hypertrophy. Vet Pathol. 10: 501-508.

18. Hayden DW, Barnes DM, Johnson KH. 1989. Morphologic changes in the mammary gland of megestrol acetate-treated and untreated cats: a retrospective study. Vet Pathol. 26(2): 104-13.

19. Wehrend A, Hospes R, Gruber AD. 2001. Treatment of feline mammary fibroadenomatous hyperplasia with a progesterone-antagonist. Vet Rec. 148(11): 346-7.

20. Enginler SÖ, Şenünver A. 2011. The Effects of Progesterone Hormone Applications Used for Suppression of Estrus on Mammary Glands in Queens. Kafkas Üniversitesi Veteriner Fakültesi Dergisi 17 (2): 277-284.

21. Seixas Travassos MA. 2006. [Feline mammary lesions: a contribute to its biopathological characterization] In portuguese. PhD thesis, Univ. de Trás-os-Montes e Alto Douro. Pp 194.

22. Sorenmo KU. 2011. Mammary gland tumors in cats: Risk factors, clinical presentation, treatments and outcome. Proceedings of the 36th World Small Animal Veterinary Congress, Jeju (Korea), 14 to 17 October. OC-I10: 764–767 (www.ivis.org/proceedings/wsava/2011/189.pdf). Accessed on the 17th September 2012.

23. Görlinger S, Kooistra HS, van den Broek A, Okkens AC. 2002 Treatment of fibro -adenomatous hyperplasia in cats with aglépristone. J Vet Intern Med. 16: 710–713

24. Pukay BP, Stevenson DA. 1983. Mammary hypertrophy in an ovariohysterectomized cat. Can Vet J. 24(5): 143-4.
25. Conneely OM, Mulac-Jericevic B, Lydon JP. 2003. Progesterone-dependent regulation of female reproductive activity by two distinct progesterone receptor isoforms. Steroids. 68(10-13): 771-8.
26. Robinson GW, Hennighausen L, Johnson PF. 2000. Side-branching in the mammary gland: the progesterone-Wnt connection. Genes Dev. 14(8): 889-94.
27. Brisken C, O'Malley B. 2010. Hormone action in the mammary gland. Cold Spring Harb Perspect Biol. 2(12): a003178. Pp.15
28. Payan-Carreira R, Martins-Bessa A. 2008. Ultrasonographic assessment of the feline mammary gland. J Feline Med Surg. 10(5): 466-71.
29. Mol JA, Gracanin A, de Gier J, Rao N, Schaefers-Okkens A, Rutteman G, Kooistra H. 2012. Molecular genetics and biology of progesterone signaling in mammary neoplasia. Proceedings of the joint meeting of the 7th International Symposium on Canine and Feline Reproduction and the 15th Congress of the European Veterinary Society for Small Animal Reproduction: 107-108 (www.ivis.org/proceedings/iscfr/2012/107.pdf?LA=1). Accessed on the 22th September 2012.
30. Millanta F, Calandrella M, Bari G, Niccolini M, Vannozzi I, Poli A. 2005. Comparison of steroid receptor expression in normal, dysplastic, and neoplastic canine and feline mammary tissues. Res Vet Sci. 79(3): 225-32.
31. Martín de las Mulas J, Millán Y, Bautista MJ, Pérez J, Carrasco L. 2000. Oestrogen and progesterone receptors in feline fibroadenomatous change: an immunohistochemical study. Res Vet Sci. 68(1): 15-21.
32. Mol JA, van Garderen E, Rutteman GR, Rijnberk A. 1996. New insights in the molecular mechanism of progestin-induced proliferation of mammary epithelium: induction of the local biosynthesis of growth hormone (GH) in the mammary glands of dogs, cats and humans. J Steroid Biochem Mol Biol. 57(1-2): 67-71.
33. Ordás J, Millán Y, de los Monteros AE, Reymundo C, de las Mulas JM. 2004. Immunohistochemical expression of progesterone receptors, growth hormone and insulin growth factor-I in feline fibroadenomatous change. Res Vet Sci. 76(3): 227-33.
34. Millanta F, Lazzeri G, Mazzei M, Vannozzi I, Poli A. 2002. MIB-1 labeling index in feline dysplastic and neoplastic mammary lesions and its relationship with postsurgical prognosis. Vet Pathol. 39(1): 120-6.
35. Dias Pereira P, Carvalheira J, Gärtner F. 2004. Cell proliferation in feline normal, hyperplastic and neoplastic mammary tissue--an immunohistochemical study. Vet J. 168(2): 180-5.
36. Schmidt PM, Chakraborty PK, Wildt DE. 1983. Ovarian activity, circulating hormones and sexual behavior in the cat. II. Relationships during pregnancy, parturition, lactation and the postpartum estrus. Biol Reprod. 28(3): 657-71.
37. Moulton J. 1990. Mammary tumors of the cat. In: Moulton J. (Ed.) Tumours in Domestic Animals. 3rd Ed. University of California Press, Berkeley. p. 547-8.

38. Ginn P, Mansell J, Rakich P. 2007. Tumours of the mammary gland. In: Maxie M. (Ed). Jubb, Kennedy, and Palmer's Pathology of Domestic Animals. Saunders, Elsevier, New York. p. 777-80.

39. Buriticá EF, Echeverry DF, Lozada AF. 2010 Hiperplasia fibroepitelial mamaria felina: reporte de un caso. Rev Ces Med Vet Zootec. 5 (1):70-76.

40. Little S. 2011. Feline reproduction: common problems you will see in practice. Proceedings of the 63rd Canadian Veterinary Medical Association Convention. Halifax, Nova Scotia, Canada, the 6 to 9 July 2011. Pp. 4. (http://canadianveterinarians.net/SpeakerNotes2011/HTML/companion/companion_little_06-Feline_Reproduction.html). Accessed on the 18th September 2012.

41. Chisholm H. 1993. Massive mammary enlargement in a cat. Can Vet J. 34(5): 315.

42. Vitásek R, Dendisová H. 2006. Treatment of Feline Mammary Fibroepithelial Hyperplasia Following a Single Injection of Proligestone. Acta Vet. Brno 75: 295-297.

43. Trummel DK. 2007. Expression of Prolactin in Feline Mammary Adenomas and Adenocarcinomas. BSc Thesis in Animal Sciences. Oregon State Univ.

44. Uçmak M, Enginler SÖ, Gündüz MG, Kirşan I, Sönmez K. 2011. Treatment of Feline Mammary Fibroepithelial Hyperplasia with the Combination of Aglepristone and Cabergoline. İstanbul Üniversitesi Veteriner Fakültesi Dergisi 37 (1): 69-73.

45. Gonzalez-Lima F, Velez D, Blanco R. 1988. Antagonism of behavioral effects of bromocriptine by prolactin in female cats. Behav Neural Biol. 49(1): 74-82.

Chapter 9

Diseases of Thyroid in Animals and Their Management

1. Introduction

Disorders of the thyroid gland are well known in companion animals but less so in livestock. In livestock, nutritional iodine deficiencies have been of greater importance than thyroid-gland diseases, particularly in the iodine-deficient areas. Thyroid hormones have many functions in the body and, in general, regulate growth, differentiation, and the metabolism of lipids, proteins and carbohydrates. The thyroid gland of animals is a bilobed structure that overlays the trachea at a point just below the larynx. Anatomical variations of the gland are quite marked between species and, to some extent, within a given species. The isthmus connecting the two lobes of the thyroid is the region that varies most markedly between species. Humans and the pig have a large discrete isthmus that forms a pyramidal lobe connecting the two lateral lobes. The cow has a fairly wide band of glandular tissue that forms the connecting isthmus. In the horse, sheep, goat, cat, and dog, the isthmus is a narrow remnant of tissue and may be nonexistent. The size of the gland relative to body weight is extremely small in all animals, approximating 0.20% of body weight. Accessory or extrathyroidal tissue is quite commonly seen in the dog, particularly near the thoracic inlet, though it may be found anywhere along the esophagus. This tissue is fully functional physiologically, synthesizes hormone, and can be located by its uptake of radionuclides. The thyroid gland is a highly vascularized tissue with a large blood flow. The functional unit of the thyroid gland is the thyroid follicle, a spherical structure composed of an outer monolayer of follicular cells surrounding an inner core of colloid, the thyroglobulin-hormone complex, which is the storage reservoir of thyroid hormone. The colloid stored in the lumen is a clear, viscous fluid. The individual follicular cells vary from 5 to 10/zm in height and the entire follicle may vary from 25 to 250/zm in diameter. The size of the follicles and the height of their cells vary according to the functional state of the gland. The cells may vary from an inactive squamous cell to the highly active, tall columnar cell. Interspersed between the follicles are the thyroid C cells, the source of calcitonin, the hypocalcemic hormone associated with calcium metabolism. A third type of hormonal tissue, the parathyroid, is embedded within the thyroid or located in close proximity. The parathyroids are the source of parathormone, the hypercalcemic hormone.

Thyroid hormones (T_4, T_3, and rT_3) immediately on entering the circulation are bound to transport proteins, mainly to thyroxine binding globulin (TBG) and in lesser amounts to thyroxine binding prealbumin (TBPA) and to albumin. There is a wide spectrum of species variation in hormone binding by serum proteins. TBG is the major binding protein for hormone, but not all species have TBG however, TBPA is present in all species. In the cat, rabbit, rat, mouse, Guinea pig, pigeon, or chicken, TBG is absent and most of the hormone is transported by albumin. In these species without TBG, albumin transports 50-80% of the hormones. T_3 (and likely rT_3) appears to bind to these transport proteins in parallel with T_4 binding.

2. Disorders of thyroid function

2.1. Hypothyroidism

This disorder is most common in dogs but also develops rarely in other species, including cats, horses, and other large domestic animals. Hypothyroidism is most common in dogs 4-10 yr old. It usually affects mid- to large-size breeds and is rare in toy and miniature breeds. Breeds reported to be predisposed include the Golden Retriever, Doberman Pinscher, Irish Setter, Miniature Schnauzer, Dachshund, Cocker Spaniel, and Airedale Terrier. There does not appear to be a sex predilection, but spayed females appear to have a higher risk of developing hypothyroidism than intact females. Clinical Hypothyroidism is usually the result of primary diseases of the thyroid gland, especially idiopathic follicular atrophy also termed "follicular collapse" and lymphocytic thyroiditis. In the adult dog, follicular atrophy is probably the most common cause of hypothyroidism. Hypothyroidism may be secondary to a pituitary insufficiency that prevents the release of either TSH or TRH. Other rare forms of hypothyroidism in dogs include neoplastic destruction of thyroid tissue and congenital (or juvenile-onset) hypothyroidism. Hypothyroidism is an extremely rare disorder in adult cats, iatrogenic hypothyroidism is the most common form congenital or juvenile-onset hypothyroidism does also occur. Hypothyroidism appears to be very rare in adult horses. In foals, congenital hypothyroidism may develop when pregnant mares graze plants that contain goitrogens, nitrate or are fed diets either deficient in or containing excessive amounts of iodine.

Clinical Findings: A deficiency of thyroid hormone affects the function of all organ systems; as a result, clinical signs are diffuse, variable, often nonspecific, and rarely pathognomonic. Slowing of cellular metabolism, results in development of mental dullness, lethargy, intolerance of exercise, and weight gain without a corresponding increase in appetite. Mild to marked obesity develops in some dogs. Difficulty in maintaining body temperature may lead to frank hypothermia; the classic hypothyroid dog is a heat-seeker. Alterations in the skin and coat are common. Dryness, excessive shedding, and retarded regrowth of hair are usually the earliest dermatologic changes. Nonpruritic hair thinning or alopecia (usually bilaterally symmetric) that may involve the ventral and lateral trunk, the caudal surfaces of the thighs, dorsum of the tail, ventral neck, and the dorsum of the nose occurs in about two-thirds of dogs with hypothyroidism. Alopecia, sometimes associated with hyperpigmentation, often starts over points of wear. Occasionally, secondary pyoderma (which may produce pruritus) is observed.

In moderate to severe cases, thickening of the skin occurs secondary to accumulation of glycosaminoglycans (mostly hyaluronic acid) in the dermis. In such cases, myxedema is most common on the forehead and face, resulting in a puffy appearance and thickened skin folds above the eyes. This puffiness, together with slight drooping of the upper eyelid, gives some dogs a "tragic" facial expression. These changes also have been described in the GI tract, heart, and skeletal muscles.

In intact dogs, hypothyroidism may cause various reproductive disturbances: in females, failure to cycle (anestrus) or sporadic cycling, infertility, abortion, or poor litter survival; and in males, lack of libido, testicular atrophy, hypospermia, or infertility. During the fetal period and in the first few months of postnatal life, thyroid hormones are crucial for growth and development of the skeleton and CNS. Therefore, in addition to the well-recognized signs of adult-onset hypothyroidism, disproportionate dwarfism and impaired mental development (cretinism) are prominent signs of congenital and juvenile-onset hypothyroidism. In primary congenital hypothyroidism, enlargement of the thyroid gland (goiter) also may be detected, depending on the cause of the hypothyroidism. Radiographic signs of epiphyseal dysgenesis (underdeveloped epiphyses throughout the long bones), shortened vertebral bodies, and delayed epiphyseal closure are common.

In dogs with congenital hypopituitarism there may be variable degrees of thyroidal, adrenocortical, and gonadal deficiency, but clinical signs are primarily related to growth hormone deficiency. Signs include proportionate dwarfism, loss of primary guard hairs with retention of the puppy coat, hyperpigmentation of the skin, and bilaterally symmetric alopecia of the trunk.

Clinical characteristics oh hypothyroidism in adult horses are poorly defined largely because of the difficulty of confirming the diagnosis and the pharmacological effect of exogenous thyroid hormone. Clinical abnormalities anecdotal attributed to hypothyroidism include exercise intolerance, infertility, weight gain, maldistribution of body fat, agalactia, anhidrosis, and laminitis among others. Congenital hypothyroid foals have a prolonged gestation but are born with a short silky hairs coat, soft pliable ears, difficulty in standing, lax joints and poorly ossified bones. The foals are referred to as dysmature. Characteristic musculoskeletal abnormalities include inferior (mandubular) prognathism, flexural deformities, ruptured common and lateral extensor tendons, and poorly ossified cubiodal bones.

Treatment: Thyroxine (T_4) is the thyroid hormone replacement compound of choice in dogs. With few exceptions, replacement therapy is necessary for the remainder of the dog's life; careful initial diagnosis and tailoring of treatment is essential. The reported replacement dosages for T_4 in dogs range from a total dose of 0.01-0.02 mg/lb (0.02-0.04 mg/kg), daily, given once or divided bid.

3. Hyperthyroidism

Among domestic animal species, disturbances of growth resulting from the production of excess thyroid hormones is most common in adult cats and often related to adenomas compared to hyperactive follicular cells. These neoplastic cells release both T_4 and T_3 at an uncontrolled rate resulting in the markedly elevated blood levels of both hormones. Cats with hyperthyroidism have elevated levels of total serum thyroxine and triiodothronine. Normal serum levels of T_4 in cats, as measure by radioimmunoassay, are approximately 1.5 to 4.5 μg/dl and serum T_3 levels are 60 to 100 ng/dl. In hyperthyroid cats the total levels of T_4 in the serum range from 5.0 to over 50 μg/dl and total levels of T_3 in the serum range from 100 to 1,000 ng/dl. Hyperthyroidism is associated with weight loss in spite of a normal or increased appetite and with restlessness and increased activity.

Dogs have a very efficient enteroheptic excretory mechanism for thyroid hormones that is difficult to overload, either from endogenous production by a tumor or by exogenous administration of thyroid hormones. Hence, thyroid tumors in the dog only occasionally secrete sufficient amount of thyroid hormone to overload the highly efficient enterohepatic excretory pathways for the thyroid hormones and produce clinical signs of hyperthyroidism. The clinical signs of hyperthyroidism in dogs with functional thyroid tumors include polyuria and polydipsia and weight loss, despite increased appetite and polyphagia, leading to muscle atrophy and weakness. The levels of T_3 and T_4 in the serum of dogs with clinical hyperthyroidism are only mildly elevated: 300-400ng/dl and 5-7 μg/dl, respectively. As compared to dogs, cats are very sensitive to phenols and phenol derivatives. They have a poor ability to conjugate phenolic compounds such as T_4 with glucuronic acid and to excrete the T_4-glucuronide into bile. In cats the capacity for conjugation of T_3 with sulfate is also limited and can easily be overloaded.

4. Goiter

Goiter is a clinical term for a non-neoplastic and non-inflamatory enlargement of the thyroid gland which develops in mammals, birds and submammalian vertebrate. The major pathogenic mechanism responsible for the development of thyroid hyperplasia include iodine-defeciant diets, goitrogenic compounds that interfere with hormone synthesis, dietary iodide-excess and genetic defects in the biosynthesis of thyroid hormone. All of these seemingly divergent factors result in deficient thyroxine and triiodothyronine synthesis and decreased blood levels of throid hormones. This is sensed by the hypothalamus and pitituary gland and lead to an increased secretion of TSH, which results in hypertrophy and hyperplasia of the follicular cells in the thyroid gland. The following subtypes of goiters are recognized: diffuse hyperplastic, colloid iodide-excess, multifocal hyperplastic, and congenital dyshormonogenetic.

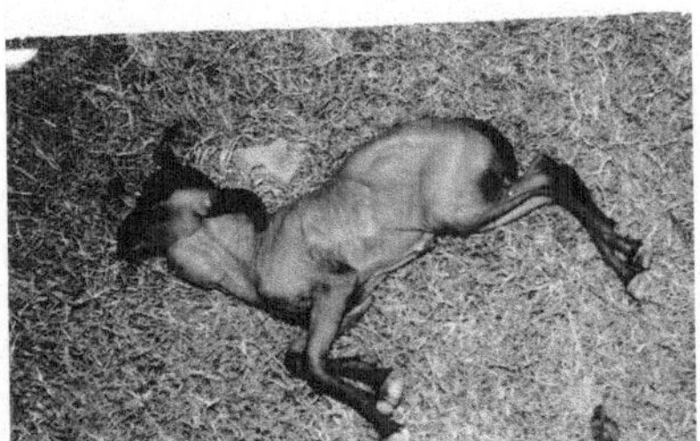

Figure 1. Goiter in a kid from Jammu region

Diffuse thyroid hyperplasia due to iodine deficiency was common in many goitrogenic areas in India before the widespread supplementation of iodized salt to animal diets. Although outbreaks of iodine-deficient goiter are now sporadic and fewer animals are affected, iodine deficiency is still responsible for most goiters seen in large domestic animals. Marginally iodine-deficient diets containing certain goitrogenic substances may result in severe thyroid hyperplasia and clinical evidence of goiter. Goitrogenic substance include thiouracil, propylthiouracil, sulfonamides, complex anions such as perchlorate (CLO4), perthecnetate(TcO4), perrhenate (ReO4) and tetrafluoroborate (TcO4). In addition, a number of plants from the genus *Brassica* contain thioglycosides which after digestion release thiocyanate and isothiocyante. A particularly potent thioglycoside, goitrin (L-5-vinyl-2 thiooxazolidone) from plants is excreted in milk. Young animals born to females on iodine-deficient diets are more likely to develop severe thyroid hyperplasia and have clinical signs of hypothyroidism including palpable enlargement of the thyroid gland. Iodine deficiency may be conditioned by other anti-thyroid compounds present in animal feed and in particular situations, these can be responsible for higher incidence of goiter. Hyperplastic goiter in ruminants is associated with prolonged low-level exposure to thiocyanates produced by the ruminal degradation of cyanogenic glucosides of plants such as white clover (*Trifolium)*, couch grass and linseed meal, and by degradation of glucosinolates of *Brassica* crops. *Leucaerne leucocephala* and other legumes of this genus are native or cultivated in many subtropical areas and contain the toxic amino acid mimosine.

Goiter in adult animals is usually of little significance and the general health of the animal is not impaired. However, goiter is of significance as a disease of the newborn, although the drastic losses of animals in endemic area are now controlled by the prophylactic use of iodized salt. Congenital hypothyroidism in domestic animals may be associated with iodine-deficient hyperplastic goiter, even though the dam shows no evidence of thyroid dysfunction. Gestation is often significantly prolonged, particularly for animals with large goiter, and there is increased incidence of dystocia with retention of fetal placenta. Foals affected with iodine-defecient goiter have moderately enlarged thyroids are waek at birth and frequently die within a few days after birth. Calves and kids with goiter are born partially or completely hairless and are either born dead or die soon after birth. Newborn goitrous pigs, goats and lambs frequently have myxedema and hair loss. The mortality rate is high in these species, with majority of offspring born dead or dying within a few hours of birth.

References

1. BelshawB. Eand RijnberkA1979Radioimmunoassay of plasma T_4 and T_3 in the diagnosis of primary hypothyroidism in dogs. J. Am. Anim. Hosp. Assoc. 15:17.
2. BroussardJ. DPetersonM. Eand FoxP. R1995Changes in clinical and laboratory findings in cats with hyperthyroidism from 1983 to 1993. J. Am. Vet. Med. Assoc. 206: 302.
3. CapenC. CBelshawB. Eand MartinS. L1975Endocrine diseases. In: Textbook of Veterinary Internal Medicine-Diseases of the dog and cat, section X, chapter 50, edited by S.J. Ettinger. Philadelphia, PA, W.B. Saunders Co., 1351
4. CarrascoN1993Iodide transport in the thyroid gland. Biochim. Biophys. Acta 1154: 65.
5. De VihlderJ. J. MVan VoorthuizenW. FVan DijkJ. E1978Hereditary congenital goiter with thyroglobulin deficiency in the breed of goats. Endocrinology 102: 1214.
6. FergusonD. C1994Update on diagnosis of canine hypothyrodism. Vet. Clin. North Am., Small Anim. Pract. 24: 515.
7. GerberHPeterHFergusonD. C1994Etiopathology of feline toxic nodular goiter. Vet. Clin. North Am., Small Anim. Pract. 24: 541.

8. GosselinS. JCapenC. Cand MartinS. L1981Biochemical and immunological investigation of hypothyroidism in dogs. Can.J.Comp.Med. 44: 158.
9. GosselinS. JCapenC. Cand MartinS. L1981Histopathologic and ultrastructural evaluation of thyroid lesions associated with hypothyroidism in dogs. Vet. Pathol. 18: 299.
10. GosselinS. JCapenC. Cand MartinS. L1981Induced lymphocytic thyroditis in dogs: Effect of intrathyroidal injection of thyroid autoantibodies. Am. J. Vet Res. 42: 1565
11. GosselinS. JCapenC. CKrakowkaS1981Lymphocytic Thyroiditis in dogs: induction with local graft-versus-host reaction. Am. J. Vet. Res. 42: 1856.
12. HogeW. RLundJ. Eand BlackmoreJ. C1974Response to thyrotropin as a diagnostic aid for canine hypothyroidism. J.Am. Vet. Med. Assoc. 10: 167.
13. HolzworthJTheranPCarpenterJ. L1980Hyperthyroidism in the cat: Ten cases. J. Am. Vet. Med. Assoc. 176: 345.
14. KamedaY1972The accessory thyroid gland of the dogs around the intrapericardial aorta. Arch. Histol. Jpn. 34: 375.
15. KapteinE. MHaysM. Tand FergusonD. C1994Thryoid hormone metabolism: A comparative evaluation. Vet. Clin. North Am., Small Anim. Prac. 24: 431.
16. MazzaferriE. L1996Radioiodine and other treatments and outcomes. In: Werner and Ingbar's the Thyroid: A Fundamental and Clinical Text, 7th edition, edited by L.E. Braverman and R.d.Utiger. Philadelphia, PA, J.b.Lipincott Co., 922
17. NachreinerR. Fand RefsalK. R1992Radioimmunoassay monitoring of thyroid hormone concentration in dogs on thyroid replacement therapy: 2,674 cases (1985-1987). J. Am. Vet. Med. Assoc. 201: 623.
18. PammenterMAlbrechtCLeibenbergW1978Afrinkander cattle congenital goiter: characteristic of its morphological and iodoprotein pattern. Endocrinology 102: 954.
19. PeterH. JGerberHStuderH1985Pathogenesis of heterogeneity in human multinodular goiter: a study on growth and function of thyroid tissue transplanted onto nude mice. J. Clin. Invest. 76: 1992.
20. PetersonM. E1984Feline hyperthyroidism. Vet. Clin. North Am., Small Anim. Prac. 14: 809.
21. RandJ. SLevineJand BestS. J1993Spontaneous adult-onset hypothyroidism in a cat. J.Vet.Intern.Med.7: 272.
22. RijnberkA1971Iodine Metabolism and thyroid disease in the dog. University of Utrecht, Utrecht, The Netherlands (thesis).
23. Scott-moncrieffJ. CNelsonR. Wand BrunerJ. M1998Comparison of serum concentrations of thyroid-stimulating hormone in healthy dogs, hypothyroid dogs, and euthyroid dogs with concurrent disease. J. Am. Vet. Med. Assoc. 212: 387.

Chapter 10

Crossregulation of the Thyroid Hormone and Corticosteroids in Amphibians and Fish: The Effects of Endocrine Disruption

1. Introduction

Thyroid hormones are involved in many physiological processes, during growth, development, behaviour, stress. Their actions are mediated by TH receptors (TR-alpha and TR-beta), which are members of the nuclear receptor (NR) superfamily and function as ligand-activated transcription factors. In amphibians, TR-alpha is expressed shortly after hatching and is maintained at a relatively constant level throughout tadpole life and metamorphosis. Then amphibian metamorphosis is dependent on thyroid hormone (TH) changes, which induces the suite of molecular and cellular changes that cause a tadpole to transform into a frog.

Hormones other than TH play important roles in amphibian metamorphosis, in part by modifying the production and actions of TH. Corticosteroids (CS), hormones produced by adrenocortical cells (interrenal glands in frogs and in fish), synergize with TH at target tissues to promote morphogenesis [1,2]. The production of CS changes with development, rising throughout metamorphosis and reaching a peak at metamorphic climax [2]. Like TH, CS actions are mediated by NRs encoded by two different genes: the glucocorticoid receptor (GR) and the mineralocorticoid receptor (MR).

In the current study we examine molecular and physiological mechanisms involved in TH and CS axes regulation. We investigate the synergy between TH and CS not only during amphibian metamorphosis, but also in fish. Indeed TH play important role in fish development. TH level is especially high in the eggs and larvae of several fish species, including the Japanese flounder (*Paralichthys olivaceus*), the zebrafish (*Danio rerio*) and the seabream (*Sparus aurata*) [3]. Darras *et al.* [4] showed that exogenous T3 increased TH levels in zebrafish embryos and accelerated development and hatching, and it seems that elevated T3 levels in culture medium regulates TR expression (for review see reference 4). Glucocorticoids are also key endocrine factors in teleost fishes, involved in metabolism, growth, reproduction [5], and GR can also regulate fish development. Hillegass *et al.* [6] showed that the embryonic zebrafish corticosteroids activate GR and modulate expression of matrix metalloproteinases during development. It seems that TH and CS can regulate each other, in a positive or negative way depending on molecular, cellular and physiologic context. This cross-regulation is important to amplify hormone signals, regulate hormone activity, and coordinate hormone action.

Due to their aqueous exposure, fish and amphibians can be used as indicators for ecotoxicological studies and for detection of endocrine disruptors (ED) *in vivo*. Endocrine disruption has become one of the major topics in environmental research, but also in public health since the ED is known to affect reproductive biology, metabolism, growth and development. The aquatic environment exposes developing embryos to all compounds present in water. After hatching, penetration of ED into aquatic organism is even easier, resulting in high bioavailability and bioaccumulation of chemicals. Amphibians (*Xenopus laevis*) and fish models (zebrafish and medaka (*Oryzias latipes*)) are species widely used for the development of new tools for ED detection and screening of chemicals in the environment. They were firstly used to study endocrine disruption of estrogenic and androgenic systems. But now, more and more studies involve chemicals in thyroid and corticosteroid disruption. Indeed, the thyroid function and corticosteroid axis are both targets for ED. Being given the involvement of both TH and CS axis in amphibian and fish development, these two species were largely used to study TH and CS disruption. The abundant knowledge about endocrinology and developmental biology in amphibian and fish, and the general scientific interest about TH and CS disruption provide evidence for using these animal models for the study of ED of these two endocrine systems [7]. For that reason, we propose to summarize the impact of endocrine disruption on TH and CS axes.

2. Thyroid hormone and corticosteroid endocrine systems: current knowledge

2.1. Thyroid hormone

Thyroid hormones (thyroxine T4 and tri-iodothyronine T3) play an important role in development, differentiation, and metabolism [8]. The lack of T3 in early human development results in growth disturbances and severe mental retardation, a disease called cretinism. TH action is also primary for developmental changes in the nervous system that occur during amphibian metamorphosis. Later in life, T3 plays an important role in metabolic balance [9]. T3 action is mediated by nuclear T3 receptors (TRs) that can bind T3 with high affinity [8]. TRs belong to the nuclear receptor superfamily that also includes the receptors for retinoids, vitamin D, fatty acids, and prostaglandins, as well as "orphan receptors" with no identified ligands [10-13]. TR is encoded by two separate genes, which are designated TR-alpha and TR-beta, located in different chromosomes (17 and 3, respectively, in humans). Like other nuclear receptors, TRs have modular structures with six regions (A–F) and three functional domains.

TR is considered as a transcription factor: it regulates target genes expression directly through DNA response elements. The thyroid hormone response element (TRE) is composed of repeated DNA sequences [14]. Although TRs can bind to TREs as monomers or homodimers, the major form of TR bound to the TRE is the heterodimer with Retinoid X Receptor (RXR). An important property of TRs is their ability to bind TREs constitutively independent of ligand occupancy [8,10,12,13]. Unliganded TR generally represses basal transcription. Ligand binding triggers a conformational change in the TR, resulting in activated transcription of its target gene. In the past few years, great progress in biochemical, functional, and structural studies has clarified the molecular mechanism of TR action.

A classical vertebrate model for thyroid hormone action in development is the amphibian tadpole. Thyroid hormone controls amphibian metamorphosis and thus plays an important role in the developmental changes in the nervous system that occur during metamorphosis. In anuran amphibians, thyroid function regulates the metamorphic process so these are one of the most commonly used *in vivo* systems for studying TH function [14]. TR mRNAs are present at very low levels in the oocyte and during embryogenesis [15-17]. High levels of TR-alpha mRNA are present after hatching and until the end of metamorphosis when levels decrease markedly, staying low in juveniles and adults [18]. TR-beta mRNA levels increase in parallel with endogenous TH levels. The promoter of TR-beta gene contains a thyroid response element, and its expression is induced by thyroid hormone itself in *X. laevis* [19]. As for TR-alpha mRNA, TR-beta mRNA levels decrease in juveniles and adults [18]. Similar profiles were observed when analyzing protein expression [20]. Furthermore, the proteins are functionally active as shown by T3 treatment inducing precocious metamorphosis [18].

Although TH effects have been mainly studied in mammals and amphibians for metamorphosis process, more and more data show that TH play important role in fish development. TH level is especially high in the eggs and larvae of several fish species [3]. In zebrafish, the thyroid gland begins to develop during early embryogenesis and begins to be active around 55 hours post fertilization (hpf) [21]. Before this developmental stage, TH comes from the maternal stock in the egg [3]. The TH receptors (TR-alpha and TR-beta) are both present in prehatch fish embryos, and allow TH functions. Prehatch embryos possess all TH function components: TR-alpha and TR-beta and TH from the maternal stock [3]. TH are synthesized and secreted by the thyroid gland after TSH stimulation. TSH is produced by thyrotropes present in the fish adenopituitary. Terminal differentiation of thyrotropes in the zebrafish adenopituitary occurs around 48hpf. The thyroid gland is active later, about 55 h post fertilization. Concerning the thyroid gland tissue organization, the zebrafish thyroid gland derives from precursor cells located in the endoderm prior to pharynx formation. During two morphogenetic phases, the thyroid primordium first adopts a position close to the cardiac outflow tract, with the first differentiated thyroid follicle, that grows afterwards along the ventral pharyngeal midline. The thyroid gland in the adult zebrafish is a loose aggregation of follicles close to the ventral aorta.

Zebrafish genome encodes two TR-alpha genes and one TR-beta gene, which are expressed at different developmental stages, suggesting that they have different function during development (for review see reference 4). Essner *et al* [22] showed that TR-alpha functions mainly as a transcriptional repressor and may repress retinoic acid signalling in zebrafish early development, and its overexpression results in a loss of the midbrain-hindbrain border and a severe disruption of the rostral hindbrain, suggesting an important role for THs in brain development. Some studies showed that a T3 exposure of embryos up-regulates TR expression and accelerates developmental rate and hatching [4,23]. This suggests that TH can exert a positive auto-regulatory feedback control on the transcription of its receptors.

2.2. Corticosteroid

Corticosteroids are implicated in many physiological process including osmoregulation, respiration, immunity, reproduction, growth and metabolism. Like thyroid hormone, corticosteroids production and action has been studied in amphibian models, for their implication in the positive control of metamorphosis [24]. In bony fishes, corticosteroids are secreted from the interrenal tissue located in the head kidney region. Cortisol is the major corticosteroid in teleost fish and its release involves the coordinated activation of the hypothalamus-pituitary-interrenal (HPI) axis. The key mediators include the release of corticotrophin-releasing factor (CRF) from the hypothalamus, and stimulating the release of adrenocorticotropic hormone (ACTH) from the pituitary. Circulating ACTH binds to melanocortin receptor 2 (MC2R) on the steroidogenic cells and activates the signalling pathway leading to cortisol biosynthesis [25].

In bony fishes, the corticosteroid receptor is a ligand-dependant transcription factor, with two major classes of receptors: the glucocorticoid receptor (GR) and the mineralocorticoid receptor (MR). Cortisol is the physiological ligand for GR. The molecular characterization of fish GR began with the cloning of rainbow trout (*Onchorynchus mykiss*) GR1 cDNA, followed by cloning of partial GR cDNA from tilapia (*Oreochromis mossambicus*) and full length GR cDNAs from Japanese flounder (*Paralichthys olivaceus*), rainbow trout GR2 and multiple GRs from cichlid fish (*Haplochromis burtoni*). The alignment of fish GR polypeptide sequences with mammalian GR showed very high homology with both C domain (DNA-binding) and E domain (hormone-binding), but the transcriptional transactivation domain has little homology. The two rainbow trout GR (rtGR1 and rtGR2) showed high sequence homology, and it has been shown phylogenetically that these two GR are a result of gene duplication common to most of teleost fishes. Expression of trout GR transcript has been found in many tissues. Fish GR showed a wide distribution in the brain, gill, and liver.

Little is known about GR and MR function in fish development. Recently, zebrafish has been used to investigate the role of corticosteroid signalling in development. It was shown that both of these receptors are present during embryogenesis [26]. Indeed, during embryogenesis, GR transcripts drops from 1.5 to 25 hpf, and then increases after hatching to the level at 1.5 hpf and was significantly higher at 25 hpf, and this level was maintained until 6 days. This study suggested a more important role for this receptor after hatch in zebrafish. It was also shown that cortisol synthesis occurred only after hatching and that maternal cortisol contributes to early developmental programming [26]. Further, Pikulkaew *et al.* [27] demonstrated that knocking down maternal GR leads to developmental defects in mesoderm formation in zebrafish. Recently, it has also been shown that GR signalling is essential for zebrafish muscle development [28].

In mammals and non-mammalian vertebrates such as amphibians, the major mineralocorticosteroid is aldosterone. However, aldosterone is not detected in fish, and deoxycorticosterone (DOC) is considered as MR ligand in fish. Like aldosterone, DOC is a selective MR agonist, that does not activate trout GR. Cortisol is also a high-affinity ligand for MR. Fish MR is distributed beyond the tissue involved in salt and water balance, especially in gills and intestine, and MR mRNA is also high in rainbow trout brain. The role of MR and its ligand remains less clear than GR, especially concerning its implication during development. MR transcripts continuously increased between 1.5 and 97 hpf and remained at the same high level at 6 days. MR has been suggested as responsible for corticosteroid signalling just after hatching, since it could be activated by maternal cortisol [26].

2.3. Relationship between TH and CR

The corticosteroid and thyroid hormone receptors possess equivalent transactivation domains and have some structural functional similarity [10,29], suggesting that these nuclear receptors may enhance transcription of target genes by similar mechanisms as summarized above. The thyroid and corticosteroid systems interact at multiple levels to influence several physiological processes like development, growth or behaviour.

Thus, the hypothalamo-pituitary-interrenal axis modulates the thyroid axis in fishes and other vertebrates. Indeed heterologous CRH potently stimulated the release of TSH from cultured pituitary cells *in vitro* [30]. Cortisol exposure also downregulates T4 plasma level in European eel (*Anguilla anguilla*), but not in trout [31,32].

Conversely, T3 seems to be involved in corticosteroid receptors regulation. Recently, Terrien *et al.* showed that 48 hours of T3 exposure increased MR and GR genes expression in one day-old zebrafish embryos [23]. In another study in common carp (*Cyprinus carpio*), experimentally induced hyperthyroidism downregulates plasma cortisol level. Kelly *et al.* [33] demonstrated a synergistic effect of thyroid hormone and cortisol on cultured *O. mykiss* pavement cell epithelia *in vitro*.

Other studies have suggested a coincident expression and synergetic action of TH and corticosteroids in other vertebrate models [34-37]. Indeed, corticosteroids and thyroid hormones act synergistically during some physiological processes such as amphibian metamorphosis, which is one of the most relevant biological models the most studied for TH and CR crossregulation [34]. Thus, it was shown that corticosteroids can synergize with thyroid hormone to accelerate tadpole metamorphosis, whether corticosteroids increase T3 binding capacity [2], or corticosteroids can increase the conversion of active T3 from T4, and decrease the degradation of T3 [38,39]. Moreover, corticosterone treatment upregulates TR-beta expression in the intestine of premetamorphic tadpoles and in tail explants cultures [37]. It is also known that GR suppresses TSH expression [40].

Like in fish models, TH seems to regulate CS in amphibians. Krain and Denver [37] showed that T3 upregulated the glucocorticoid receptor expression in tadpoles tail, and this regulation might be consistent with a physiological regulatory relationship, given the developmental pattern of thyroid hormone production and GR mRNA in the tail. In contrast, T3 has been shown to downregulate GR expression in the brain.

The coincident increase in cortisol and TH during flounder metamorphosis [35] and the regulation of GR mRNA expression after T3 treatment in *X. laevis* [37] support the idea of possible crosstalk between the thyroid hormones and the corticoid signalling system and are in agreement with previous studies highlighting the relationship between TH and the corticoid signalling system. More recently, corticosteroids have been shown to synergize with TH to promote morphogenesis [1], and that the synergistic actions of TH and corticosteroids occurs at the level of the TR-beta expression and deiodinase type 2, which converts T4 to T3 [34].

3. Use of aquatic organisms to investigate endocrine disruption

Many natural or synthetic chemicals are now routinely observed in water. Evidence revealed that these compounds might interfere with the endogenous endocrine systems of wildlife and humans. Thus, it is now essential to monitor their presence in the environment. Aquatic organisms as amphibians and fish models (zebrafish and medaka) are species widely used in ecotoxicology and for the development of transgenic techniques. These techniques allow development of new tools to detect and screen chemicals in the environment. The zebrafish has numerous technical advantages, so that it can be considered as a model organism: its complete embryogenesis occurs during the first 72 hours post-fertilization and most of the internal organs develop rapidly in the first 24-48 hours. They are easy to observe because embryos are transparent, which allows to easily track their development and expression of fluorescent proteins in transgenic fishes *in vivo*, until advanced stages [41]. In addition to rapid development (adult zebrafish can start to breed after 4 months), there are several other advantages of using zebrafish for assay development, including: small size, low cost to maintain, and easily bred in large numbers. Furthermore, a pair of zebrafish can produce over 100-200 eggs per day. Finally, single embryos can be maintained in small volumes during first days of development until hatching so that zebrafish can be used for automatic reading in 96-well plates. Chemicals can then be tested directly in the solution in which the embryos develop, facilitating high throughput screening [42]. These significant advantages over other species are making the zebrafish as a fully relevant biological model for detecting the effects of pollutants present in the water.

Zebrafish embryo bioassay has been extensively employed in drug and chemical screening [43,44] and the advantages promoting the use of the embryo assay for those purposes should also promote its use for endocrine disruptors phenotypic screening. Zebrafish embryos and larvae express hormones and receptors, and they possess all molecular actors to respond to exposure to endocrine disruptors.

Moreover, transgenesis in zebrafish is fast and routinely used. For these reasons, the zebrafish is now used to develop simple, rapid, cost-effective and innovative methods for screening environmental pollutants [45,46]. Some stable transgenic zebrafish lines have recently been used for screening chemicals that can mimic the action of estrogens [47], and for developing automated image acquisition and analysis in 96-well plates [46]. Recently, a fluorescent transient fluorescent transgenic zebrafish model has been developed to easily and rapidly screen compounds capable of disrupting thyroid function [23].

Another fish species, the medaka (*Oryzias latipes*) has evolved as an alternative model organism for rapid screening of endocrine activities. Indeed, the medaka has the same advantages than zebrafish (transparent embryos, fishes easy to breed, a short life cycle, easy reproduction and regular renewal of a large number of experiments). In addition to these technical advantages, the medaka has been widely used as a vertebrate model for the study of organogenesis and embryogenesis, and is now increasingly used as a model for conducting toxicity studies [48]. The growing interest in studies on the model of medaka was accompanied by a strong development of tools and methods available to study genetic aspects of such development. In this context, it is not surprising that medaka is now used to study the impact of endocrine disruptors, particularly for the characterization of the stress response and its genetic components [49]. Unlike other models of fish (zebrafish, stickelback), the medaka is more robust, easily exposable to environmental samples, while also the tools of transgenesis are more effective in this model. It is also one of the fish models referenced by the OECD for the detection of estrogenic disruptors.

Finally, amphibians are also used as indicators for ecotoxicological potencies of several environmental stressors. The aquatic larvae are continuously exposed to chemicals compounds present in water because the eggs are lacking a protective eggshell or membrane. After hatching, the skin of amphibians' larvae is still very permeable, allowing an easy penetration of all compounds leading to high bioavailability and bioaccumulation of endocrine disruptors. This development stage of amphibians is the most sensitive and the most used to study effects of environmental pollutants. Thus, Fini *et al.* used *in vivo X. laevis* tadpoles to monitor heavy metal pollution in water in continuous flow systems [50]. The same team already used *X. laevis* to detect the thyroid disrupting effect of BPA *in vivo* [51].

4. Impact of endocrine disruptors on thyroid hormone and corticosteroids systems in fish

Many natural and man-made chemicals (plasticizers, pesticides, detergents and pharmaceuticals) interfere with the endocrine system and can result in adverse health effects in humans, mammals and fish. Wildlife living in or in closer association with the aquatic environment are especially impacted by these endocrine disruptors, because water act as sinks for chemical discharges. Thus, fish and amphibians are the main potential targets for endocrine disruption at multiple levels, either direct or indirect, through ingestion and accumulation of endocrine disruptor, the exposition or through the food chain. Chronic exposure to endocrine disruptors, such as the oestrogenic compounds used in birth control, can feminize male fish and decrease their capacity to reproduce. In the opposite, masculinised female specimens were found in effluent containing androgenic chemicals [52]. Endocrine disruption on thyroid hormone and corticosteroids in fish was also studied.

Endocrine disruptors may impact corticosteroid signalling system in a direct manner (competition with endogenous ligand) or indirect manner (alteration in accessory proteins, kinases, cytoskeleton...). Among corticosteroids disruptors, chemicals including Polychlorinated Biphenyls (PCB) and heavy metals were the most studied. For example, it has been shown that Arsenic affects GR signalling and one mechanism involves the downregulation of GR content in trout hepatocytes [53]. Another study showed that Copper exposure during 5 days *in vivo* reduced GR-immunoreactivity in rainbow trout gill cells [54].

Cadmium is another metal that is widely distributed in the aquatic environment and is toxic to fish at sublethal concentrations [55]. Due to its long half-life and low excretion rate, Cadmium can also accumulate in various organs, primarily within the liver, kidney and reproductive and respiratory systems in fish [56]. This metal is known to disrupt head kidney corticosteroid production in fish. Vijayan *et al* [57] showed recently that Cadmium exposure leads to suppression of the ACTH-stimulated cortisol production. This study suggested that MC2R signalling, the primary step in ACTH-induced cortocosteroidogenesis, is a key target for Cadmium-mediated disruption of cortisol production in trout.

Because Polybrominated Diphenyl Ethers (PBDE), used as flame retardants, are similar in structure to thyroxine T4 and tri-iodothyronine T3 [58], several teams have studied their effect on thyroid function. Biologic effects of PBDEs in rodent are similar to those of PCB, increasing risks for reproductive and endocrine disruption. In 2011, Yu *et al.* [59] exposed zebrafish to low levels of PBDEs for most their lives. While the fish did accumulate different types of PBDE in their tissues, there was no toxicity. But the PBDEs were present in the eggs, and the chemicals and their associated toxic effects passed along the progeny and reduced hatch rates and altered thyroid hormone system of the next generation. This study is important because it shows that PBDEs trigger thyroid hormone disruption not only in the exposed population but also in the subsequent generation.

Due to its structural homology with thyroid hormone, Bisphenol A (BPA) is also frequently studied as endocrine disruptor for thyroid function. Is has been shown that BPA can interact with TR and it can be considered as a TR antagonist [60,61]. First, transgenic *X. laevis* were used to test *in vivo* whether BPA interferes with TH and to create an *in vivo* detection system for BPA endocrine disruptive properties [62]. More recently, Terrien *et al.* [23] used zebrafish receiving transient transgenesis of TR-sensitive reporter systems to study BPA disrupting effects. In this fish model, the green fluorescent protein (GFP) is expressed under the control of the TH/bZip promoter from *X. laevis* known to contain two thyroid hormone responsive elements (TRE). Exposure to T3 increased the GFP fluorescence in these transient transgenic fish. When tested alone, Bisphenol A did not modify fluorescence, but when tested with T3, it significantly reduced T3-induced fluorescence suggesting disruption of the thyroid function by BPA [23]. Many other natural (Rotenone) or synthetic (Malathion, Endosulfan) chemicals present in the environment produce thyroid disruption in fish, with varied responses (for review see reference 7).

Because of the close relationship between thyroid and corticosteroid axis in fish and amphibians, alteration of one of these axes could affect the other one. Indeed endocrine disruption due to chemicals present in the environment affects these two endocrine systems, separately or concomitant. Further studies have to investigate the final effect of disruption of one of these endocrine axes on the other one.

5. Conclusion

Nuclear receptor crossregulation are important mechanisms for amplifying hormone signals, regulating hormone activity through negative feedback, and coordinating hormone action in a temporal and tissue-specific-manner. In this chapter, we were interested in crossregulation between thyroid hormone and corticosteroids. These two endocrine systems are keys actors of many physiological processes. Their coincident expression and synergetic action were studied in different models (amphibian metamorphosis, stress response in fish). Corticosteroids are known to synergize with thyroid hormone to promote metamorphosis, and links between the thyroid and corticosteroid axes are present at multiple levels. Understanding the interactions between TH and CS will allow us to better understand the effects of endocrine disruptors.

The use of fish species as model organism for research on endocrine disruption is interesting the identification of potential new endocrine disruptors because of endocrine system and hormone signalling pathways are sufficiently similar to other vertebrates. In this context, we should observe more and more studies leading to a large development of screening tools based on these aquatic animals in a next future. However the consequences of the molecular, physiological or organisms' effects for the population may be different between species. Confirmation in higher vertebrates or in humans of the effects observed in fish is necessary if we want to clearly identify new endocrine disruptors. For instance, the use of aquatic organisms in endocrine disruption studies is relevant, because of their closeness with water-soluble chemicals. And the vast technical possibilities offered by the zebrafish and the medaka models for functional genomics studies justify their use in ED research.

References

1. Denver RJ. Stress hormones mediate environment-genotype interactions during amphibian development. General and Comparative Endocrinology 2009;164(1) 20-31.
2. Kikuyama S, Niki K, Mayumi M, Shibayama R, Nishikawa M, Shintake N. Studies on corticoid action on the toad tadpole tail in vitro. General and Comparative Endocrinology 1983;52(3) 395-9.
3. .Power DM, Llewellyn L, Faustino M, Nowell MA, Bjornsson BT, Einarsdottir IE, et al. Thyroid hormones in growth and development of fish. Comparative Biochemistry and Physiology Part C: Toxicology & Pharmacology 2001;130(4) 447-59.
4. .Darras VM, Van Herck SL, Heijlen M, De Groef B. Thyroid hormone receptors in two model species for vertebrate embryonic development: chicken and zebrafish. Journal of Thyroid Research 2011;2011(402320) 1-8.
5. .Prunet P, Sturm A, Milla S. Multiple corticosteroid receptors in fish: from old ideas to new concepts. General and Comparative Endocrinology 2006;147(1) 17-23.
6. .Hillegass JM, Villano CM, Cooper KR, White LA. Glucocorticoids alter craniofacial development and increase expression and activity of matrix metalloproteinases in developing zebrafish (Danio rerio). Toxicological Science 2008;102(2) 413-24.
7. .Peter VS, Peter MC. The interruption of thyroid and interrenal and the inter-hormonal interference in fish: does it promote physiologic adaptation or maladaptation? General and Comparative Endocrinology 2011;174(3) 249-58.
8. .Lazar MA. Thyroid hormone receptors: multiple forms, multiple possibilities. Endocrine Reviews 1993;14(2) 184-93.
9. .Utiger RD. Recognition of thyroid disease in the fetus. New England Journal of Medicine 1991;324(8) 559-61.
10. .Evans RM. The steroid and thyroid hormone receptor superfamily. Science 1988;240(4854) 889-95.
11. .Glass CK. Differential recognition of target genes by nuclear receptor monomers, dimers, and heterodimers. Endocrine Reviews 1994;15(3) 391-407.

12. .Mangelsdorf DJ, Thummel C, Beato M, Herrlich P, Schutz G, Umesono K, et al. The nuclear receptor superfamily: the second decade. Cell 1995;83(6) 835-9.

13. .Ribeiro RC, Kushner PJ, Baxter JD. The nuclear hormone receptor gene superfamily. Annual Review of Medicine 1995;46443-53.

14. .Morvan-Dubois G, Demeneix BA, Sachs LM. Xenopus laevis as a model for studying thyroid hormone signalling: from development to metamorphosis. Molecular and Cellular Endocrinology 2008;293(1-2) 71-9.

15. .Banker DE, Bigler J, Eisenman RN. The thyroid hormone receptor gene (c-erbA alpha) is expressed in advance of thyroid gland maturation during the early embryonic development of Xenopus laevis. Molecular and Cellular Biology 1991;11(10) 5079-89.

16. .Havis E, Le Mevel S, Morvan-Dubois G, Shi DL, Scanlan TS, Demeneix BA, et al. Unliganded thyroid hormone receptor is essential for Xenopus laevis eye development. Embo Journal 2006;25(20) 4943-51.

17. .Oofusa K, Tooi O, Kashiwagi A, Kashiwagi K, Kondo Y, Watanabe Y, et al. Expression of thyroid hormone receptor betaA gene assayed by transgenic Xenopus laevis carrying its promoter sequences. Molecular and Cellular Endocrinology 2001;181(1-2) 97-110.

18. .Yaoita Y, Brown DD. A correlation of thyroid hormone receptor gene expression with amphibian metamorphosis. Genes and Development 1990;4(11) 1917-24.

19. .Tata JR. Autoregulation and crossregulation of nuclear receptor genes. Trends in Endocrinology and Metabolism 1994;5(7) 283-90.

20. .Eliceiri BP, Brown DD. Quantitation of endogenous thyroid hormone receptors alpha and beta during embryogenesis and metamorphosis in Xenopus laevis. Journal of Biological Chemistry 1994;269(39) 24459-65.

21. .Alt B, Reibe S, Feitosa NM, Elsalini OA, Wendl T, Rohr KB. Analysis of origin and growth of the thyroid gland in zebrafish. Developmental Dynamics 2006;235(7) 1872-83.

22. .Essner JJ, Johnson RG, Hackett PBJr. Overexpression of thyroid hormone receptor alpha 1 during zebrafish embryogenesis disrupts hindbrain patterning and implicates retinoic acid receptors in the control of hox gene expression. Differentiation 1999;65(1) 1-11.

23. .Terrien X, Fini JB, Demeneix BA, Schramm KW, Prunet P. Generation of fluorescent zebrafish to study endocrine disruption and potential crosstalk between thyroid hormone and corticosteroids. Aquatic Toxicology 2011;105(1-2) 13-20.

24. .Kikuyama S, Kawamura K, Tanaka S, Yamamoto K. Aspects of amphibian metamorphosis: hormonal control. International Review of Cytology 1993;145105-48.

25. .Aluru N, Vijayan MM. Molecular characterization, tissue-specific expression, and regulation of melanocortin 2 receptor in rainbow trout. Endocrinology 2008;149(9) 4577-88.

26. .Alsop D, Vijayan MM. Development of the corticosteroid stress axis and receptor expression in zebrafish. American Journal of Physiology - Regulatory, Integrative and Comparative Physiology 2008;294(3) R711-R719.

27. .Pikulkaew S, Benato F, Celeghin A, Zucal C, Skobo T, Colombo L, et al. The knockdown of maternal glucocorticoid receptor mRNA alters embryo development in zebrafish. Developmental Dynamics 2011;240(4) 874-89.

28. .Nesan D, Kamkar M, Burrows J, Scott IC, Marsden M, Vijayan MM. Glucocorticoid receptor signaling is essential for mesoderm formation and muscle development in zebrafish. Endocrinology 2012;153(3) 1288-300.

29. .Thompson CC, Evans RM. Trans-activation by thyroid hormone receptors: functional parallels with steroid hormone receptors. Proceedings of the National Academy of Sciences of the United States of America 1989;86(10) 3494-8.

30. .Larsen DA, Swanson P, Dickey JT, Rivier J, Dickhoff WW. In vitro thyrotropin-releasing activity of corticotropin-releasing hormone-family peptides in coho salmon, Oncorhynchus kisutch. General and Comparative Endocrinology 1998;109(2) 276-85.

31. .Leatherland JF. Thyroid response to ovine thyrotropin challenge in cortisol- and dexamethasone-treated rainbow trout, Salmo gairdneri. Comparative Biochemistry and Physiology A: Comparative Physiology 1987;86(2) 383-7.

32. .Redding JM, deLuze A, Leloup-Hatey J, Leloup J. Suppression of plasma thyroid hormone concentrations by cortisol in the European eel Anguilla anguilla. Comparative Biochemistry and Physiology A: Comparative Physiology 1986;83(3) 409-13.

33. .Kelly SP, Wood CM. The physiological effects of 3,5',3'-triiodo-L-thyronine alone or combined with cortisol on cultured pavement cell epithelia from freshwater rainbow trout gills. General and Comparative Endocrinology 2001;123(3) 280-94.

34. .Bonett RM, Hoopfer ED, Denver RJ. Molecular mechanisms of corticosteroid synergy with thyroid hormone during tadpole metamorphosis. General and Comparative Endocrinology 2010;168(2) 209-19.

35. .de Jesus EG, Inui Y, Hirano T. Cortisol enhances the stimulating action of thyroid hormones on dorsal fin-ray resorption of flounder larvae in vitro. General and Comparative Endocrinology 1990;79(2) 167-73.

36. .de Jesus EG, Hirano T, Inui Y. Changes in cortisol and thyroid hormone concentrations during early development and metamorphosis in the Japanese flounder, Paralichthys olivaceus. General and Comparative Endocrinology 1991;82(3) 369-76.

37. .Krain LP, Denver RJ. Developmental expression and hormonal regulation of glucocorticoid and thyroid hormone receptors during metamorphosis in Xenopus laevis. Journal of Endocrinology 2004;181(1) 91-104.

38. .Galton VA. Deiodination of thyroxine and related compounds. Thyroid 1990;1(1) 43-8.

39. .Galton VA. Mechanisms underlying the acceleration of thyroid hormone-induced tadpole metamorphosis by corticosterone. Endocrinology 1990;127(6) 2997-3002.

40. .Pamenter RW, Hedge GA. Inhibition of thyrotropin secretion by physiological levels of corticosterone. Endocrinology 1980;106(1) 162-6.

41. .Goldsmith JR, Jobin C. Think small: zebrafish as a model system of human pathology. Journal of Biomedicine and Biotechnology 2012;2012817341.

42. .Westerfield M. The Zebrafish Book. A Guide for the Laboratory Use of Zebrafish (Danio Rerio*), 4th ed. Univ of Oregon Press, Eugene 2007; Available from: URL: http://zfin.org/zf_info/zfbook/zfbk.html

43. .Shi X, Du Y, Lam PK, Wu RS, Zhou B. Developmental toxicity and alteration of gene expression in zebrafish embryos exposed to PFOS. Toxicology and Applied Pharmacology 2008;230(1) 23-32.

44. .Zon LI, Peterson RT. In vivo drug discovery in the zebrafish. Nature Reviews Drug Discovery 2005;4(1) 35-44.

45. .Raldua D, Babin PJ. Simple, rapid zebrafish larva bioassay for assessing the potential of chemical pollutants and drugs to disrupt thyroid gland function. Environmental Science and Technology 2009;43(17) 6844-50.

46. .Vogt A, Codore H, Day BW, Hukriede NA, Tsang M. Development of automated imaging and analysis for zebrafish chemical screens. Journal of Visualized Experiments 2010;401-3.

47. .Chen H, Hu J, Yang J, Wang Y, Xu H, Jiang Q, et al. Generation of a fluorescent transgenic zebrafish for detection of environmental estrogens. Aquatic Toxicology 2010;96(1) 53-61.

48. .Zeng Z, Shan T, Tong Y, Lam SH, Gong Z. Development of estrogen-responsive transgenic medaka for environmental monitoring of endocrine disrupters. Environmental Science and Technology 2005;39(22) 9001-8.

49. Iguchi T, Watanabe H, Katsu Y. Application of ecotoxicogenomics for studying endocrine disruption in vertebrates and invertebrates. Environmental Health Perspectives 2006;114(S1) 101-5.

50. .Fini JB, Pallud-Mothre S, Le Mevel S, Palmier K, Havens CM, Le Brun M, et al. An innovative continuous flow system for monitoring heavy metal pollution in water using transgenic Xenopus laevis tadpoles. Environmental Science and Technology 2009;43(23) 8895-900.

51. .Fini JB, Le Mevel S, Turque N, Palmier K, Zalko D, Cravedi JP, et al. An in vivo multiwell-based fluorescent screen for monitoring vertebrate thyroid hormone disruption. Environmental Science and Technology 2007;41(16) 5908-14.

52. .Drysdale DT, Bortone SA. Laboratory induction of intersexuality in the mosquitofish, Gambusia affinis, using paper mill effluent. Bulletin of Environmental Contamination and Toxicology 1989;43(4) 611-7.

53. .Baumann H, Paulsen K, Kovacs H, Berglund H, Wright AP, Gustafsson JA, et al. Refined solution structure of the glucocorticoid receptor DNA-binding domain. Biochemistry 1993;32(49) 13463-71.

54. .Dang ZC, Flik G, Ducouret B, Hogstrand C, Wendelaar Bonga SE, Lock RA. Effects of copper on cortisol receptor and metallothionein expression in gills of Oncorhynchus mykiss. Aquatic Toxicology 2000;51(1) 45-54.

55. .Lacroix A, Hontela A. Role of calcium channels in cadmium-induced disruption of cortisol synthesis in rainbow trout (Oncorhynchus mykiss). Comparative Biochemistry and Physiology Part C: Toxicology & Pharmacology 2006;144(2) 141-7.

56. .Hollis L, McGeer JC, McDonald DG, Wood CM. Effects of long term sublethal Cd exposure in rainbow trout during soft water exposure: implications for biotic ligand modelling. Aquatic Toxicology 2000;51(1) 93-105.

57. .Sandhu N, Vijayan MM. Cadmium-mediated disruption of cortisol biosynthesis involves suppression of corticosteroidogenic genes in rainbow trout. Aquatic Toxicology 2011;103(1-2) 92-100.

58. .Hamers T, Kamstra JH, Sonneveld E, Murk AJ, Kester MH, Andersson PL, et al. In vitro profiling of the endocrine-disrupting potency of brominated flame retardants. Toxicological Science 2006;92(1) 157-73.

59. .Yu L, Lam JC, Guo Y, Wu RS, Lam PK, Zhou B. Parental transfer of polybrominated diphenyl ethers (PBDEs) and thyroid endocrine disruption in zebrafish. Environmental Science and Technology 2011;45(24) 10652-9.

60. .Moriyama K, Tagami T, Akamizu T, Usui T, Saijo M, Kanamoto N, et al. Thyroid hormone action is disrupted by bisphenol A as an antagonist. Journal of Clinical Endocrinology and Metabolism 2002;87(11) 5185-90.

61. .Zoeller RT. Environmental chemicals as thyroid hormone analogues: new studies indicate that thyroid hormone receptors are targets of industrial chemicals? Molecular and Cellular Endocrinology 2005;242(1-2) 10-5.

62. .Fini JB, Dolo L, Cravedi JP, Demeneix B, Zalko D. Metabolism of the endocrine disruptor BPA by Xenopus laevis tadpoles. Annals of the New York Academy of Sciences 2009;1163394-7.

Chapter 11

Acute Toxicity Profiles of Aqueous and Ethanolic Extracts of Capsicum annum Seeds from South Western Uganda

1. Introduction

Capsicum annum belongs to the Kingdom Plantae plants, subkingdom of Tracheobiota (vascular plants), super-division of Spermatophyta (seed plants), division of Magnoliophyta (flowering plants), class Magnoliopsida (dicotyledons), subclass Asteridae, order Solanels, family Solanaceae (potato family), genus Capsicum L. (pepper), species *Capsicum annum* L. (Cayenne pepper) and variety *Capsicum annum* L. var annum (Cayenne pepper).

Capsicuma annum is a perennial shrub growing up to 2 m (6') in height, having a woody trunk. It has green fruits that ripen to red. The active ingredient in the plant is *capsaicin* that is used for the management of various medical conditions. The varieties of this "fruit" vary greatly in size, colour and pungency. The plant extract that provides therapeutic action is the seed oil.

Globally, *Capsicum annum* has many uses. It is used as a feed additive and as spices. The corrosive nature of capsaicin, its gross irritating effects and its toxicities are well documented. A qualitative assessment of bioactive chemical compounds in *Capsicum annum* established the presence of reducing compounds, saponins, alkaloid salts, alkaloids, quarternary bases, anthracenosides, flavanosides, flavonds, coumourin derivatives, steroid glycosides and anthocyanosides

It is indeed true that *Capsicum annum* possesses many medicinal plant bioactive substances that are active against certain bacteria, viruses and protozoa [1-3]. In-vitro studies indicated that *Capsicum annum* fruits are efficacious against common bacteria e.g. Staphylococcus, Streptococcus species etc. The widespread use of *Capsicum annum* as an herbal remedy by smallholder poultry farmers is based on a wide range of doses [3]. A wide range of medicinal plant users do not believe that plant extracts can be toxic, yet standard laboratory tests [1, 3-5] indicate profound toxicity from some medicinal plants.

The smallholder farmers in the South Western Agro-ecological Zone of Uganda (SWAEZ) use *Capsicum annum* [6] as a medicinal plant for controlling various poultry diseases like Newcastle disease. They would pick 3-4 seeds of Capsicum annum seeds from their gardens or neighbours gardens and crush the harvested seeds in a cup and then mixed it in various proportions of water, from half a litre to up to two litres. The mixed extract is then given to the suspected sick birds infected with Newcastle disease. The birds may be assisted to drink the extract or the birds may drink it freely at will. The shelf life of the prepared extracts is usually one to at least two days then fresh mixtures are constituted depending on the severity and improvements in the health conditions of the bird(s).

Despite the plant and its compounds being used by the farmers, the acute toxicities of *Capsicum annum* extracted under aqueous and ethanolic solvent systems are not yet known. The study hypothesized that medicinal plant with unknown acute toxicity levels exist in the SWAEZ of Uganda. The study assessed the acute toxicity levels of *Capsicum annum* in the SWAEZ under aqueous and ethanolic solvent systems.

2. Materials and methods

2.1. Plant seed collection and preparation

The *Capsicum annum* seeds were collected from Rubindi Sub County of Mbarara district in the South Western Agro-Ecological Zone (SWAEZ). A total of 2 kilograms of the sample was harvested and labelled with the laboratory number (CA 001 Lag), date and kept in black a polythene bag in a cupboard. The seeds were packed in a paper box wrapped in polythene and taken to the Division of Pharmacology and Physiological Sciences, College of Veterinary Medicine, Animal Resources and Bio-security (COVAB), Makerere University (Uganda). The seeds were then dried at room temperature of 25^0C for 7 days. Afterwards, 200 gr were weighed for water extraction and another 200 gr for ethanolic extraction. The seeds were manually ground to fine powder using a mortar and pestle.

Weighing and extraction process: A total of 160 gr of the powdered sample was weighed and soaked in a dark bottle containing 1 litre of 70% ethanol with intermittent shaking for 72 hours. Similarly, 160 gr were weighed for extraction in 1 litre of water. After three days of extraction the extract was filtered using cotton wool fixed within a funnel. The filtrate was collected in a glass conical flask and labelled, and the residue discarded. The filtrate was then subjected to a rotary evaporator at reduced pressure and temperature for concentration to a constant volume. After concentration the extract was put in an oven at 45^0c until a semi-solid form of extract was obtained. This was put in bijous bottle, well labelled, and kept in a refrigerator at 4^0c for future use. The percentage yield (%yield) $=10g\times100/160=6.25\%$. The percentage yield (%yield) was 6.25% of the fruit extract.

2.2. Acute toxicity study protocol

The ethical committee of Mbarara University of Science and Technology (MUST) approved the use of experimental animals for the experiments.

Swiss albino mice of 16-25 gr bodyweight from both sexes were selected and labelled using tail markers of different colours. The animals (n=30) were divided into five groups of six mice each and kept in different cages for easy observation.

The dose levels were determined after a preliminary acute toxicity trial, which had been carried out earlier. The doses rates were as shown in table 1.

Table 1. Preliminary acute toxicity levels of crude extracts of *Capsicum annum*

Groups	Extracts Dose levels (mg/kg)		*n*	Nº dead	
	Aqueous (a)	*Ethanolic (b)*		Aqueous (a)	*Ethanolic (b)*
Group 1	10,000	3500	6	0	0
Group 2	12,000	5000	6	2	2
Group 3	14,000	6500	6	4	4
Group 4	16,000	8000	6	6	6
Control	1ml dH_20		6	0	0

The volumes of the drug doses administered to the mice were calculated using the following formula [4]: Volume (ml) = body weight (kg) x dose levels (mg/kg)/stock drug concentration (mg/ml). The extracts were administered by gavage orally.

The derived dose levels for ethanolic extracts were 3,500, 5000, 6500 and 8,000 mg/kg and for aqueous extracts were 10,000, 12,000, 14,000 and 16,000 mg/ml.

Postmortem procedure: The numbers of mice which died after being subjected to the medicinal plant crude extracts were noted. Randomly selected animals (n=2) from each group were submitted to necropsy for organ collection. The surviving mice were sacrificed at the end of the experiment after observation for 7 days and subjected to post mortem analysis. Within 24hrs, organs from mice that died or were sacrificed were collected and fixed in jars containing formalin (10% formaldehyde) and subsequently submitted to routine paraffin embedding. The liver, kidney, lungs, intestines and brain were collected for histopathology analysis. Four (4) micrometer sections of the collected organs were routinely stained with haematoxylin and eosin for histological examination, performed by a Pathologist. Putative histopathological changes in the structural organization of the liver, kidney, lungs, intestines and brain were observed and recorded.

Data collection and analysis: Mortality (number of dead mice) were counted in each group and recorded. The median lethal dose that killed 50% of the test animals was determined using the graphical and Probit analysis. Any signs of toxicity observed in the collected organs were also recorded.

Quality assurance: The calyces were shade dried to prevent loss of essential chemical components and the voucher specimen were taken to the herbarium (Biology Department, Mbarara University of Science and Technology) for identification and also to ensure the quality of the techniques adopted from world Health Organization (WHO) guidelines on herbal quality control.

Distilled water was used for extraction to prevent contamination of the extract. Both the aqueous and ethanolic extracts of *Capsicum annum* seeds were kept in sterilized bottles and placed in a refrigerator at 4°C to prevent mould formation. All the reagents used were analytical grade.

The Swiss albino mice of the same age were used for the study to minimize variation in the test results. The control group given 1 ml of distilled water was used for comparison with the groups given the plant extract.

3. Results

3.1. Aqueous acute toxicity profile of *Capsicum annum* seeds

The aqueous acute toxicity profile of *Capsicum annum* seeds under various dose levels is shown in table 2.

Table 2. Acute toxicity profile of aqueous and ethanolic *Capsicum annum extracts*

Extracts	Group	Dose (mg/kg)	log dose	dead/total	dead%	Probit
Aqueous	1	10,000	4.00	0/6	0	3.04
	2	12,000	4.08	2/6	33.33	4.53
	3	14,000	4.15	3/6	50.00	4.95
	4	16,000	4.20	4/6	66.66	5.36
	5	18,000	4.26	6/6	100.00	6.75
Ethanolic	1	3500	3.54	0/6	0	3.04
	2	5000	3.70	2/6	33.33	4.53
	3	6500	3.81	4/6	66.67	5.36
	4	8000	3.90	6/6	100	6.75

It was observed that it would take 12043 mg/kg to kill 50% of the test animals (Graph 1). This gives a wide safety margin for the lethal dose of *Capsicum annum* fruits extracts in test animals. This is the LD 50 for the aqueous extract; which is the most commonly method used by the local farmers.

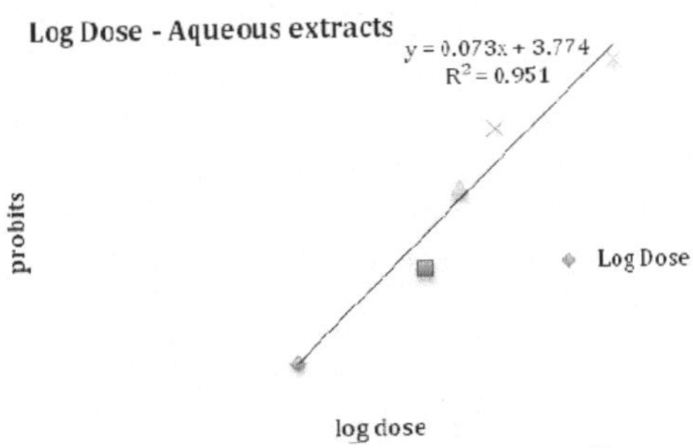

Graph 1. Probit for aqueous *Capsicum annum* extracts. From the equation 1Y=mx-c,where: Y=0.0737(4.15)+3.7749 = 0.305855+ 3.7749 = 4.080755; Ld_{50} = antilog of 4.080755 =12,043.563 mg/kg.

3.2. Toxicity signs observed with dose increase within the groups

There were notable side effects associated to higher doses of *Capsicum* extracts, such as limb movements, gut irritation, loss of balance, GIT muscle twitching. Hyperactivity was noted within 2 minutes after administration. Vocalization, urination, drowsiness, reddening of lips, dyspnoea and circling movement were noted and convulsions occurred before death.

3.3. Acute toxicity of 70% ethanolic extract of *Capsicum annum*

The ethanolic acute toxicity profile of *Capsicum annum* seeds under various dose levels is shown in table 2. The LD50 was calculated according to Fisher's and Yates as in Table 2. The lethal dose was established to be 5,492mg/kg (Graph 2).

3.4. Signs of acute toxicity observed

For the ethanolic extracts at a dosage of 3500mg/kg and 5000mg/kg, the following signs were observed: irritation shown by the use of forelimbs to scratch the areas of the mouth, gasping for air and dyspnoea. For aqueous extracts at a dosage of 6500mg/kg and 8000mg/kg there were observed twitching of GIT muscles, urination, dry mouth, reddening of lips and convulsions.

3.5. Comparison of key histo-pathological findings due to aqueous and ethanolic extracts

The key histopathological findings due to the effects of aqueous and 70% ethanolic extracts of *Capsicum annum* are detailed in table 3.

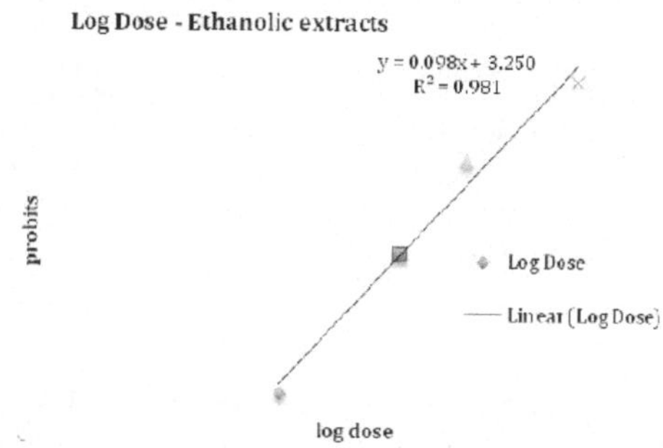

Graph 2. Probit for 70% ethanolic *Capsicum annum* extracts. From the equation 2y=bx-c, where Y=0.0989 (4.945) + 3.2507 = 0.4890605 + 3.2507 = 3.7397605..Ld_{50} = antilog (3.7397605) = 5492.3790

3.6. Histopathology findings

Table 3. Comparison of key histopathological findings of aqueous and 70% ethanolic extracts for the collected organs

Organs examined	Control group	Toxic effects associated to Capsicum annum aqueous extracts	Toxic effects associated to Capsicum annum 70% alcohol extracts
Brain	A	B	C
	A –Brain (Control). The scale bar is 100μm	B –No significant effects on the brain at 10,000mg/kg. The scale bar is 100μm	C –Slight congestion of the meninges at 3500mg/kg. The scale bar is 100μm
Kidney (Medulla)	D	E	F
	D –Kidney (Control) Medulla. The scale bar is 100μm	E –Kidney renal haemorrhages, congestion and tissue degeneration at 12,000mg/kg. The scale bar is 100μm	F –Haemorrhages and congestion at 5,00mg/kg. The scale bar is 100μm
Lungs	G	H	I

Organs examined	Control group	Toxic effects associated to Capsicum annum aqueous extracts	Toxic effects associated to Capsicum annum 70% alcohol extracts
	G –Lungs (Control). The scale bar is 100μm	H –Mild Lung emphysema noted at 10,000mg/kg. The scale bar is 100μm	I –Lungs haemorrhages and congestion at 5,000mg/kg. The scale bar is 100μm
Small intestine	J	K	L
	J –Small intestine (Control). The scale bar is 100μm	K –Erosions of the small intestine at 14,000mg/kg. The scale bar is 100μm	L –Intestines villus sloughing off and mucosal erosion at 6,500mg/kg. The scale bar is 100μm
Liver	M	N	O
	M –Liver (Control). The scale bar is 100μm	N –Hepatic degeneration and congestion of the liver at 14,000mg/kg. The scale bar is 100μm	O –Liver wide necrosis and tissue degeneration at 6,500mg/kg. The scale bar is 100μm
Heart	P	Q	R
	P –Heart (Control). The scale bar is 100μm	Q –Myocardial haemorrhages at 12,000mg/kg. The scale bar is 100μm	R –Wide spread haemorrhages on the myocardium at 5,000mg/kg. The scale bar is 100μm

4. Discussion

4.1. Lethal dose (LD50) levels

The lethal dose (LD50) of aqueous extracts of *Capsicum annum* was found to be12043 mg/kg. The 70% ethanolic extracts of *Capsicum annum* had a lethal dose (LD50) of 5492 mg/kg. Consequently the *Capsicum annum* is classified as practically non-toxic because the LD50 results fall in the dose range of 5-15g/kg of body weight [4].

Local smallholder farmers are using aqueous extracts of *Capsicum annum* seeds to manage various disorders. This study has confirmed that the use of the aqueous extract of *Capsicum annum* by the local poultry farmers is safe. Save to note here that the smallholder farmer's dose levels greatly vary from one farmer to another and in varying levels of concoctions [6]. The estimate dose for local farmers range between 4014-6022mg/kg for aqueous extracts. The farmers' dose levels are two-three times below the determined LD50 of 12043mg/Kg body weight for aqueous extracts.

The Organization for Economic Cooperation Development (OECD) Guidelines for the Testing of Chemicals [7] recommended that the maximum dose levels for any chemical compounds should not exceed 5000 mg/kg of the animal body weight. The ethanolic extraction of Capsicum annum has advantages compared to the aqueous because ethanol is better solvent for extraction of bioactive compounds.

The extracts derived from ethanolic solvents have lower LD50 of 5492mg/kg because ethanol is less polar. The ethanolic extracts have yet another advantage: the longer shelf life for use because of the preservative effects of alcohol on the extracts when compared to that of the water in aqueous extracts [5]. It can be noted here that extracts, which seem to show high toxicity in many circumstances, have no traditional uses, which is in agreement with previous findings [1,8].

After administration of the higher extract dosages there were often observed notable clinical signs in test animals, due to the side effects of the extracts. Key clinical signs noted were irritation, evidenced by the use of fore limbs to scratch the areas of the mouth, gasping for air, dyspnoea, twitching of GIT muscle, urination, dry mouth, reddening of lips and convulsions. The effects of bioavailability of the drugs on major organs like the intestines, liver, lungs, kidneys and brain showed clear manifestations of the presence of the active substances. Bioavailability is the rate and extent to which the active drug ingredient is absorbed from a drug product and becomes available at the site of drug action. The effects of the active substances in the body of the mice could affect by the rate of disintegration of the drug product, dissolution of the drug in the fluids at the absorption site or the transfer of drug molecule across the membrane lining the gastrointestinal tract into the systemic circulation.

The key physiologic factors that could affect the availability of the active substances in the body include: variations in absorption power along GI tract, variations in pH of GI fluids, gastric emptying rate, intestinal motility, perfusion of GI tract, presystemic and first-pass metabolism, age, sex, weight and disease states. The interactions with other substances like food, fluid volume and other drugs or chemicals could also play an important role.

There exist some reports of seeds side effects by *Capsicum annum* on chickens reared under the traditional use system. This finding concurs with the experimental trials. Aware of this fact, is to note that mice, chickens compared to other mammals hence exhibit a large surface area compared to other mammals.

The histopathological findings showed significant effects on brain, kidney, lungs, small intestines, liver and heart. Studies in India indicated that necropsy examination is paramount in linking the general and target organ specific toxic effects of phytomedicine [9]. Many others are in agreement OECD [10-12]. Absence of any significant gross pathological lesions in treated rats and mice at the terminal sacrifice indicates the justifiable harmless nature of the phytomedicine [9].

5. Conclusion

Results of study indicated that the lethal dose (LD50) of aqueous extracts of *Capsicum annum* was12043 mg/kg compared with 5,492mg/kg for 70% ethanolic extracts. The clinical signs noted depended on the level of concentration of the plant extracts.The study concludes that 70% ethanol extracts of *Capsicum annum and aqueous extracts* of capsicum annum are safe to use and are classified as practically non-toxic (5-15g/kg body weight). Both extracts are suitable for traditional poultry disease management by farmers. Further toxicity studies using chicken as animal species are necessary. Sub-acute and chronic toxicity tests are recommended in order to determine the long-term effects of the extract.

Appendix

Table 4. Probit conversion tables. Source: [4]

%	0	1	2	3	4	5	6	7	8	9
0		2.67	2.95	3.12	3.25	3.36	3.45	3.52	3.59	3.66
10	3.72	3.77	3.82	3.87	3.92	3.96	4.01	4.05	4.08	4.12
20	4.16	4.19	4.23	4.26	4.29	4.33	4.36	4.39	4.42	4.45
30	4.48	4.50	4.53	4.56	4.49	4.61	4.64	4.67	4.69	4.72
40	4.75	4.77	4.80	4.82	4.85	4.87	4.90	4.92	4.95	4.97
50	5.00	5.03	5.05	5.08	5.10	5.13	5.15	5.18	5.20	5.23
60	5.25	5.28	5.31	5.33	5.36	5.39	5.41	5.44	5.47	5.50
70	5.52	5.55	5.58	5.61	5.64	5.67	5.71	5.74	5.77	5.81
80	5.84	5.88	5.92	5.95	5.99	6.04	6.08	6.13	6.18	6.23
90	6.28	6.34	6.41	6.48	6.55	6.64	6.75	6.88	7.05	7.33
The percentage dead for 0 and 100 will be corrected before determination of LD50 using the following formula [4]: *For 0% dead: 100(0.25/n); for 100% dead: 100(n-0.25/n).*										

References

1. Chandra P, Sachan N, Ghosh A K and Kishore K (2010).Acute and Sub-chronic Oral Toxicity Studies of a Mineralo-herbal Drug Amlena on Experimental Rats.International Journal of Pharmaceutical Research and Innovation, Vol. I: 15-18, 2010
2. Atsamo, A. D., Nguelefack, T. B., Datte, J.Y and Kamanyi, A (2011).Acute and subchronic oral toxicity assessment of the aqueous extract from stem bark of Erythrinasenegalensis DC (Fabaceae) in rodents. J. Ethnopharmacology. (2011).
3. Wang Cuina, Zhang Tiehua, Liu Jun, Lu Shuang, Zhang Cheng, Wang Erlei, Wang Zuozhao, Zhang Yan, Liu Jingbo (2011).Subchronic toxicity study of corn silk with rats.J.Ethnopharmacol. (2011).
4. Ghosh, M.N.1984.Fundamentals of Experimental Pharmacology.2nd Edition.Culcutta: Scientific Book Agency; 1984. pp. 153–158.
5. BussmannR.W.., Malca G., Glenn A., Sharon D., Nilsen B., Parris B. , Dubose D., Ruiz D., Saleda J., Martinez M., Carillo L. , Walker K., Kuhlman A., Townesmith (2011). Toxicity of medicinal plants used in traditional medicine in Northern Peru. J. Ethnopharmacol. (2011).
6. Lagu C and Kayanja F I B 2010: Medicinal plant extracts widely used in the control of Newcastle disease (NCD) and helminthosis among village chickens of South Western Uganda. Livestock Research for Rural Development.Volume 22, Article #200.http://www.lrrd.org/lrrd22/11/lagu22200.htm (accessed 2 November, 2011).
7. Organization for Economic Co-operation and Development (OECD), 1995 Guidelines for the Testing of Chemicals (No. 407, Section 4: Health Effects) "Repeated Dose 28-Day Oral Toxicity in Rodents" (Adopted on 12 May 198 1 and Updated on 27 July 1995.)

8. Bizimenyera E.S., Swam G.E., Samdumu F. B., McGaw L.J and Eloff J. N (2007). Safety profiles of peltophorumafricanumsond. (Fabaceae) extracts. PhD thesis, University of Pretoria; 2007.

9. Joshua A.J., Goudar K.S., Sameera N., Pavan Kumar G., Murali B., Dinakar N. and Amit A (2010).Safety Assessment of Herbal Formulations, Rumbion™ and Tyrel™ in Albino Wistar Rats.American Journal of Pharmacology and Toxicology 5 (1): 42-47, 2010 ISSN 1557-4962.

10. Organization for Economic Co-operation and Development (OECD), 2000. Guidance document on the recognition, assessment and use of clinical signs as humane endpoints for experimental animals used in safety evaluation.Environmental Health and Safety Monograph Series on Testing and Assessment No.

11. Gad, S.C., 2007.The Rat. In: Animal Models in Toxicology, Gad, S.C. (Ed.). CRC Press, Boca Raton, FL, ISBN: 10: 0824754077, pp: 193-195.

12. Hayes, A.W., 2007. Principles of Pathology for Toxicological Studies In: Principles and Methods of Toxicology, Hayes, A.W. (Ed.), 5th Edn., CRC Press, New York, ISBN: 084933778X pp: 592.

Chapter 12

The in vitro Antihelminthic Efficacy of Erythrina Abyssinica Extracts on Ascaridia galli

1. Introduction

Helminth Infestation can lead to reduced growth and egg production in poultry. Coupled with high costs in 'wasted feeding' and demand for de-worming, this result in considerable economic losses in poultry enterprises and directly affects livelihood of small holder farmers [1]. In the birds, there is slow growth rate hence reduced body weight, delayed market weight attainment because of competition for nutrients by the bird and parasites. For the farmer, there is loss of income, reduced employment, and compromised household welfare, difficulty to raise educational fees, health fess, and social security activities.

Though an important veterinary practice, helminths control is largely neglected in village-level chicken production. The situation demands for alternative and inexpensive helminths control measures. Locally available medicinal plants have traditionally been used by small holder farmers to manage various livestock and human ailments [1-4], However, scientific data on the efficacy of these plants in helminthic control is lacking [5-8], It has been reported that local communities in the south-western agro-ecological zone (SWAEZ), Uganda, use *Erythrina abyssinica* (Leguminocae) extracts to deworm village chicken [9].

Ascaridiasis is a common disease of poultry (especially chicken and turkeys) in Uganda; it's caused by a nematode, *Ascaridia galli. A. galli* is a highly pathogenic worm residing in small intestines and is transmitted through eggs.

Ascaridiasis lead to weight depression and in severe cases causes intestinal blockage, loss of blood, reduced sugar content, retarded growth and mortality. It was noted that the age of the host and severity of exposure play a role in *A. galli* infections. Chickens older than 3-months are largely resistant to *A. galli* infection. *A galli* larvae undergo little to no development in older chicken. Larval development is arrested in the third stage at high dose rates as a result of resistance rather than a density-dependent phenomenon. Also, heavier broiler breeds are known to be more resistant to Ascarid infections than lighter white leghorn chicken [1,4],

The study hypothesized that plants with known but undocumented anthelmintic activity exist in the SWAEZ of Uganda. The efficacy of medicinal plant varies with the location in the SWAEZ. This study aimed to investigate the efficacy of *Erythrina abyssinica* under in vitro conditions and to compare its efficacy with that of a conventional drug, the piperazine citrate.

2. Materials and methods

a. Collection and maintenance of the worms

Ascarid worms have a large, thick, yellowish white head with 3 large lips. The male is 50-76 mm long, 490-1.21 mm wide. It has a preanal sucker oval or circular, with strong chitinous wall with a papilliform interruption on its posterior rim; tail with narrow caudal alae or membranes and 10 pairs of papillae. The female is 60-116 mm long, 900-1.8mm wide; the vulva is the anterior part of the body, and eggs are elliptical, thick Shelled and not embryonated at time of deposition [10].

The worms used in this study were collected from fresh intestines taken from slaughtered indigenous chicken from the Bwaise market. The intestines were grossly evaluated and the worms removed and preserved in Goodwin's solution at a temp of 37°c in an incubator.

The Goodwin's physiological solution was prepared as following [11,12,13,14, 15]. The constituents of Goodwin's physiological solution were calcium chloride (0.20g), glucose (5g), magnesium chloride (0.10g), potassium chloride (0.2g), sodium bicarbonate (0.15g), sodium chloride (8g) and sodium hydrogen phosphate (0.5g), all quantities dissolved in one (1) litre of distilled water. Calcium chloride was added later after dissolving other salts to discourage its precipitation. The solution was pre warmed to 37^0C before placing in the worms.

b. *Erythrina abysinnica* selection and extraction procedures

Erythrina abyssinica (local and Luganda names: *Muyigiti;* Runyakole name:*Ekiko*) (Figure 1), is a deciduous savannah species. It grows in open woodland and grassland. It has characteristic red overflowing flowers. It can be propagated through seedlings, cuttings and truncheons. In the south-western rangelands of Uganda, it is sometimes planted along fences of paddocks to support barbed wires. It has various traditional medicinal applications in livestock. It is also used in traditional human medicine [2, 14].

The leaves, stem and root barks of the plant *Erythrina abyssinica* were collected in the four districts of southwestern agro-ecological zone of Uganda. The Rubare subcounty in Ntungamo, the Rubindi subcounty in Mbarara, the Bugongi subcounty in Bushenyi and the Lugusulu subcounty in Rakai districts.

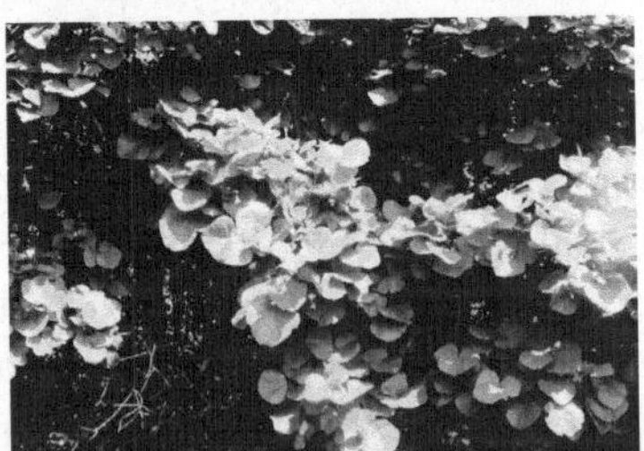

Figure 1. Picture of Erythrina abyssinica

The collected *Erythrina abyssinica* materials were pressed and voucher specimen deposited with the Botany Department at Mbarara University of Science and Technology.

The remaining plant materials were taken to Mbarara Zonal Agricultural Research and Development Institute (Mbarara ZARDI) for drying. The plants were dried in the shade at 25⁰C for one week. The plant materials were then pounded into powder (in a mortar) for chemical extraction at the Uganda Natural Chemotherapeutics Research laboratories (UNCRL).

Two hundred fifty grams (250gr) of freshly dried powdered root, stem barks and leaves were macerated in 2000 ml of 70% ethanol for 72 hours with intermittent shaking. Filtration through cotton wool was done to remove coarse particles (residues) and filter paper 12.5mm (Whitman®, No.1). The filtrate was concentrated on rota-vapour under reduced pressure at 40⁰C. The concentrated extracts were later dried on weighed kidney dishes to a constant weight at 50⁰C. The above procedures were repeated with water as solvent. The dried extracts were packed into universal bottles and kept at 4⁰C until needed for bioassays.

c. Preparation of piperazine citrate stock concentration

A 100% *Piperazine citrate* powder was bought from a known Veterinary pharmacy in Kampala. Of this 30gr were weighed and dissolved in 600mls of Goodwin's solution to make a stock concentration of 50mg/ml of the drug as the highest concentrated dose level. The stock concentration was then serially diluted to make final concentrations of 25.00mg/ml, 12.50mg/ml and 6.25mg/ml for the experiment.

d. Experimental design

The conical flasks of 250ml capacity were labelled according to the different extracts and piperazine doses namely 0, 6.25, 12.5, 25 and 50 mg/ml. In each of the dose rate concentrations 200, 187.5, 175, 150 and 100 mls respectively of Goodwin solutions were added. The extracts added were 0, 12.5, 25, 50 and 100 mls respectively. The final volume per conical flask is 200mls of a solution containing Godwin solution and extracts. Ten worms were placed in each flask and these were incubated at 37°C in water bath. The worms were monitored every 12hrs for a period of 48hrs (table 1).

The experiment had the following treatment groups: Negative control (N), Positive control involving three replicates of Piperazine citrate (P1,P2,P3), and the testing extracts, involving three replicates of Root bark (RB1, RB2, RB3), of Stem barks (SB1, SB2, SB3) and of Leaves (L1, L2,L3).

3. Worm motility assessment

In preliminary experiments, a criteria used for assessing the effects of crude plant extracts on the motility of adult *Ascaridia galli* was developed, combining the procedures previously described in literature [14], [28]. Worm motility was assessed at 12hours, 24hours, 36 hours and 48hours post treatment.

After 12, 24, 36 and 48 hours of incubation at 37⁰C, the worms were gently removed from the testing treatment and re-suspended in Goodwin's physiological solution at the same temperature for 30 seconds for possible recovery of parasite motility. The worms were assessed for death or paralysis. A worm was considered to be motile if it moved in a sinusoidal motion when stimulated by water at 40-50°C. Similarly it was considered paralyzed if on stimulating it by water at 50⁰C only part of the body responded either by raising the head and whether some parts showed autolysis and change of colour to pale white. Motility was also assessed by pressing the worm with an index finger, or using water at 50 - 60°C to differentiate dead from paralyzed worms.

The percentage of immotile or dead worm was calculated as the number of dead worms divided by the total number of worms per flask multiplied by 100 to represent percentage paralyzed or dead.

4. Data analysis

The data collected were first entered in a laboratory counter book and then entered in a computer database (Microsoft Excel). The bioassay data was analyzed by the General Linear Model Procedures with multiple comparisons (Bonferroni method) and regression, using the Graph Pad Prism Version 5.01 software, Inc San Diego, CA USA. P value <0.05 was taken for significance level. The differences between the controls and treated means were analysed using one-way analysis of variance (ANOVA). Student t-test was used to separate means where ANOVA showed significant difference. Graphs were drawn to illustrate the trends in activity by the *Erythrina* extracts and *Piperazine citrate* against *Ascaridia galli.*

The Comparison among specific plant extracts (Root-R, Stem-S and Leaves-L) and Districts (B-Bushenyi, M-Mbarara, N-Ntungamo, R-Rakai) was carried out using one way Anova then Post tested using Tukey test followed by Bonferroni post hoc *t*-test. P-value = 0.05 was used for significance level. The comparison in variations within concentrations of different extracts were conducted using Newman-Keuls Multiple Comparison Test P- value = 0.05 was used for significance level. The following parameters were tested: districts (Bushenyi, Mbarara, Ntungamo and Rakai), log transformation of the dose levels 0, 6.25, 12.5, 25 and 50 mg/ml, corresponding to 0.000, 0,796, 1.097, 1.398, 1.699.

5. Results presentation

The mean of action irrespective of the districts for Piperazine (P), Rootbark (R), Stem bark (S) and Leaves (L) at different concentrations 0, 6.25, 12.5, 25 and 50 mg/ml of the extracts. The *A. galli* were subjected to extracts for 48hours, monitored at each 12 hours interval, and results are detailed in Table 1.

Table 1. Mean of action irrespective of the districts (Generally for Piperazine (P), Rootbark (R), Stem bark (S) and Leaves (L) for different concentrations of the extract

Concentrations (mg/ml)	Total No. of worms used	Total No. of worms immobilized (paralysed +dead) after 48 hours			
		Piperazine	Root barks	Stem barks	Leaves
0	10	0	0	0	0
6.25	10	2.67±0.14	1.42±0.48	1.83±0.27	3.58±0.96
12.5	10	6.25±0.33	3.42±0.39	3.58±0.45	7.75±0.60
25	10	8.75±0.28	6.50±0.75	5.00±0.55	8.08±0.38
50	10	10.00	7.92±0.98	7.17±0.91	9.46±0.53

The rank correlation coefficient for the different extracts Piperazine (P), Root bark (R), Stem bark (S) and Leaves (L) at concentrations 0, 6.25,12.5,25,50 mg/ml are detailed in

Figures 2 to 5. The *Piperazine citrate* has a rank correlation coefficient of R^2=0.7701; Root bark (R) R^2=0.8966, Stem bark (S) R^2=0.924 and Leaves R2=0.721

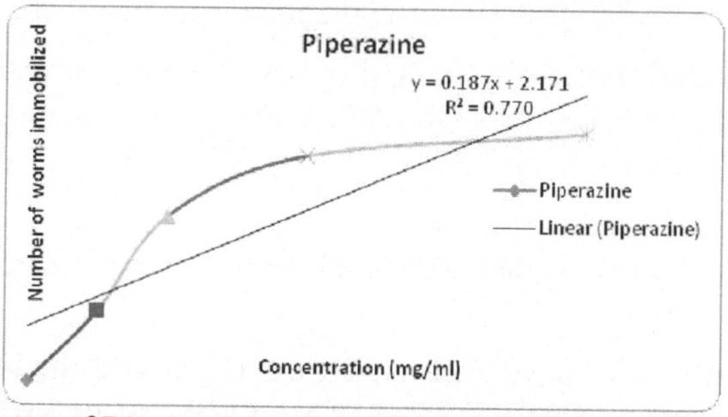

Figure 2. The effects of Piperazine citrate on the number of worms immobilized (paralysed +dead)

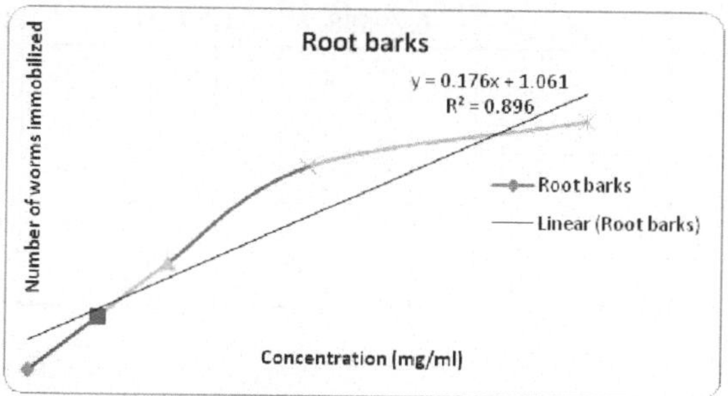

Figure 3. The effects of Root barks on the number of worms immobilized (paralysed +dead)

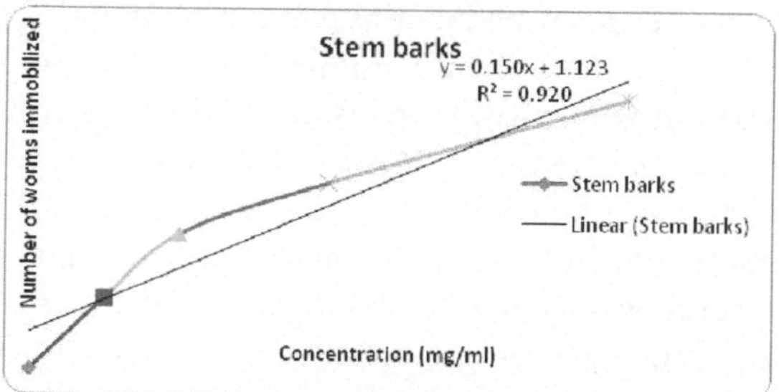

Figure 4. The effects of Stem barks on the number of worms immobilized (paralysed +dead)

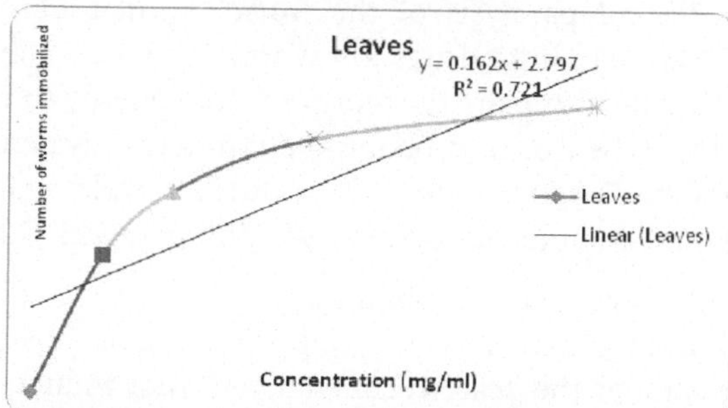

Figure 5. The effects of Leaves on the number of worms immobilized (paralysed +dead)

The study established the existence of a statistical significant relationship (P<0.05) between the Positive control (*Piperazine citrate*) at different concentrations and the extracts from different parts (root, stem and leaves) of the plant irrespective of the plant origin.

Further, the results found statistically insignificant differences (p>0.05) in activity against *A.galli* among specific plant extracts (Root-R, Stem-S and Leaves-L) and their location (Bushenyi, Mbarara, Ntungamo and Rakai)

The activity of the leaf extracts from Bushenyi, Mbarara, Ntungamo and Rakai districts were comparable to the conventional drug in the management of *Ascaridia galli as detailed* in Table 2.

Table 2. Details the concentration of the extracts and the levels of worm immobilization (paralysed +dead) after 48 hours (R – Root barks; S – Stem barks; L – Leaves)

Concentration mg/ml	0			0.79588			1.09691			1.39794			1.69897		
Plant parts	R	S	L	R	S	L	R	S	L	R	S	L	R	S	L
Bushenyi	0	0	0	0	2	3	2	4	4	5	5	6	7	8	10
Mbarara	0	0	0	1	2	2	2	5	4	5	7	6	7	7	8
Ntungamo	0	0	0	1	2	3	2	4	5	5	5	7	7	8	9
Rakai	0	0	0	2	2	2	3	3	6	6	6	8	9	7	9

6. Discussion

The research showed that the leaves, stem barks and root barks of *Erythrina abyssinica* may be useful in poultry helminthosis control. This information supports its used as antihelminthic in ethno-veterinary medicine as previously defended [2-3]. The percentage of motility inhibition is an estimate of anthelmintic efficacy by comparing worm motility before and after incubation with plant extracts and *Piperazine citrate*. In this study the *Ascaridia galli* motility was assessed at 12, 24, 36 and 48 hours post treatment. The motility decreased with increasing extract concentration and increase in the incubation period. The anthelmintic property of plants is dependent on secondary plant metabolites [16-17] which in turn may depend on solvent of extraction [18] Paralyses of *Ascaridia galli* were very evident in treated groups that progressed till death of the parasite.

Piperazine is a GABA receptor agonist. Piperazine binds directly and selectively to muscle membrane GABA receptors, presumably causing hyperpolarization of nerve endings, resulting in flaccid paralysis of the worm. Similar observations have been reported showing that anthelmintic drugs kill worms either by starving them to death or by causing paralysis, which impairs the worm to store energy to meet their metabolic energy requirements [19]. The worms probably died from energy deficiencies (starvation) since they became paralyzed and fail to feed. It was further explained that interfering with feeding for up to 24 hours is sufficient to kill most adult parasites [12].

It is very crucial to note here that immobilization of the worms is ideal but it may lead to stenosis of the intestinal lumen. Thus it is important that a substance possess laxative properties in order to remove the dead worm load, or it may induce the death of the host as a consequence of toxic syndromes.

It has been reported that some plant metabolites like tannins bind to glycoprotein on the cuticle of the parasite and disturb the physiological functions like motility [20].

The crude extracts yielded significant positive activity on *A.galli* as detailed in Table 1 within 48 hours. The study established that there were insignificant differences in plant parts in the various localities viz; Ntungamo, Mbarara, Bushenyi and Rakai. The differences between the therapeutic potential for root, stem and leaf vary between regions in a similar way/proportion. The South Western Agro-ecological Zone of Uganda in which Ntungamo, Mbarara, Bushenyi and Rakai districts lies in the same agro ecological conditions, similar rainfall, temperature, humidity, soil ingredients and other biotic factors.

However, it has been found that ecological, genetic and environmental differences of plants harvested from the wild may vary in quality, consistency of active bio-compounds [21]. The variation in medicinal plants may also be linked to age of the plant, seasonal variation and geographical deviation at harvest site.

The study also indicated both plant extracts, in particular the leaves, and *Piperazine citrate* response did not differ significantly (Figures 2 to 5). The use the plant leaves crude extract as alternative de-wormer but dosages need to be standardized. This would make farmers save on cost of livestock production. These findings agree with previous farmer's claims that the plant is useful in the treatment of helminthosis [4,9,14].Repeated exposure to insufficient crude extract concentration could lead to worm resistance. This would explain the continued reports of helminthosis and low livestock productivity despite farmers use of medicinal plants to contain the parasites.

Ethanolic extraction was selected in this work to extract active substances from the root bark, stem bark and leaves of *Erythrina abyssinica*. Farmers use water to extract the active substances. There may be variation in extraction potential using aqueous and ethanol solvent systems due to the kind of bioactive substances extracted by the two solvents since different solvents extract different compounds depending on type of substances and polarity [22].

Further, alcohol is a "good for all-purpose" solvent for preliminary extraction [12,22]. In this study the use of ethanol has an added advantage of extract preservation and increasing the shelf life of the medicinal plant extracts. This would not only reduce labour of repeated preparation but also promote the plant species conservation.

The anthelmintic activities observed might be due the *Erythrina* condensed tannins, though synergy by other compounds could have enhanced the activity. The role of condensed tannins in helminth control has been demonstrated [23-24].

Chemically, tannins are polyphenolic compounds [30] and some synthetic phenolic anthelmintics, like niclosamide and oxyclozanide are said to interfere with energy generation in helminth parasites by uncoupling oxidative phosphorylation. It is possible that tannins contained in the extracts of *Erythrina abyssinica* produced similar effects. It was also suggested that tannins bind to free proteins in the gastrointestinal tract of host animal [2,25] or glycoprotein on the cuticle of the parasite disturbing the physiological functions like motility, feed absorption and reproduction [20,26-27,] or by interference with morphology and proteolytic activity of microbes [13,28] and cause death.

Alternatively, the presence of alkaloids salts which are physiologically active with sedative and analgesic properties could have contributed to the paralysis and consequent death of the worms. Alkaloids are toxic due to their stimulatory effects, leading to excitation of cells and neurological dysfunction.

7. Conclusion and recommendations

The study validates the farmers efforts, who have been using for long these medicinal plants and stem barks for management of diverse ailments in poultry and other livestock diseases. The findings of the current study provide evidence that *Erythrina abyssinica* can be used by local farmers to control poultry helminthosis. Our study found that leaves had very good activity on *Ascaridia galli* comparable with the conventional *piperazine citrate.* This finding provides a new innovation in the utilization of plants parts to solve helminthes problems in local chicken. The use of leaves is important for sustainable conservation of plants. Plants where the community use the root barks are more endangered than plants whereby the community use plant leaves. The use of leaves is an opportunity to conservation of *Erythrina abyssinica* without tampering with the root barks.

Nevertheless, there is the need to conduct acute toxicity test to establish safety of the plant extracts. The use *Erythrina abyssinica* leaves other than root or stem is sustainable way of conserving the medicinal plants.

References

1. Masimba E S, Mbiriri D T, Kashangura M T and Mutibvu T 2011: Indigenous practices for the control and treatment of ailments in Zimbabwe's village poultry. Livestock Research for Rural Development. Volume 23, Article #257. Retrieved September 4, 2012, from http://www.lrrd.org/lrrd23/12/masi23257.htm
2. Kotze, A. C., Clifford, S., O'Grady, J., Behnke, J. M. and McCarthy, J. S., 2004. An in vitro larval motility assay to determine anthelmintic sensitivity for human hookworm and strongyloides species. American Journal of Tropical Medicine and Hygiene, 71, 5, 608-616.
3. Mathias, E., D.V. Rangnekar, and C.M. McCorkle, 1999. Ethnoveterinary Medicine: Alternatives for Livestock Development. Proceedings of an International Conference held in Pune, India, on November 4-6, 1997. Volume 1: Selected Papers. BAIF Development Research Foundation, Pune, India.
4. Nalule A S, Mbaria J M, Olila D and Kimenju J W , 2011: Ethnopharmacological practices in management of livestock helminthes by pastoral communities in the drylands of Uganda. Livestock Research for Rural Development. Volume 23, Article #36.Retrieved May 18, 2011, from http://www.lrrd.org/lrrd23/2/nalu23036.htm
5. Athanasiadou S, Githiori J and Kyriazakis I, 2007 Medicinal plants for Helminth parasite control: facts and fictions. Animal (2007), 1:9, pp1397-1400.
6. Gakuya D .W, 2001. Pharmacological and clinical evaluation of the anthelmintic activity of Albizia anthelmintica Brogn, Maerua edulis De wolf and Maerua subcordata De wolf plant extracts in sheep and mice. PhD thesis. University of Nairobi, Clinical Sciences Department; 2001.

7. Githiori J B, 2004. Evaluation of anthelmintic properties of ethno veterinary plant preparations used as livestock dewormers by pastoralists and small holder farmers in Kenya. PhD thesis, Uppsala 2004. Acta Universitatis Agriculturae Sueciae Veterinaria 173.

8. Hammond J A, Fieding D and Bishop S C, 1997 Prospects for plant anthelmintics in tropical veterinary medicine. Veterinary Research Communications 2: 213-228.

9. Lagu C and Kayanja F I B ,2010: Medicinal plant extracts widely used in the control of Newcastle disease (NCD) and helminthosis among village chickens of South Western Uganda. Livestock Research for Rural Development. Volume 22, Article #200.Retrieved May 18, 2011, from http://www.lrrd.org/lrrd22/11/lagu22200.htm

10. Anonymous (2011). Ascaridia galli infection. http://www.worldpoultry.net/diseases/ascaridia-galli-infection-d58.html retrieved on 30th June, 2011

11. Lamson, P.D and Brown, H. W., 1936. Methods of testing the anthelmintic properties of ascaricides, American Journal of Hygiene, 23, 85-103.

12. Nalule A S, Mbaria J M, Kimenju J W and Olila D 2012: Ascaricidal activity of Rhoicissus tridentata root-tuber ethanolic and water extracts. Livestock Research for Rural Development. Volume 24, Article #144. Retrieved September 4, 2012, from http://www.lrrd.org/lrrd24/8/nalu24144.htm.

13. Waghorn, G.C., and McNabb, W.C., 2003. Consequences of plant phenolic compounds for productivity and health of ruminants. Proceedings of the Nutrition Society, 62, 383–392.

14. Wasswa P and Olila D (2006). The in-vitro Ascaricidal activity of selected indigenous medicinal plants used in Ethno Veterinary practices in Uganda. African Journal of Traditional Complementary and alternative Medicines (2006) 3 (2).

15. Donahue, M. J., Yacoub, N.J., Kaeini, M. R., Masaracchia, R. A., Harris, B .G., 1981. Glycogen metabolizing enzymes during starvation and feeding of A. suum maintained in a perfusion chamber. Journal of Parasitology, 67, 4, 505-510.

16. Brookes, K.B and Katsoulis, L. C., 2006. Bioactive components of Rhoicissus tridentata: a pregnancy-related traditional medicine. South Africa Journal of Science, 102, 5-6, 267-272.

17. Naido, V., 2005. Screening of four major plants commonly used in ethno veterinary medicine for antimicrobial and protozoal and antioxidant activity. Unpublished Master of Science thesis, University of Pretoria Ltd.

18. Malu S. P., ObochI G. O., Edem C. A. and Nyong B. E. 2009. Effect of methods of extraction on phytochemical constituents and antibacterial properties of tetracarpidium conophorum seeds. Global journal of pure and applied sciences Vol 15, no. 3, 2009: 373-376

19. Schoenian, S., 2008. Understanding anthelmintics (dewormers). Small Ruminant Info Series. Western Maryland Research & Education Center, University of Maryland Cooperative Extension.

20. Thompson, D. P. and Geary, T. G., 1995. The structure and function of helminth surfaces. In: Marr J.J, (Edn). Biochemistry and Molecular Biology of Parasites. 1st Ed. New York: Academic Press 203–32.

21. Street R.A., Stirk W.A and Staden Van (2008). South African Medicinal plant trade-Challenges in regulating quality, safety and efficacy. Journal of Ethnopharmacology 119 (2008) 705-710.

22. Harborne, J. B. 1973. Phytochemical Methods. Chapman and Hall, London p. 113.

23. Cenci F.B., Louvandini, H., McManus, C.M., DellPorto, A., Costa, D.M., Araújo, S.C., Minho, A.P., and Abdalla, A.L., 2007. Effects of condensed tannin from Acacia mearnsii on sheep infected naturally with gastrointestinal helminthes Veterinary Parasitology, 144, 1-2,132-137.

24. Molan, A. L., Waghorn, G .C., Min, B .R. and McNabb, W. C., 2000.The effect of condensed tannins from seven herbages of Trichostrongylus columbriformis larval migration in vitro. Folia Parasitological, 47, 39-44.

25. Athanasiadou, S., Kyriazakis, I., Jackson, F., Coop, R. L., 2001. Direct anthelmintic effects of condensed tannins towards different gastrointestinal nematodes of sheep: In vitro and in vivo studies. Veterinary Parasitology, 99, 205–19.

26. Aerts, R.J., Barry, T.N., McNabb, W. C., 1999. Polyphenols and agriculture: beneficial effects of proanthocyanidins in forages. Agricultural Ecosystems Environment, 75, 1-12.

27. Githiori, J.B., Athanasiadou, S. and Thamsborg, S. M. 2006. Use of plants in novel approaches for control of gastrointestinal helminths in livestock with emphasis on small ruminants. Veterinary Parasitolology.

28. Min, B. R., Barry, T. N., Attwood, G. T., and McNabb, W. C., 2003. The effect of condensed tannins on the nutrition and health of ruminants fed fresh temperate forages: a review. Animal Feed Science and Technology, 106, 3–19.

29. Nanyingi.M. O., Mbaria J.M, Lanyasunya.A.L., Wagate.C.G .,Koros.K.B., Kaburia.H.F., Munenge. R.W and Ogara W.O (2008). Ethnopharmacological survey of Samburu district, Kenya. Journal of Ethnobiology and Ethnomedicine 2008, 4:14

30. Bate-Smith, E. C., 1962. The phenolic constituent of plants and their taxonomic significance, dicotyledons. Journal of the Linnean Society of London, Botany, 58, 95–103.

Index

D

E

F

9 789387 695979

Printed at Repro India Ltd.